T0290272

Inherited Gastrointestinal Cancers: Identification, Management, and the Role of Genetic Evaluation and Testing

Editor

FAY KASTRINOS

GASTROINTESTINAL ENDOSCOPY CLINICS OF NORTH AMERICA

www.giendo.theclinics.com

Consulting Editor
CHARLES J. LIGHTDALE

January 2022 • Volume 32 • Number 1

ELSEVIER

1600 John F. Kennedy Boulevard • Suite 1800 • Philadelphia, Pennsylvania, 19103-2899

http://www.theclinics.com

GASTROINTESTINAL ENDOSCOPY CLINICS OF NORTH AMERICA Volume 32, Number 1
January 2022 ISSN 1052-5157, ISBN-13: 978-0-323-84958-6

Editor: Kerry Holland
Developmental Editor: Jessica Cañaberal

Gastrointestinal Endoscopy Clinics of North America (ISSN 1052-5157) is published quarterly by Elsevier Inc., 360 Park Avenue South, New York, NY 10010-1710. Months of issue are January, April, July, and October. Business and Editorial Offices: 1600 John F. Kennedy Blvd., Suite 1800, Philadelphia, PA, 19103-2899. Periodicals postage paid at New York, NY and additional mailing offices. Subscription prices are $370.00 per year for US individuals, $837.00 per year for US institutions, $100.00 per year for US and Canadian students/residents, $407.00 per year for Canadian individuals, $862.00 per year for Canadian institutions, $486.00 per year for international individuals, $862.00 per year for international institutions, and $245.00 per year for international students/residents. To receive student/resident rate, orders must be accompanied by name of affiliated institution, date of term, and the *signature* of program/residency coordinator on institution letterhead. Orders will be billed at individual rate until proof of status is received. Foreign air speed delivery is included in all *Clinics* subscription prices. All prices are subject to change without notice. **POSTMASTER:** Send address change to *Gastrointestinal Endoscopy Clinics of North America*, Elsevier Health Sciences Division, Subscription Customer Service, 3251 Riverport Lane, Maryland Heights, MO 63043. **Customer Service: 1-800-654-2452 (US). From outside the United States, call 1-314-447-8871. Fax: 1-314-447-8029. E-mail: JournalsCustomerService-usa@elsevier.com (for print support) or JournalsOnlineSupport-usa@elsevier.com (for online support).**

Reprints. For copies of 100 or more, of articles in this publication, please contact the Commercial Reprints Department, Elsevier Inc., 360 Park Avenue South, New York, NY 10010-1710. Tel. 212-633-3874; Fax: 212-633-3820; E-mail: reprints@elsevier.com.

Gastrointestinal Endoscopy Clinics of North America is covered in *Excerpta Medica, MEDLINE/PubMed (Index Medicus),* and *MEDLINE/MEDLARS.*

Contributors

CONSULTING EDITOR

CHARLES J. LIGHTDALE, MD
Professor of Medicine, Division of Digestive and Liver Diseases, Columbia University Medical Center, New York, New York

EDITOR

FAY KASTRINOS, MD, MPH
Associate Professor of Medicine, Division of Digestive and Liver Diseases, Herbert Irving Comprehensive Cancer Center, Columbia University Irving Medical Center, Vagelos College of Physicians and Surgeons, New York, New York

AUTHORS

CAROL A. BURKE, MD
Departments of Gastroenterology, Hepatology, and Nutrition, and Colorectal Surgery, Sanford R. Weiss MD Center for Hereditary Gastrointestinal Neoplasia, Digestive Disease and Surgical Institute, Cleveland Clinic, Cleveland, Ohio

LEAH H. BILLER, MD
Dana-Farber Cancer Institute, Instructor of Medicine, Harvard Medical School, Brigham & Women's Hospital, Boston, Massachusetts

RANDALL E. BRAND, MD
Professor of Medicine, Division of Gastroenterology, Hepatology, and Nutrition, Department of Medicine, University of Pittsburgh, Pittsburgh, Pennsylvania

SIOBHAN A. CREEDON, RN, NP
Dana-Farber Cancer Institute, Boston, Massachusetts

JEREMY L. DAVIS, MD
Center for Cancer Research, National Cancer Institute, National Institutes of Health, Bethesda, Maryland

CHRISTINE DROGAN, MS, CGC
Section of Gastroenterology, Hepatology and Nutrition, Department of Medicine, University of Chicago, Chicago, Illinois

BETH DUDLEY, MS, MPH
Certified Genetic Counselor, Division of Gastroenterology, Hepatology, and Nutrition, Department of Medicine, University of Pittsburgh, Pittsburgh, Pennsylvania

YICHUN FU, MD
Samuel Bronfman Department of Medicine, Icahn School of Medicine at Mount Sinai, New York

LAUREN A. GAMBLE, MD
Center for Cancer Research, National Cancer Institute, National Institutes of Health, Bethesda, Maryland

MAHNUR HAIDER, MD
Assistant Professor of Medicine, Section of General Internal Medicine & Geriatrics, John W. Deming Department of Medicine, Tulane University School of Medicine, New Orleans, Louisiana

KIMBERLY J. HILFRANK, MS, MPH, CGC
Lecturer in Genetic Counseling, Division of Digestive and Liver Diseases, Columbia University Irving Medical Center, New York, New York

KAREN HURLEY, PhD
Department of Psychiatry and Psychology, Neurologic Institute and Sanford R. Weiss MD Center for Hereditary Gastrointestinal Neoplasia, Digestive Disease and Surgical Institute, Cleveland Clinic, Cleveland, Ohio

GREGORY IDOS, MD, MS
City of Hope Comprehensive Cancer Center, Duarte, California

MATTHEW F. KALADY, MD
Professor of Surgery, Division of Colorectal Surgery, The Ohio State University Wexner Medical Center, Columbus, Ohio

FAY KASTRINOS, MD, MPH
Associate Professor of Medicine, Division of Digestive and Liver Diseases, Herbert Irving Comprehensive Cancer Center, Columbia University Irving Medical Center, Vagelos College of Physicians and Surgeons, New York, New York

BRYSON W. KATONA, MD, PhD
Division of Gastroenterology and Hepatology, Department of Medicine, University of Pennsylvania Perelman School of Medicine, Philadelphia, Pennsylvania

TRILOKESH KIDAMBI, MD
City of Hope Comprehensive Cancer Center, Duarte, California

ALEX C. KIM, MD
Assistant Professor of Surgery, Division of Surgical Oncology, The Ohio State University Wexner Medical Center, Columbus, Ohio

WOOJIN KIM, MD
City of Hope Comprehensive Cancer Center, Duarte, California

MARGARET KLEHM, RN, MPH, MSN, FNP
Dana-Farber Cancer Institute, Boston, Massachusetts

SONIA S. KUPFER, MD
Section of Gastroenterology, Hepatology and Nutrition, Department of Medicine, University of Chicago, Chicago, Illinois

JAMES LIN, MD, MPH
City of Hope Comprehensive Cancer Center, Duarte, California

JESSICA M. LONG, MS, CGC
Division of Hematology/Oncology, Department of Medicine, University of Pennsylvania, Philadelphia, Pennsylvania

AIMEE L. LUCAS, MD, MS
Associate Professor, Samuel Bronfman Department of Medicine, Henry D. Janowitz
Division of Gastroenterology, Icahn School of Medicine at Mount Sinai, New York

CAROLE MACARON, MD
Assistant Professor of Medicine, Cleveland Clinic Lerner College of Medicine of Case
Western Reserve University, Department of Gastroenterology, Hepatology and Nutrition,
Sanford R. Weiss MD Center for Hereditary Gastrointestinal Neoplasia, Digestive Disease
and Surgical Institute, Cleveland Clinic, Cleveland, Ohio

GAUTAM N. MANKANEY, MD
Department of Gastroenterology and Hepatology, Virginia Mason Franciscan Health,
Seattle, Washington

JENNIFER K. MARATT, MD, MS
Assistant Professor, Division of Gastroenterology and Hepatology, Indiana University
School of Medicine, Richard L. Roudebush Veterans Affairs Medical Center, Regenstrief
Institute, Inc, Indianapolis, Indiana

MOHAMAD MOUCHLI, MD
Department of Gastroenterology, Hepatology, and Nutrition, Digestive Disease and
Surgical Institute, Cleveland Clinic, Cleveland, Ohio

JACQUELYN M. POWERS, MS, CGC
Division of Hematology/Oncology, Department of Medicine, University of Pennsylvania,
Philadelphia, Pennsylvania

SHEILA D. RUSTGI, MD
Assistant Professor of Medicine, Division of Digestive and Liver Diseases, Columbia
University Irving Medical Center, New York, New York

PETER P. STANICH, MD
Associate Professor of Medicine, Division of Gastroenterology, Hepatology and Nutrition,
The Ohio State University Wexner Medical Center, Columbus, Ohio

ELENA STOFFEL, MD, MPH
Associate Professor, Division of Gastroenterology, Department of Internal Medicine,
University of Michigan, Rogel Cancer Center, Ann Arbor, Michigan

BRIAN SULLIVAN, MD, MHS
Assistant Professor of Medicine, Division of Gastroenterology, Duke University Medical
Center, Durham, North Carolina

MATTHEW B. YURGELUN, MD
Dana-Farber Cancer Institute, Assistant Professor of Medicine, Harvard Medical School,
Brigham & Women's Hospital, Boston, Massachusetts

Contents

> Pancreatic cancer (PC) is a highly lethal cancer and projected to be the second leading cause of cancer death by 2030. Multigene panel testing has facilitated the identification of germline variants associated with an increased risk of PC. Precision treatment has led to improved outcomes for patients with these findings. Because of these improved outcomes as well as the implications for at-risk family members who may benefit from additional cancer screening, the NCCN recommends universal genetic testing for newly diagnosed PC patients. This review describes the most common heritable conditions associated with PC and those who may benefit from screening.

> Individuals with a genetic susceptibility to pancreatic ductal adenocarcinoma (PDAC) may benefit from surveillance to increase the likelihood of early detection. Currently, candidates for surveillance are identified based on genetic test results and family history of PDAC, and surveillance is accomplished through imaging of the pancreas (endoscopic ultrasound or MRI). Novel methods that incorporate personalized risk, biomarkers, and radiomics are being investigated in an attempt to improve identification of at-risk individuals and to increase detection of precursor and early-stage lesions.

> Hereditary pancreatitis (HP) is a rare inherited chronic pancreatitis (CP) with strong genetic associations, with estimated prevalence ranging from 0.3 to 0.57 per 100,000 across Europe, North America, and East Asia. Apart from the most well-described genetic variants PRSS1, SPINK1, and CFTR, many other genes, such as CTRC, CPA1, and CLDN2 and CEL have been found to associate with HP, typically in one of the 3 main mechanisms including altered trypsin activity, pancreatic ductal cell secretion, and calcium channel regulation. The current mainstay of management for patients with HP comprises genetic testing for eligible

genetic testing options, and expected outcomes from genetic testing in these individuals. In more recent years, adenomatous colonic polyposis has evolved beyond the more robustly characterized familial adenomatous polyposis (FAP) and MUTYH-associated polyposis (MAP) now encompassing more newly described genes and associated syndromes. Technological innovation, from whole-exome sequencing to multigene panel testing, has dramatically increased the amount of genotypic and phenotypic data amassed in adenomatous polyposis cohorts, which has contributed greatly to informing diagnosis and clinical management of affected individuals and their families.

Familial adenomatous polyposis (FAP) is characterized by numerous adenomatous colorectal polyps. Colonoscopy screening is recommended to start at age 10 to 12 with intervals of 1 to 2 years. Colectomy is indicated for malignancy, colorectal symptoms or significant progression. Even after colectomy, endoscopic surveillance remains critical. Duodenal and gastric polyposis is also common in FAP. Screening with upper endoscopy and ampullary visualization is recommended at age 20 to 25. The interval is determined by duodenal polyposis, but guidelines are increasingly factoring in ampullary and gastric manifestations. Surgical management for advanced upper tract polyps or malignancy may also be needed.

Prevention of colorectal neoplasia with chemoprevention is a long-studied research area and of clinical use in patients with the 2 commonest hereditary colorectal cancer syndromes, Lynch syndrome and familial adenomatous polyposis. No medication is currently approved for administration to prevent colorectal neoplasia. We provide a review of available evidence on the efficacy of chemoprevention in individuals with a hereditary colorectal cancer syndrome. Emerging data in animal models and limited data in humans suggest vaccines may be a breakthrough in these populations. Clinicians must acknowledge chemoprevention is an adjunct to management and does not supplant endoscopic and surgical intervention.

Although environmental factors such as Helicobacter pylori, tobacco, and diet are major contributors to the development of gastric cancer (GC) worldwide, it is estimated that up to 5% to 10% of GC cases are due to an underlying hereditary susceptibility caused by germline pathogenic variants. Hereditary diffuse gastric cancer (HDGC) caused by germline pathogenic variants in the CDH1 gene is the principal familial GC syndrome.

However, other well-established hereditary gastrointestinal syndromes have been associated with an increased risk of GC. In this review, we will discuss the latest insights and advances in our understanding of GC associated with Lynch syndrome (LS), familial adenomatous polyposis (FAP), gastric adenocarcinoma and proximal polyposis of the stomach (GAPPS), Li-Fraumeni syndrome (LFS), Peutz–Jeghers syndrome (PJS), and juvenile polyposis syndrome (JPS). We will also discuss the emergence of new associations of the homologous recombination pathway genes (BRCA1, BRCA2) with GC.

Lauren A. Gamble and Jeremy L. Davis

Inactivating germline variants in the CDH1 tumor suppressor gene cause the hereditary diffuse gastric cancer syndrome. Total gastrectomy is recommended for prevention, although it is associated with adverse outcomes and chronic health risks. Gastric cancer surveillance is an alternative to surgery; however, upper gastrointestinal endoscopy is limited by poor sensitivity. Cancer surveillance requires accurate detection of early carcinoma and patient-specific disease penetrance estimates. Current clinical care should incorporate up-to-date information on variable disease penetrance, which does not seem to correlate with CDH1 genotype. Affected patients and families warrant a balanced presentation of options for cancer surveillance and prophylaxis.

GASTROINTESTINAL ENDOSCOPY CLINICS OF NORTH AMERICA

RELATED CLINICS SERIES

Gastroenterology Clinics
(www.gastro.theclinics.com)
Clinics in Liver Disease
(www.liver.theclinics.com)

THE CLINICS ARE AVAILABLE ONLINE!
Access your subscription at:
www.theclinics.com

Foreword

Inherited Gastrointestinal Cancer in the New Era of Genetic Testing

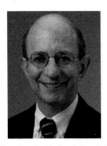

Charles J. Lightdale, MD
Consulting Editor

Gastrointestinal (GI) endoscopists are usually at the front line in the tissue diagnosis of malignancies involving the GI tract. Based on careful evaluation of family history and often early onset of these cancers, an inherited predilection may be suspected. In the modern age of personalized or precision medicine, the cancer tissue itself is often tested for somatic genetic mutations that may be a pathway for specific new oncology therapies. When inherited syndromes are a concern, with all body cells affected, germ-line genetic analysis can be carried out usually using blood or cheek mucosa cells to identify genetic mutations passed from one generation to the next. Such testing generally has targeted a single or small number of genes known to be involved in specific syndromes. Recently, the ability to screen for abnormal genes has grown exponentially in power, and at the same time, the cost has been reduced to the point where multi-gene testing panels are now available, practical, and affordable.

Specialists in inherited cancer syndromes and genetic counselling can be increasingly found in academic medical centers and larger community hospitals. In gastroenterology, the big three organs involved with inherited cancer are the colon, the pancreas, and the stomach. Multiple non-GI organs may also be involved in some of these cancer syndromes (eg, in Lynch syndrome which often presents first in the colon). The specific gene abnormalities involved are not only important for the affected individual but also important for other family members, who may be or may not be at risk. For those identified at risk by genetic testing, strategies for cancer prevention and surveillance for early diagnosis may be key to their survival.

GI endoscopists involved in the management of patients and families when a possibly inherited cancer is diagnosed must be well informed in how to proceed. This issue of the *Gastrointestinal Endoscopy Clinics of North America* is designed exactly for this purpose. I am delighted that Fay Kastrinos, a gastroenterologist and a leader in the field of inherited GI cancer, has agreed to be the Editor of this issue

Gastrointest Endoscopy Clin N Am 32 (2022) xiii–xiv
https://doi.org/10.1016/j.giec.2021.10.002
1052-5157/22/© 2021 Published by Elsevier Inc.

giendo.theclinics.com

of the *Gastrointestinal Endoscopy Clinics of North America*. She has assembled an extraordinary group of specialists, who have covered the topic "Inherited Gastrointestinal Cancers and the Role of Genetic Evaluation and Testing" with great breadth and depth. Gastroenterologists, surgeons, and oncologists should all be interested in reading this issue, which illuminates current progress in this field of high importance to patients with GI cancer and their families.

Charles J. Lightdale, MD
Department of Medicine
Columbia University Medical Center
161 Fort Washington Avenue
New York, NY 10032, USA

E-mail address:
CJL18@columbia.edu

Preface

Inherited Gastrointestinal Cancers and the Role of Genetic Evaluation and Testing

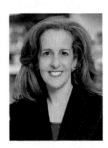

Fay Kastrinos, MD, MPH
Editor

Genetic evaluation and testing for familial risk of gastrointestinal cancers have rapidly evolved over recent decades. Advancements in DNA-sequencing technologies have allowed for more consistent use of tumor testing to determine therapeutic selection and germline testing to assess for the inherited risk of cancer. Traditionally, the decision to pursue germline genetic testing involved a detailed review of personal and family cancer history and the use of clinical criteria that relied heavily on cancer burden and young ages of cancer diagnoses in families. When clinical criteria were met, subsequent phenotype-driven genetic testing was pursued, where only one or a small number of genes were tested. However, the decreasing costs of next-generation sequencing technologies and the widespread use of multigene panel testing have led to improved accessibility and increased uptake of germline testing, across all cancer types. This approach to genetic evaluation also extends beyond the patient with cancer to individuals with family but no personal cancer history, who can benefit from intensive screening and risk-reducing strategies for cancer prevention.

For the gastroenterologist, results of germline testing can guide recommendations for endoscopic and radiographic surveillance in identified carriers of pathogenic variants in cancer-susceptibility genes associated with gastrointestinal malignancies. However, the growing use of multigene panel testing has (and will continue to) redefined gene-cancer associations, and in turn, cancer risk estimates that vary from low to high penetrance. Cancer screening recommendations and preventive strategies tailored by genotype, in addition to other individual risk factors, afford us the ability to improve clinical outcomes for patients at highest risk of cancer and their families.

In this issue of the *Gastrointestinal Endoscopy Clinics of North America*, we focus on the genetic evaluation and testing, clinical management, and preventive strategies for

Gastrointest Endoscopy Clin N Am 32 (2022) xv–xvi
https://doi.org/10.1016/j.giec.2021.10.001
1052-5157/22/© 2021 Published by Elsevier Inc.

inherited pancreatic cancer and pancreatitis, inherited colorectal cancer, including Lynch syndrome and polyposis-related conditions, and inherited gastric cancer, including hereditary diffuse gastric cancer.

Fay Kastrinos, MD, MPH
Division of Digestive and Liver Diseases
Herbert Irving Comprehensive Cancer Center
Columbia University Irving Medical Center
and the Vagelos College of Physicians and Surgeons
630 West 168th Street; P&S 318
New York, NY 10032, USA

E-mail address:
Fk18@columbia.edu

Familial Predisposition and Genetic Risk Factors Associated with Pancreatic Cancer

Sheila D. Rustgi, MD, Kimberly J. Hilfrank, MS, MPH, CGC,
Fay Kastrinos, MD, MPH*

KEYWORDS

- Hereditary pancreatic cancer • Familial pancreatic cancer • Genetic testing
- Genetic risk assessment • Pancreatic cancer screening

KEY POINTS

- The prevalence and impact of germline variants on treatment options and outcomes for pancreatic cancer has led to recommendations for universal genetic testing for newly diagnosed pancreatic cancer patients.
- Herein, we describe the most common hereditary cancer syndromes associated with pancreatic cancer, their clinical features and risks for other cancers.
- Affected family members with these syndromes may benefit from pancreatic cancer screening for early detection.

INTRODUCTION

Pancreatic ductal adenocarcinoma (PDAC) is the ninth most common cancer diagnosis and yet is projected to be the second leading cause of cancer death in the United States by 2030.[1] Although most patients present with metastatic disease, the overall survival after a PDAC diagnosis has improved across all stages. The largest improvement in survival has been for early-stage PDAC, as the only potential cure must include surgical resection. In addition, neoadjuvant treatment for those with localized disease has increased surgical candidacy and substantially improved 5-year survival rates to 39%. Precision treatment, informed by tumor and germline genetic testing, can also optimize therapeutic regimens and outcomes for those diagnosed with PDAC. Because of this, the National Comprehensive Cancer Network now recommends genetic testing for all newly diagnosed PDAC patients or their first-degree relatives if the

Division of Digestive & Liver Diseases, Columbia University Irving Medical Center, 630 West 168th Street, Box 83, Room P&S 3-401, New York, NY 10032, USA
* Corresponding author.
E-mail address: Fk18@cumc.columbia.edu

Gastrointest Endoscopy Clin N Am 32 (2022) 1–12
https://doi.org/10.1016/j.giec.2021.09.001
1052-5157/22/© 2021 Elsevier Inc. All rights reserved.
giendo.theclinics.com

initial patient cannot be tested.[2] Understanding these results is important for the patients and the providers treating them.

In recent years, much of the natural history of PDAC has been elucidated including precursor lesions that can be targeted for screening. PDAC screening is currently limited to a small subset of the population that has a familial or genetic risk where annual imaging of the pancreas has demonstrated improvements in mortality, with early disease or precursor lesions can potentially be surgically resected. This article reviews inherited risk factors for the development of PDAC and identifies high-risk individuals (HRIs) who can be considered for PDAC screening.

FAMILIAL PANCREATIC CANCER

Family history of PDAC confers an increased risk for the development of pancreatic cancer. The magnitude of this risk is influenced by the number of relatives affected by PDAC and their degree relation. Individuals with 2 first-degree relatives experience an elevated PDAC risk ratio of 6.4-fold, or a lifetime risk of 8% to 12%, whereas those with 3 first-degree relatives are related to an elevated risk ratio of 32-fold with a lifetime risk of 40%.[3] In addition, earlier age of PDAC confers an increased risk, where kindreds with PDAC diagnosed at younger than 50 years have a relative risk of 9.3.[4]

Familial pancreatic cancer (FPC) is a more specific term used to define a kindred with 2 or more family members with PDAC who share a first-degree relationship,[5] in the absence of other hereditary cancer syndromes. Data from the National Familial Pancreas Tumor Registry (NFPTR) suggest that familial clustering of PDAC cases is not due to chance alone, and that both genetic factors and environmental exposures, such as cigarette use, play a role.[3] The standardized incidence ratio of PDAC in FPC kindreds was 9.0, meaning that the risk of PDAC was 9 times that of the average population among FPC kindreds. In sporadic cases, the standardized incidence ratio was 1.8, suggesting that the risk for developing PDAC increases with an increasing burden of pancreatic cancer among family members.[3]

Next-generation sequencing and the availability of germline multigene panel testing, which allows for multiple cancer susceptibility genes to be evaluated simultaneously from the same patient sample, provides additional information regarding genetic association and cancer risk assessment. When undergoing multigene panel testing, approximately 20% of FPC kindreds that are defined by clinical criteria solely reliant on family history, will be redefined as having an inherited cancer syndrome.[6] When comparing the prevalence of pathogenic variants detected by multigene panel testing among individuals with PDAC who met clinical criteria for FPC versus those who did not, 13.5% with FPC had a detected germline alteration versus 9.4% of individuals from a non-FPC kindred. Although this difference was not statistically significant, the study may have been underpowered to detect small differences.[7] Approximately, 12% of the detected pathogenic variants among the individuals from FPC kindreds were related to known cancer syndromes associated with PDAC (such as BRCA1, BRCA2, ATM, PALB2), in contrast to only 4.3% detected in the non-FPC subjects (P = .02).[7] A limitation of this study was related to ascertainment bias, where the cohort was an enriched population with increased family cancer history and the results may not be generalizable to other populations with PDAC. Furthermore, although there was a difference in frequency of germline pathogenic variants between those with and without FPC, the result was not statistically significant, likely due to inadequate power to detect small differences. However, the study highlights that the genetic basis of much of the inherited susceptibility to PDAC remains unexplained.

INHERITED CANCER SYNDROMES WITH INCREASED RISK OF PDAC

Family history of pancreatic cancer is reported in approximately 10% of patients with PDAC, with at least one first-degree or second-degree relative also being affected.[8] Previous estimates of PDAC heritability ranged from 9.8% to 18%, whereas a more recent estimate from results of multigene panel testing was as high as 21.2%.[9] The germline pathogenic variants most often associated with PDAC are *BRCA2, PALB2, ATM,* and *CDKN2A;*[10] however, multigene panel testing has provided additional information regarding the spectrum of associated pathogenic variants and their correlating inherited syndrome **(Table 1)**. In addition, pathogenic germline variants have been detected in individuals with PDAC but without a family history of PDAC, with small cohort estimates ranging from 3.9% to 13.5% of patients with PDAC.[11,12]

In a recent case-control study of 3030 subjects diagnosed with PDAC and 123,136 reference controls, the frequency of 21 cancer predisposition genes detected by multigene panel testing was evaluated.[13] The panel included candidate genes for several cancer types beyond those related to PDAC.[13] This PDAC cohort was predominantly non-Hispanic white (95.6%), 5.5% had a personal history of breast, ovarian, colorectal, or nongynecologic cancer, and 11.3% had a first-degree or second-degree relative with PDAC. When compared to controls, 6 genes were significantly associated with PDAC and detected in 5.5% of patients with PDAC: *CDKN2A, TP53, MLH1, ATM, BRCA1,* and *BRCA2.*[13] Of patients who had a family history of PDAC, 7.9% had a mutation in 1 of the 6 significant genes, as did 5.2% of patients without a family history.[13] The odds ratio of cancer compared to controls ranged from 2.58 for *BRCA1* to 12.33 for *CDKN2A.* This significant difference in mutation rates between patients and controls highlights the expanding number of inherited syndromes related to PDAC. In addition, 25.7% of the pathogenic variants identified were associated with conditions involving multiple other cancer risks, many of which are prevalent malignancies and could be prevented or detected early with cancer screening strategies. This emphasizes the need for cascade germline genetic testing in family members of newly identified PDAC patients in whom a familial pathogenic variant is detected.[13] Family members unaffected by cancer who are found to harbor the same germline alteration through cascade screening may elect to begin screening and take other preventative measures for cancer control, including screening for the early detection of PDAC.

GENETIC CONDITIONS AND RELATED PATHOGENIC VARIANTS ASSOCIATED WITH PANCREATIC CANCER

Several hereditary cancer syndromes confer an increased risk of PDAC; most genes involve tumor suppression that includes homologous recombination and mismatch repair systems.

Familial Atypical Multiple Mole Melanoma

Familial atypical multiple mole melanoma (FAMMM), an autosomal dominant condition, is caused by germline mutations in the tumor suppressor gene, *CDKN2A,* and is associated with an increased risk for both PDAC and melanoma. The lifetime risk of developing PDAC in individuals with FAMMM is more than 15%, making *CDKN2A* one of the genes most strongly associated with increased risk for PDAC.[14] In particular, there is a specific founder mutation in the Netherlands, a deletion denoted *p16*-Leiden, which confers a 20% to 25% lifetime risk for pancreatic cancer as well as 53% to 100% lifetime risk of melanoma.[15,16] Even among those carrying this alteration, PDAC was noted to cluster within 7 of the 19 families, suggesting the presence of family history also increased PDAC risk.[16] Although *CDKN2A* was initially described

Table 1
Inherited cancer syndromes associated with PDAC

Gene	Syndrome	Predominant Cancers	Gene Function	Pancreatic Cancer Risk
ATM	Ataxia-Telangiectasia (biallelic)	Female breast	DNA double-stranded break repair	~5%[45]
BRCA1	Hereditary Breast and Ovarian Cancer	Male and female breast, ovarian, Fallopian tube, primary peritoneal, prostate, melanoma	Homologous recombination repair	~5%[14]
BRCA2	Hereditary Breast and Ovarian Cancer	Male and female breast, ovarian, Fallopian tube, primary peritoneal, prostate, melanoma	Homologous recombination repair	5%–10%[14]
CDKN2A	Familial Atypical Multiple Mole Melanoma Syndrome	Melanoma	Tumor suppressor	17% at age 75 y[45]
MLH1	Lynch Syndrome	Colorectal, endometrial, ovarian, urothelial, gastric, small bowel, biliary, brain	Mismatch repair	6.2%[22]
MSH2/EPCAM	Lynch Syndrome	Colorectal, endometrial, ovarian, urothelial, gastric, small bowel, biliary, brain	Mismatch repair	0.5%–1.6%[22]
MSH6	Lynch Syndrome	Colorectal, endometrial, ovarian, urothelial, gastric, small bowel, biliary, brain	Mismatch repair	1.4%–1.6%[22]
PMS2	Lynch Syndrome	Colorectal, endometrial, ovarian	Mismatch repair	<1%–1.6%[22]
PALB2	None	Female breast	Homologous recombination repair	5%–10%[14]
STK11	Peutz-Jeghers Syndrome	Female breast, colorectal, stomach, small intestine, cervical	Tumor suppressor	36%[22] 8%–11% by age 70 y[45]
TP53	Li-Fraumeni Syndrome	Female breast, soft tissue sarcoma, osteosarcoma, colorectal, adrenocortical carcinoma, leukemia, brain and CNS tumors	Tumor suppressor	5%–10%[14]

From Hilfrank KJ, Rustgi SD and Kastrinos F. Inherited predisposition to pancreatic cancer. Semin Oncol 2021 2021/03/29.

among white patients with a family history of melanoma and pancreatic cancer, a recent case-control study of African-American patients identified a moderately penetrant, pathogenic rare coding variant in *CDK2NA*[17] that was more frequently detected in African-Americans with PDAC than others; this finding may possibly contribute to the increased cancer risk for PDAC in this group.[17]

Hereditary Breast Ovarian Cancer Syndrome

There are several germline mutations and syndromes associated with a combination of breast, ovarian, and pancreatic cancers. Pathogenic mutations in *BRCA1* and *BRCA2* result in hereditary breast and ovarian cancer syndrome (HBOC), in which the lifetime risk for breast cancer ranges from 41% to 90%, and the lifetime ovarian cancer risk is estimated to be up to 62%.[14] The *BRCA1*, *BRCA2,* and *PALB2* genes are essential to initiate double-stranded break repair and successful homologous recombination of chromosomes. *PALB2* works alongside *BRCA1* and *BRCA2* in the DNA repair pathway to correct DNA double-stranded breaks.[18] The cancers observed with *PALB2* are similar to those of *BRCA1* and *BRCA2* and the increased lifetime risk for female breast cancer and ovarian cancer is between 41% to 60% and 3% to 5%, respectively.[14]

With respect to PDAC risk in HBOC, *BRCA2* mutations are the most commonly identifiable genetic factor, identified in 5%–17% of FPC kindreds and confer a relative risk of 3.5 to 6.2[19]; *PALB2* mutations are estimated to confer similar risk and *BRCA1*, albeit slightly lower. It was historically thought that up to 11% of PDAC cases harbored a *BRCA1* mutation and up to 17% had a *BRCA2* mutation.[14] However, these studies were subject to ascertainment bias as the cohorts described generally had a history of FPC or were of Ashkenazi Jewish ancestry. More recent studies using broader and more general population samples estimated that up to 3% of pancreatic cancer cases have a *BRCA1* mutation and up to 6% have a *BRCA2* pathogenic variant.[14] Mutations in the *PALB2* gene confer a lifetime risk of pancreatic cancer of 5% to 10%.[14]

In addition, the *ATM* gene is also instrumental in DNA double-stranded break repair, as it codes for a protein kinase that activates various enzymes that can identify and correct the breaks, thus making it an integral component of the DNA repair process.[20] It is prevalent among PDAC patients with germline mutations and was present in 2.30% of the unselected cohort of PDAC patients previously described.[13] Like the aforementioned homologous recombination repair genes, the estimated lifetime PDAC risk for *ATM* mutation carriers is between 5% and 10%.[14] Additional cancer risks include female breast cancer and ovarian cancer, with the risk for breast cancer at between 15% and 40% and the ovarian cancer risk of up to 3%.[14]

Lynch Syndrome

Lynch syndrome is a hereditary cancer syndrome that is present in 1 in 300 Americans. It results from a pathogenic variant in one of the following four mismatch repair genes: *MLH1, MSH2, MSH6, PMS2,* and *EPCAM*, which causes epigenetic silencing of *MSH2*.[21] Lynch syndrome is the most common cause of hereditary colon cancer, as it accounts for 2% to 4% of all colorectal cancer cases.[21] Although colorectal and endometrial cancer carry the highest cancer risks associated with Lynch syndrome, additional malignancies with increased risk include ovarian, urothelial, gastric, small bowel, biliary tract, and pancreatic cancers.[22] Similar to other Lynch syndrome–associated cancers, the risk for developing pancreatic cancer varies by gene.[22] The risk varies from 6.2% by age 80 years for those with a pathogenic variant in the *MLH1* gene to 0.5% to 1.6% for *MSH2* and *EPCAM* carriers, to 1.6% for *MSH6* carriers.[22] Pathogenic variants in *PMS2* are associated with a weaker phenotype in comparison with the other Lynch syndrome mismatch repair genes and carriers of this variant do not appear to have an increased risk of PDAC.[22]

Peutz-Jeghers Syndrome

Peutz-Jeghers syndrome is characterized by the development of hamartomatous polyps in the colon and results from mutations in the *STK11/LKB1* tumor suppressor gene.[22] In addition to the development of polyps and mucocutaneous hyperpigmentation around the mouth, lips, and nose, Peutz-Jeghers syndrome is linked to an increased risk for several cancer types. In a cohort study composed of 144 Peutz-Jeghers patients, 7 developed PDAC with a median age of onset of 54 years.[23] Studies have shown an increased relative risk for PDAC in carriers of Peutz-Jeghers syndrome with a lifetime risk estimated to be between 11% and 36% and a relative risk of 132-fold compared with the general population.[22–24]

Li-Fraumeni Syndrome

Li-Fraumeni syndrome is caused by pathogenic mutations in the tumor suppressor gene, *TP53*, which plays an imperative role in cell cycle regulation and apoptosis. Owing to this important role, Li-Fraumeni syndrome is autosomal dominant and highly penetrant; recent studies demonstrated the lifetime cancer risk to be near 100%.[14] This syndrome has childhood onset and includes a wide array of cancer types such as sarcomas, early-onset breast cancer, gastric cancer, colon cancer, leukemia, melanoma, and brain tumors.[14] However, soft tissue sarcomas, osteosarcomas, adrenocortical tumors, brain tumors, and breast cancer are considered to be the hallmark cancer types of Li-Fraumeni Syndrome.[14] In addition to developing cancers in childhood, individuals with Li-Fraumeni syndrome are also more likely to develop multiple primary cancers over their lifetime.[14] Although PDAC is not a core cancer of Li-Fraumeni syndrome, *TP53* carriers are believed to be at a 7.3 relative risk of developing PDAC.[25]

Hereditary Pancreatitis

Hereditary pancreatitis is a syndrome characterized by recurrent acute and chronic pancreatitis starting at an early age, insufficiently explained by other more common causes of pancreatitis. Hereditary pancreatitis, defined as pancreatitis within a family affecting 2 or more generations, is associated with a cumulative risk of 40% for the development of PDAC or a standardized incidence ratio that is 53 times that of the average population.[26] Familial pancreatitis is a less strict definition wherein pancreatitis occurs in families more commonly than in the typical population and may or may not have an underlying genetic mutation.[27] Hereditary pancreatitis is associated with germline mutations in *PRSS1*,[28,29] *SPINK1*, *CTRC*, and *CFTR* and is inherited in an autosomal dominant manner with incomplete penetrance. Mutations in these genes lead to premature activation of pancreatic enzymes.[30,31] Genetic testing for hereditary pancreatitis among patients with chronic pancreatitis allows for a better assessment of pancreatic cancer risk. Current recommendations highlight the importance of PDAC surveillance only in PRSS1 carriers who have the highest risk of developing chronic pancreatitis and a potentially accelerated course of neoplastic progression.

NOVEL INHERITED SUSCEPTIBILITY GENE

Given that most FPC cases are not attributed to known inherited cancer syndromes, studies are ongoing to identify additional genes that may have a potential association with PDAC among families with an increased burden of this cancer. In a whole-genome sequencing study, the oncogene *RABL3* was detected among multiple family members with PDAC from an FPC kindred.[32] In this family, an autosomal dominant pattern of inheritance was appreciated where 5 individuals had PDAC and additional malignancies were reported among relatives. Multigene panel testing did not identify germline pathogenic variants in known risk genes associated with cancer susceptibility but whole genome sequencing in 2 family members detected a nonsense mutation in *RABL3*, denoted p.Ser36*. Additional family members were tested for this mutation and this analysis demonstrated cosegregation of the *RABL3* allele with cancer. In addition, the p.Ser36* mutation's impact on cancer development was validated using an in-vivo zebrafish model. However, further validation of these results is warranted before *RABL3* is included in multigene panel testing for PDAC susceptibility.

GENETIC RISK ASSESSMENT AND TESTING FOR INHERITED PANCREATIC CANCER

The indications for genetic testing related to PDAC have recently changed given that certain germline mutation carriers have improved outcomes with targeted chemotherapeutic agents.[33,34] Previously, only PDAC with a family history consistent with a pattern for an inherited cancer syndrome, such as hereditary breast and ovarian cancer or Lynch syndrome, met criteria for germline genetic testing.[35] However, these criteria were limiting, and it was demonstrated that 50% of PDAC patients with actionable gene mutations would be missed using such guidelines.[35] In 2019, the National Comprehensive Cancer Network recommended that all individuals diagnosed with PDAC, regardless of age, family history, or ancestry, undergo multigene panel testing[14] (**Fig. 1**). In addition, genetic counseling and comprehensive germline testing with a multigene panel were recommended for first-degree relatives of individuals diagnosed with pancreatic cancer and individuals of an FPC kindred.[14] If a germline pathogenic variant is identified in an inherited cancer predisposition gene of which PDAC is but one manifestation, family members can benefit from earlier and enhanced screenings for the range of cancer risks conferred. In a recent study of 213 individuals

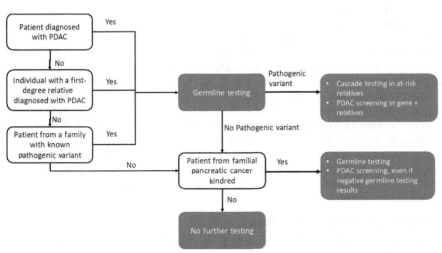

Fig. 1. Approach to genetic testing for personal or family history of PDAC. Shaded boxes denote testing; white boxes denote patient population; FDR, first-degree relative; PC, pancreatic cancer. (*From* Hilfrank KJ, Rustgi SD and Kastrinos F. Inherited predisposition to pancreatic cancer. *Semin Oncol* 2021 2021/03/29.)

with PDAC who underwent multigene panel testing, 8.6% were found to carry mutations in genes with implications for breast, ovarian, and colorectal cancer.[35] Thus, in addition to obtaining information surrounding their family's history of PDAC, asymptomatic individuals who test positive for an inherited cancer syndrome may learn of their increased risk for other cancers, and can take steps to reduce those risks.

GENOME-WIDE ASSOCIATION STUDIES AND POLYGENIC RISK SCORES

As an increased number of genome-wide association studies have been performed, there has been increased attention to the interplay between multiple changes in the genetic code and its impact on cancer risk. One method of evaluation is with polygenic risk scores, whereby several single nucleotide polymorphisms (SNPs) are identified that may be associated with risk of a disease. Using the number of SNPs present, as well as some environmental factors, researchers can create a risk score to identify patients at risk of PDAC, even if they do not carry monogenic inherited cancer syndromes, such as the conditions described earlier. Recently, the PANcreatic Disease ReseArch consortia (PANDORA) created and validated a polygenic score using 30 known SNPs and reported the risk of PDAC in a cohort of 839 PDAC cases and 2040 controls.[36] The score was significantly associated with PDAC and the risk increased when tobacco use and diabetes were also included. Although this score requires further validation, it has the potential to be used as a risk stratification tool to identify additional patients at high risk of PDAC who do not carry pathogenic variants associated with the monogenic syndromes currently known to be associated with PDAC.

RATIONALE FOR PDAC SCREENING IN HRIs

Screening is not currently recommended for patients with an average risk of pancreatic cancer[37] and the United States Preventive Services Task Force has found no evidence that screening or treatment of screen-detected pancreatic cancer improves disease-specific morbidity or mortality, or all-cause mortality. Given the low incidence of PDAC in the general population, and therefore the low positive predictive value of any screening test because of the high rate of false-positive results, screening can carry risks, including complications from invasive procedures and unnecessary treatment, that may outweigh any projected benefits.[38]

However, experts have called for surveillance of HRIs defined as those who generally have at least a 5-fold relative risk of PDAC, which predominantly includes those with a familial or genetic predisposition.[4,38–40] Of note, this does not include those with only one first-degree relative with PDAC as their risk is less than 5-fold. The benefits of surveillance in a high-risk population allow for the possibility of downstaging the cancer, which is an important consideration given how often it is diagnosed at a metastatic stage without the possibility of cure. The goals of a surveillance program are that, once a patient is identified as being at high risk for PDAC, they should be offered testing to identify high-grade dysplasia and early neoplasia when it can be resected and before it progresses.[41–43]

Individuals Eligible for PDAC Screening

The International Cancer of the Pancreas Screening (CAPS) Consortium is a panel of multidisciplinary experts that developed consensus recommendations for screening selected high-risk populations, including screening techniques, age at initiation interval of screening, with reports of clinical and surgical management.[41] HRIs include those with Peutz-Jeghers syndrome; those with both at least one first-degree relative and FAMMM, BRCA1, BRCA2, PALB2, Lynch (MLH1/MSH2/MSH6, specifically), ATM; or those with FPC defined as at least 2 affected relatives, one of whom is an FDR to the individual being considered for surveillance. The prospective clinical trial of these HRIs is ongoing at various US centers (https://clinicaltrials.gov; identifier NCT02000089) and also by the PRECEDE Consortium, another international collaboration aimed at the early detection of PDAC. The current CAPS recommendations for PDAC screening are similar to and supported by other groups including the American Society of Clinical Oncology,[44] American Gastroenterological Association,[19] the American College of Gastroenterology,[40] and the National Comprehensive Cancer Network.[14]

FUTURE CONSIDERATIONS

Given the current National Comprehensive Cancer Network guidelines for universal germline testing of all patients diagnosed with PDAC and multigene panel testing in first-degree relatives of these patients, an increased pool of germline mutation carriers will be identified who will be eligible for PDAC screening. Although recent studies support screening of HRIs for the early detection of PDAC or high-risk precursor lesions, additional data are needed regarding the optimal surveillance intervals and the potential of alternative or complementary modalities for screening.

SUMMARY

Further investigation of potential screening modalities, better assessment and incorporation of additional risk factors to personalize surveillance, and evaluation of ongoing long-term surveillance data will help improve the management of HRIs for the prevention and early detection of PDAC.

CLINICS CARE POINTS

- Precision treatment, informed by tumor and germline genetic testing, can optimize treatment regimens and outcomes for those newly diagnosed with PC.
- Previously genetic testing was performed only for those with a significant family history of cancer. However, recent evidence suggests up to 50% of PC patients with actionable gene mutations would be missed.
- New guidelines now recommend genetic testing for all newly diagnosed PC patients or their first-degree relatives if the affected patient cannot be tested.
- If a mutation is identified, cascade testing should be offered to all at-risk relatives, and those who also carry the gene should be offered PC screening.
- If no pathogenic variant is identified but a patient is from a familial pancreatic cancer kindred (defined as two family members with PC who are first-degree relatives), at-risk family members should be offered PC screening.
- Polygenic risk scores, where a number of single nucleotide polypmorphisms may increase risk of PC, are an emerging tool that needs further validation but may be useful for risk stratification.

DISCLOSURE

The authors have nothing to disclose.

REFERENCES

1. Rahib L, Smith BD, Aizenberg R, et al. Projecting cancer incidence and deaths to 2030: the unexpected burden of thyroid, liver, and pancreas cancers in the United States. Cancer Res 2014;74:2913–21.
2. Tempero MA, Malafa MP, Chiorean EG, et al. Pancreatic adenocarcinoma, version 1.2019. J Natl Compr Canc Netw 2019;17:202–10.
3. Klein AP, Brune KA, Petersen GM, et al. Prospective risk of pancreatic cancer in familial pancreatic cancer kindreds. Cancer Res 2004;64:2634–8.
4. Brune KA, Lau B, Palmisano E, et al. Importance of age of onset in pancreatic cancer kindreds. J Natl Cancer Inst 2010;102:119–26.
5. Canto MI, Almario JA, Schulick RD, et al. Risk of neoplastic progression in individuals at high risk for pancreatic cancer undergoing long-term surveillance. Gastroenterology 2018;155:740–751 e2.
6. Hruban RH, Canto MI, Goggins M, et al. Update on familial pancreatic cancer. Adv Surg 2010;44:293–311.
7. Chaffee KG, Oberg AL, McWilliams RR, et al. Prevalence of germ-line mutations in cancer genes among pancreatic cancer patients with a positive family history. Genet Med 2018;20:119–27.
8. Brand RE, Lerch MM, Rubinstein WS, et al. Advances in counselling and surveillance of patients at risk for pancreatic cancer. Gut 2007;56:1460–9.
9. Chen F, Childs EJ, Mocci E, et al. Analysis of heritability and genetic architecture of pancreatic cancer: a PanC4 study. Cancer Epidemiol Biomarkers Prev 2019; 28:1238–45.
10. Zhen DB, Rabe KG, Gallinger S, et al. BRCA1, BRCA2, PALB2, and CDKN2A mutations in familial pancreatic cancer: a PACGENE study. Genet Med 2015;17: 569–77.
11. Hu C, Hart SN, Bamlet WR, et al. Prevalence of pathogenic mutations in cancer predisposition genes among pancreatic cancer patients. Cancer Epidemiol Biomarkers Prev 2016;25:207–11.
12. Shindo K, Yu J, Suenaga M, et al. Deleterious germline mutations in patients with apparently sporadic pancreatic adenocarcinoma. J Clin Oncol 2017;35:3382–90.
13. Hu C, Hart SN, Polley EC, et al. Association between inherited germline mutations in cancer predisposition genes and risk of pancreatic cancer. JAMA 2018;319: 2401–9.
14. Daly M, Pal T, Berry M, et al. *Genetic/Familial High-Risk Assessment: Breast, Ovarian, and Pancreatic, Version 2.2021, NCCN Clinical Practice Guidelines in Oncology.* J Natl Compr Canc Netw 2021;19(1):77-102.
15. Ibrahim IS, Wasser MN, Wu Y, et al. High growth rate of pancreatic ductal adenocarcinoma in CDKN2A-p16-Leiden mutation carriers. Cancer Prev Res (Phila) 2018;11:551–6.
16. Vasen HF, Gruis NA, Frants RR, et al. Risk of developing pancreatic cancer in families with familial atypical multiple mole melanoma associated with a specific 19 deletion of p16 (p16-Leiden). Int J Cancer 2000;87:809–11.
17. McWilliams RR, Wieben ED, Chaffee KG, et al. CDKN2A germline rare coding variants and risk of pancreatic cancer in minority populations. Cancer Epidemiol Biomarkers Prev 2018;27:1364–70.
18. Hofstatter EW, Domchek SM, Miron A, et al. PALB2 mutations in familial breast and pancreatic cancer. Fam Cancer 2011;10:225–31.

19. Aslanian HR, Lee JH, Canto MI. AGA clinical practice update on pancreas cancer screening in high-risk individuals: expert review. Gastroenterology 2020;159: 358–62.
20. Roberts NJ, Jiao Y, Yu J, et al. ATM mutations in patients with hereditary pancreatic cancer. Cancer Discov 2012;2:41–6.
21. Provenzale D, Gupta S, Ahnen DJ, et al. Genetic/familial high-risk assessment: colorectal version 1.2016, NCCN clinical practice guidelines in oncology. J Natl Compr Canc Netw 2016;14:1010–30.
22. Gupta S, Weiss J, Axell L, et al. *NCCN Guidelines Insights: Genetic/Familial High-Risk Assessment: Colorectal, Version 2.2019.* J Natl Compr Canc Netw, 2019;17(9):1032-41.
23. Korsse SE, Harinck F, van Lier MG, et al. Pancreatic cancer risk in Peutz-Jeghers syndrome patients: a large cohort study and implications for surveillance. J Med Genet 2013;50:59–64.
24. Resta N, Pierannunzio D, Lenato GM, et al. Cancer risk associated with STK11/LKB1 germline mutations in Peutz-Jeghers syndrome patients: results of an Italian multicenter study. Dig Liver Dis 2013;45:606–11.
25. Ruijs MWG, Verhoef S, Rookus MA, et al. TP53 germline mutation testing in 180 families suspected of Li–Fraumeni syndrome: mutation detection rate and relative frequency of cancers in different familial phenotypes. J Med Genet 2010;47:421.
26. Lowenfels AB, Maisonneuve P, DiMagno EP, et al. Hereditary pancreatitis and the risk of pancreatic cancer. J Natl Cancer Inst 1997;89:442–6.
27. Hasan A, Moscoso DI, Kastrinos F. The role of genetics in pancreatitis. Gastrointest Endosc Clin N Am 2018;28:587–603.
28. Comfort MW, Steinberg AG. Pedigree of a family with hereditary chronic relapsing pancreatitis. Gastroenterology 1952;21:54–63.
29. Whitcomb DC, Gorry MC, Preston RA, et al. Hereditary pancreatitis is caused by a mutation in the cationic trypsinogen gene. Nat Genet 1996;14:141–5.
30. Witt H, Luck W, Hennies HC, et al. Mutations in the gene encoding the serine protease inhibitor, Kazal type 1 are associated with chronic pancreatitis. Nat Genet 2000;25:213–6.
31. Zielenski J. Genotype and phenotype in cystic fibrosis. Respiration 2000;67: 117–33.
32. Nissim S, Leshchiner I, Mancias JD, et al. Mutations in RABL3 alter KRAS prenylation and are associated with hereditary pancreatic cancer. Nat Genet 2019;51: 1308–14.
33. Lowery MA, Wong W, Jordan EJ, et al. Prospective evaluation of germline alterations in patients with exocrine pancreatic neoplasms. J Natl Cancer Inst 2018; 110:1067–74.
34. Golan T, Hammel P, Reni M, et al. Maintenance Olaparib for Germline BRCA-mutated metastatic pancreatic cancer. N Engl J Med 2019;381:317–27.
35. Young EL, Thompson BA, Neklason DW, et al. Pancreatic cancer as a sentinel for hereditary cancer predisposition. BMC Cancer 2018;18:697.
36. Galeotti AA, Gentiluomo M, Rizzato C, et al. Polygenic and multifactorial scores for pancreatic ductal adenocarcinoma risk prediction. J Med Genet 2021;58: 369–77.
37. Force UPST. Screening for Pancreatic cancer: US preventive services task force reaffirmation recommendation statement. JAMA 2019;322:438–44.
38. Lucas AL, Kastrinos F. Screening for pancreatic cancer. JAMA 2019;322:407–8.

39. Canto MI, Harinck F, Hruban RH, et al. International Cancer of the Pancreas Screening (CAPS) Consortium summit on the management of patients with increased risk for familial pancreatic cancer. Gut 2013;62:339–47.
40. Syngal S, Brand RE, Church JM, et al. ACG clinical guideline: Genetic testing and management of hereditary gastrointestinal cancer syndromes. Am J Gastroenterol 2015;110:223–62 [quiz 263].
41. Goggins M, Overbeek KA, Brand R, et al. Management of patients with increased risk for familial pancreatic cancer: updated recommendations from the International Cancer of the Pancreas Screening (CAPS) Consortium. Gut 2020;69:7–17.
42. Overbeek KA, Cahen DL, Canto MI, et al. Surveillance for neoplasia in the pancreas. Best Pract Res Clin Gastroenterol 2016;30:971–86.
43. Lorenzo D, Rebours V, Maire F, et al. Role of endoscopic ultrasound in the screening and follow-up of high-risk individuals for familial pancreatic cancer. World J Gastroenterol 2019;25(34):5082-96.
44. Stoffel EM, McKernin SE, Brand R, et al. Evaluating susceptibility to pancreatic cancer: ASCO provisional clinical opinion. J Clin Oncol 2019;37:153–64.
45. Llach J, Carballal S, Moreira L. Familial pancreatic cancer: current perspectives. Cancer Manag Res 2020;12:743–58.

Pancreatic Cancer Surveillance and Novel Strategies for Screening

Beth Dudley, MS, MPH, Randall E. Brand, MD*

KEYWORDS

- Hereditary pancreatic cancer • Familial pancreatic cancer
- Pancreatic cancer surveillance • Pancreatic cancer screening

KEY POINTS

- Individuals with a genetic susceptibility to pancreatic cancer may benefit from surveillance to increase the likelihood of early detection.
- Currently, candidates for surveillance are identified based on genetic test results and family history of pancreatic ductal adenocarcinoma (PDAC), and surveillance is accomplished through imaging of the pancreas (endoscopic ultrasound or MRI).
- Novel methods that incorporate personalized risk, biomarkers, and radiomics are being investigated in an attempt to improve identification of at-risk individuals and to increase detection of precursor and early-stage lesions.

INTRODUCTION

Pancreatic ductal adenocarcinoma (PDAC) accounts for 3.2% of all cancer diagnoses in the United States, but is responsible for 7.9% of all cancer deaths, with a 5-year survival of 10.8%.[1] The dismal survival is due in large part to a lack of early detection, with more than half of cases being metastatic at time of diagnosis.[1] The lifetime risk for PDAC in the United States is 1.7%.[1] Screening in the general population is not performed, in part because of the disease's rarity and the lack of a reliable, cost-effective screening tool. Approximately 10% of PDAC is attributed to genetic susceptibility,[2] either because of an identified pathogenic variant in a cancer susceptibility gene[3–11] or a combination of shared genetic, environmental, and lifestyle risk factors, resulting in a familial predisposition.[12,13] Family members of individuals with hereditary or familial PDAC have an increased risk for this cancer and therefore may benefit from surveillance to increase the likelihood of early detection. Currently, imaging of the

R.E.B. has received research funding from Immunovia and Freenome related to biomarker development for the early detection of pancreatic cancer.

Division of Gastroenterology, Hepatology, and Nutrition, Department of Medicine, University of Pittsburgh, 5200 Centre Avenue, Suite 409, Pittsburgh, PA 15232, USA

* Corresponding author.

E-mail address: brandre@upmc.edu

pancreas, usually by endoscopic ultrasound (EUS) or MRI, is the standard surveillance modality for individuals at increased risk for PDAC, but several novel strategies to increase early detection are being explored through research.

DEFINITIONS

Familial pancreatic cancer (FPC) is the term used to describe a family in which 2 individuals who are first-degree relatives to each other have been diagnosed with PDAC with no identified genetic cause.

Screening is testing performed in the asymptomatic general population.
Surveillance is testing performed in asymptomatic high-risk individuals.
Diagnostic is testing performed in the setting of symptoms.

DISCUSSION
Candidates for Pancreatic Ductal Adenocarcinoma Surveillance

Several organizations have published recommendations regarding high-risk PDAC surveillance, including the American College of Gastroenterology (ACG),[14] the American Society of Clinical Oncology (ASCO),[15] the International Cancer of the Pancreas Screening (CAPS) Consortium,[16] and the National Comprehensive Cancer Network (NCCN).[17] These recommendations have some mostly minor variations, but there is general consensus that surveillance should be considered in the setting of pathogenic variants in BRCA1, BRCA2, the mismatch repair genes, STK11, CDKN2A, ATM, and PALB2. With the exception of NCCN, these organizations also recommend surveillance in FPC families. ACG, the International CAPS Consortium, and NCCN provide parameters for family history requirements and propose an age to begin surveillance, as illustrated in **Table 1**.

The magnitude of increased PDAC risk varies by gene and depending on whether an individual has an identified pathogenic variant or is from an FPC family (Chapter x, see **Table 1**).[1,3–13,18,19] Consequently, the parameters for surveillance vary as well. For individuals with pathogenic variants in STK11 or CDKN2A, which confer the highest risks for PDAC, no family history is required to be eligible for surveillance, and surveillance begins at an earlier age.

Because the increased PDAC risk is more modest for individuals with pathogenic variants in BRCA1/2, the mismatch repair genes, ATM, and PALB2 and because it has been suggested that risk is more significant for pathogenic variant carriers who have a family history of PDAC,[20] these individuals are currently considered eligible for surveillance only if they have a family history of the disease. The International CAPS Consortium recommends surveillance for these individuals if they have at least 1 affected first-degree relative, whereas ACG and NCCN also include second-degree relatives. Some experts think that the family history requirement results in missed opportunity for early detection and have proposed that PDAC surveillance be offered to all individuals with pathogenic variants in BRCA1/2, the genes in this group with the most data regarding PDAC risk.[21]

The risk for PDAC is variable for individuals in an FPC family depending on the number of affected family members, but risk has only been estimated for individuals who have affected first-degree relatives.[12,13] As such, ACG, ASCO, and the International CAPS Consortium recommend surveillance for individuals in an FPC family who have at least 1 affected first-degree relative. The more restrictive parameters seem to be supported by recent data that suggest individuals undergoing surveillance are more likely to be diagnosed with PDAC, high-grade dysplasia, or high-risk features if they have a pathogenic variant than if they are from an FPC family.[22]

Table 1
Pancreatic cancer surveillance guidelines by organization

	Organization								
	ACG,[14] 2015			International CAPS Consortium,[16] 2020			NCCN,[17] 2020		
Syndrome or Gene	Is FH Required?	FH Specifications	Age to Begin, y	Is FH Required?	FH Specifications	Age to Begin, y	Is FH Required?	FH Specifications	Age to Begin, y
HBOC (BRCA1/2)	Yes	≥1 FDR or SDR	50[a]	Yes	≥1 FDR	45–50[a]	Yes	≥1 FDR or SDR	50[a]
Lynch syndrome (MLH1, MSH2, MSH6, PMS2)	Yes	≥1 FDR or SDR	50[a]	Yes	≥1 FDR (excludes PMS2)	45–50[a]	Yes	≥1 FDR or SDR (excludes PMS2)	50[a]
Peutz-Jeghers syndrome (STK11)	No	—	35	No	—	40	No	—	30–35[a]
FAMMM (CDKN2A)	No	—	50[a]	No	—	40	No	—	40[a]
ATM	Yes	≥1 FDR or SDR	50[a]	Yes	≥1 FDR	45–50[a]	Yes	≥1 FDR or SDR	50[a]
PALB2	Yes	≥1 FDR or SDR	50[a]	Yes	≥1 FDR	45–50[a]	Yes	≥1 FDR or SDR	50[a]
FPC	Yes	≥1 FDR	50[a]	Yes	≥1 FDR	50–55[a]	—	—	—

Abbreviations: FAMMM, familial atypical multiple mole melanoma; FDR, first-degree relative; FH, family history; HBOC, hereditary breast and ovarian cancer; SDR, second-degree relative.
[a] Or 10 y before the earliest age of diagnosis in the family if before age 60.

In a 2016 publication, Bartsch and colleagues[23] established that high-risk lesions are uncommon in individuals before age 50 and suggest that surveillance before age 50 is unlikely to be beneficial in most individuals. As such, surveillance has typically been recommended to begin at age 50 for most at-risk individuals. Exceptions include CDKN2A and STK11 pathogenic variant carriers, where initiation of testing begins between the ages of 30 and 40, and those individuals who have a family history of PDAC diagnosed before age 60 (see **Table 1**). The suggestion by Bartsch and colleagues for not beginning PDAC surveillance before age 50 for other pathogenic variants has not been widely adopted as illustrated in the recent CAPS International consensus recommendations, whereby an age range of 45 to 50 to commence surveillance was given for these groups.[16]

Current Pancreatic Ductal Adenocarcinoma Surveillance Modalities

To date, there is no biomarker with sufficient sensitivity or specificity to rely on for PDAC screening or surveillance, although this has long been the goal of early detection research and is discussed in more detail later in this article. As a result, PDAC surveillance is currently accomplished through imaging of the pancreas that allows for visualization of abnormalities.

The target abnormalities for pancreatic cancer surveillance are advanced precursor neoplasia or early-stage PDAC (T1N0).[20,24] PDAC arises from 1 of 3 pathways, involving the following precursor lesions: pancreatic intraepithelial neoplasia (PanIN), intraductal papillary mucinous neoplasms (IPMN), or mucinous cystic neoplasms (MCNs).[20] The first 2 pathways comprise most cases, with MCNs being less common. PanINs are microscopic lesions that originate from pancreatic ducts, whereas IPMNs and MCNs are mucin-producing cystic neoplasms. IPMNs originate from the main pancreatic duct or its side branches, whereas MCNs do not connect with the duct system.[25] High-grade PanIN lesions (PanIN3) and IPMNs with high-risk features are the ideal advanced precursor lesions that surveillance aims to detect.[20] At present, high-grade PanIN lesions are challenging to detect through surveillance given their microscopic nature. High-risk IPMN features include size larger than 3 cm, main pancreatic duct measurement greater than or equal to 10 mm, presence of enhancing mural nodules, thickened/enhancing cyst walls, lymphadenopathy, accompanying jaundice, rapid growth rate (>5 mm in 2 years or >10 mm during follow-up), and the presence of high-risk mutations through molecular analysis of cyst fluid (TP53, PIK3CA, PTEN, AKT1, SMAD4).[26,27]

Imaging options include MRI/magnetic resonance cholangiopancreatography and EUS. Computed tomography is not currently used for surveillance, as it detects fewer lesions than other imaging modalities and results in radiation exposure.[28] The organizational recommendations discussed in the previous section all offer the option of MRI or EUS, with no preference for 1 modality over the other.[14–17] As a result, the decision is largely made based on clinician preference or patient-specific restrictions; for example, altered gastric anatomy resulting from procedures like gastric bypass may preclude complete visualization of the pancreas by EUS, whereas MRI may be contraindicated in individuals who have metal or electronic devices in their body.

Harinck and colleagues[29] published a comparison of MRI and EUS in 2015, which suggests that the 2 modalities could have complementary purposes. The investigators reported 55% agreement between EUS and MRI in the reporting of clinically relevant lesions, with MRI better at cyst detection and EUS better at small solid lesion detection. Two small solid lesions, one of which was an early-stage PDAC, were only detected by EUS, whereas 3 of 9 cystic lesions greater than 10 mm in size were only found on MRI. The other solid lesions identified only by EUS was 2 adjacent 3-

mm PanIN2 foci, which is of unknown clinical significance because the natural history of PanIN2 lesions is not well described.

Regardless of whether surveillance is performed through EUS, MRI, or a combination of the two, PDAC surveillance recommendations generally agree that it should be performed in expert centers, ideally in conjunction with research protocols, and after a frank conversation regarding its risks, benefits, uncertainties, and limitations.[14–17]

Pancreatic Ductal Adenocarcinoma Surveillance Outcomes

Historically, expert clinicians who offer PDAC surveillance to high-risk individuals have done so with the caveat that data proving its benefit are lacking. Although that caveat is still true to some extent, several studies published over the last few years have begun to show that individuals diagnosed with PDAC while undergoing surveillance are more likely to have resectable disease, which results in a stage-shift that should translate to improved survival.

One of the first studies to suggest improved outcomes was published by Vasen and colleagues[30] in 2016. This prospective study documented surveillance outcomes of individuals undergoing annual EUS or MRI across 3 European centers; they reported that 13 of 178 individuals with a pathogenic variant in *CDKN2A* were diagnosed with PDAC, with a 75% resection rate and a 24% 5-year survival.

The seminal paper regarding the potential success of PDAC surveillance was published by Canto and colleagues in 2018.[31] In this study, the investigators provide data from 354 individuals undergoing surveillance over a period of 16 years. In total, 14 individuals were diagnosed with PDAC, and 10 individuals were found to have high-grade dysplasia during this time, a total of 7% of the patient cohort. Ten of the PDAC diagnoses were found in individuals undergoing routine surveillance; the remaining 4 were diagnosed during a period of noncompliance. Nine of the 10 individuals diagnosed with surveillance-detected PDAC were resectable and had a 3-year survival rate of 85%. The 4 noncompliant individuals had a 25% 3-year survival rate. The investigators calculated in their cohort an annual progression rate of 1.6% per year for developing an invasive PDAC or high-grade dysplasia, with a median follow-up time of 5.6 years.

In 2019, the International CAPS Consortium published outcome data, including approximately 1700 individuals undergoing PDAC surveillance in 11 international centers.[32] They reported that 32 individuals underwent surgery for early-stage PDAC (19) or high-risk precursor lesions (main duct IPMN [4], branch duct IPMN [4], or PanIN3 [5]), whereas only 5 individuals had been diagnosed with inoperable PDAC. An additional 39 patients underwent resection for a low-risk or benign lesion. Similar to the Canto study, there was a significant stage shift seen as compared with a nonscreened general population with approximately 85% of patients identified at a resectable stage. As expected, survival rates were greatest in patients with high-risk precursor lesions as compared with invasive PDAC, with the former group having similar survival rates to those 39 individuals with low-risk or benign lesions.

A meta-analysis of studies reporting on PDAC surveillance in high-risk individuals was published in 2020.[33] In total, 24 studies representing 2112 individuals undergoing surveillance were included in the analysis. The investigators reported that 111 individuals needed to be screened in order to detect 1 case of high-grade dysplasia or T1N0 PDAC and concluded that surveillance programs are successful, with no significant differences between screening modality (EUS or MRI).

Cost-effectiveness studies provide insight into the required performance characteristics for successful PDAC surveillance. For example, a 2019 study published by Corral and colleagues[34] found that PDAC surveillance through MRI or EUS was cost-effective in high-risk individuals younger than age 76 years; they reported that MRI was more cost-effective for moderate risk (5-fold) individuals, whereas EUS was favored for high-risk (20-fold) individuals. A study from 2021 by Kumar and colleagues[35] reported on the threshold analysis of the cost-effectiveness of EUS in high-risk subjects for developing PDAC enrolled in the Cancer of the Pancreas Screening 5 (CAPS5) multicenter study. Their model of a one-time index EUS demonstrated excellent cost-effectiveness if lifetime PDAC probability is greater than 10.8%. Other variables that contributed to the cost-effectiveness included the probability of a missed lesion on index EUS, future PDAC development after normal index EUS, or length of survival following pancreatic lesion resection. The following limitations highlighted in the study by Kumar and colleagues underscore the value of collaborative PDAC surveillance registries, such as CAPS5 and the PRECEDE (Pancreatic Cancer Early Detection Consortium) and identify future areas of research focus. These limitations are "(1) long-term follow-up of those who undergo resection, (2) development of PDAC outside screening, (3) the risk to patients with mutations and a family history of PDAC, and (4) the survival benefit conferred by early detection."[35]

Despite the emergence of promising data regarding improved outcomes with PDAC surveillance in high-risk individuals, current options for surveillance have their limitations. First, the ability to identify high-risk individuals for surveillance is currently limited to those individuals who have a single-gene cancer predisposition or individuals from an FPC family. Thus, the majority (~90%) of individuals who develop a PDAC do not qualify for surveillance.

Another concern is that surveillance can lead to surgery for screen-detected findings that ultimately prove to be low-risk lesions. For example, a 2020 publication addressing surgical outcomes of high-risk PDAC surveillance found that 42% of individuals who underwent surgery were found to have only low-grade precursor lesions.[36] In addition, the previously cited International CAPS Consortium study that reported on high-risk individuals who underwent surgery included 71 individuals who had surgery, only 32 (45%) of whom had high-risk lesions.[32]

Last, some individuals undergoing surveillance are still diagnosed with interval unresectable PDACs. A recent Dutch study found that 10 of 165 pathogenic variant carriers undergoing annual EUS or MRI surveillance were diagnosed with PDAC over an average follow-up period of 63 months; 4 of these individuals presented with symptomatic interval cancers, and the median survival of the 10 individuals was 18 months.[37] These limitations indicate a need for improvement in the ability to identify high-risk individuals, as well as more sensitive and specific methods of early detection.

Novel Strategies for Risk Stratification

As mentioned previously, current surveillance candidates include patients with a genetic predisposition for developing PDAC, which only make up 10% of PDAC patients. In order to increase the number of candidates for PDAC surveillance, novel enrichment strategies are needed, aiming for a lifetime risk of 5% to 10%, as opposed to general population lifetime rate in the United States of 1.7%.[38] **Table 2** provides a summary of current and potential future candidates for PDAC surveillance.

Polygenic risk scores

Cancer is a multifactorial disease. Even for individuals who have identified pathogenic variants in cancer predisposition genes, other smaller genetic risk factors, environmental exposures, and lifestyle choices play a role in cancer development. In recent years, these multifactorial components have been an active area of research regarding

Table 2	
Current and potential future candidates for pancreatic ductal adenocarcinoma surveillance	
Current PDAC Surveillance Indications	**Potential Future PDAC Surveillance Indications**
Pathogenic variant in *CDKN2A* or *STK11*	Chronic pancreatitis
Pathogenic variant in *ATM*, *BRCA1/2*, MMR gene, or *PALB2* with affected FDR or SDR	New-onset diabetes
FPC with at least one affected FDR	Increased risk based on polygenic risk score
Hereditary pancreatitis	
Incidentally detected cystic lesions in the pancreas	

Abbreviation: MMR, mismatch repair (*MLH1, MSH2, MSH6, PMS2*).

cancer risk estimates. Polygenic risk scores (PRS) have been developed for a variety of cancer types and use several different single nucleotide polymorphisms (SNPs) to stratify risk among study participants. In some cases, PRS are combined with lifestyle or medical risk factors to further tailor risk. A recent publication explores the development of a PRS for PDAC in a European population.[39] These investigators created a PRS using data from 3619 PDAC cases and 5790 controls. Their PRS included 28 individual SNPs that have been previously shown to impact PDAC risk, as well as 2 SNPs that allow for inference of blood type because that has been shown to impact PDAC risk. They also combined the PRS score with information about smoking status and type 2 diabetes to create a multifactorial score. Although the investigators were pleased that their model could predict different levels of risk with statistical significance, they ultimately thought that the poor area under the curve values generated by the data indicated that more PDAC risk SNPs need to be identified and that more nongenetic risk factors need to be incorporated to allow for clinical use.

Although PRS and multifactorial risk predictors hold promise in allowing for expanded and more tailored identification of at-risk individuals, more research is needed in this area, especially for populations that are not of European ancestry. Once optimized, these tools could identify new individuals who would benefit from PDAC surveillance and could help provide a better understanding of individual risks for people who are currently eligible for surveillance.

New-onset diabetes
Approximately 0.5% to 1% of individuals diagnosed with type 2 diabetes after age 50 will be diagnosed with PDAC within 3 years.[40,41] As such, individuals with new-onset diabetes (NOD) may represent an enriched population to target for early diagnosis of PDAC. A study published in 2018 outlined a model that could allow for further stratification of risk in individuals with NOD.[42] These investigators used knowledge that PDAC-related NOD was more likely to be associated with weight loss, rapid change in fasting blood glucose levels, and older age of diagnosis than traditional type 2 diabetes. These 3 factors were incorporated into a model called ENDPAC, which stratifies risk for PDAC as high, intermediate, and low. The investigators recommend that individuals with high-risk scores undergo further evaluation for PDAC. Currently, a large multicenter study is underway to further investigate the development of PDAC in NOD patients, with the hopes that the resulting data will provide a useful clinical tool.[43]

Given the data about NOD and PDAC risk, some experts have proposed using serial measurement of fasting blood glucose or hemoglobin A1c as a surveillance tool for high-risk individuals. For example, 75% of experts in the International CAPS Consortium thought that routine testing for diabetes should be included in the surveillance protocol for high-risk individuals.[16] As a result, their updated 2018 guidelines include measurement of fasting blood glucose or hemoglobin A1c at baseline evaluation and during follow-up.

Chronic pancreatitis

Initial reports described a significant risk of developing pancreatic cancer in patients with chronic pancreatitis.[44,45] Subsequent studies reported a significantly lower risk, with an odds ratio of less than 3 when excluding those patients diagnosed with chronic pancreatitis within 2 years of the PDAC diagnosis.[46,47] Recent International Consensus Guidelines on Surveillance for Chronic Pancreatitis concluded that surveillance was only warranted in affected individuals with hereditary pancreatitis owing to *PRSS1* pathogenic variants because the risk was deemed high enough to justify surveillance starting at age 40 in pancreatic specialist centers.[48] There was no consensus reached on how to perform surveillance.

Novel Strategies for Surveillance

Although the number of patients is small, the aforementioned studies do lend support that advanced precursor lesions are the ideal surveillance target based on excellent long-term survival rates for patients undergoing pancreatectomies with these findings.[31,32] Because most advanced precursor lesions are PanINs, which are not consistently visualized by current imaging modalities, innovative approaches are required to identify them. One potential use for these approaches is to decrease the cost of surveillance by using them for initial evaluation in high-risk individuals and only proceeding to costlier imaging tests if positive.[49] Some promising strategies currently under investigation are discussed.

Biomarkers

For years, PDAC early detection researchers have sought a biomarker that has sufficient sensitivity and specificity to be used in high-risk individuals and even in the general population. Thousands of publications have been generated on the topic, but an acceptable screening tool has yet to be identified. In an effort to further this research, the Early Detection Research Network encourages consortia and multilaboratory studies to increase large-scale validation of proposed biomarkers and has created reference sets of human specimens that are collected, processed, and stored under standardized processes.[49]

The best-known biomarker associated with PDAC is CA19-9. Although sometimes useful to assess treatment response and progression in individuals with PDAC, it is not a reliable screening or diagnostic tool, at least when used alone.[50] The most promising biomarker studies combine CA19-9 with 1 or more novel biomarkers to create a panel. Some of these biomarkers include thrombospondin-2, MUC5AC, sTRA, and trefoil factors (TFF1, TFF2, and TFF3).[51–54]

Most biomarker work is not performed in high-risk individuals. One exception is the PanFAM-1 study, which is investigating the utility of a previously developed biomarker panel in high-risk individuals undergoing surveillance for PDAC.[55,56] This study recently completed data collection and is in the process of analysis. Once reported, more should be known about biomarker research in the high-risk setting.

Circulating tumor DNA

Building on the idea of using protein biomarkers to detect PDAC, some researchers have begun to investigate the addition of circulating tumor DNA to their algorithms. In

2017, a study was published that described the development of a screening panel that included testing for KRAS mutations, which are commonly found in PDAC, as well as measurement of 4 proteins: CA19-9, CEA, HGF, and OPN.[57] The investigators reported that this panel detected 64% of stage I and II PDACS in their study group.

These researchers continued their work, later reporting the development of a test that they named CancerSEEK, designed to detect 8 cancer types, including PDAC.[58] Ninety-three PDACs were included in their data set; most of these were stage II at diagnosis (89%), with a smaller proportion of stage I (4%) and stage III (6%) cancers. Stage IV cancers were not included. This test measures 8 protein levels, including CA19-9, and identifies the presence or absence of mutations in 1933 genomic positions. It detected 75% of PDACs in their study cohort.

Radiomics

Current PDAC surveillance is centered on imaging tests that detect pancreatic abnormalities, but as illustrated above, even individuals undergoing routine surveillance are sometimes diagnosed with advanced interval cancers.[37] This fact suggests that improving the ability of imaging tests to identify precursor lesions could be useful in improving early detection. To that end, radiomics is an emerging field that holds promise. Traditionally, interpretation of radiographic images has been performed qualitatively by trained clinicians. The concept behind radiomics is to incorporate quantitative assessment of images by artificial intelligence, which allows for the identification of patterns not detectable visibly.

The use of radiomics in pancreatic disease is in its infancy, but there are some published studies. In 2019, Chu and colleagues[59] reported the successful differentiation between PDAC and normal pancreas using radiomic features. In addition, a handful of studies have been published regarding the use of radiomics in evaluating pancreatic cystic lesions.[60]

SUMMARY

Early detection efforts require the identification of individuals at increased risk for PDAC. Likewise, continued research to improve strategies for the early detection of PDAC is critical in order to benefit these individuals.

CLINICS CARE POINTS

- Individuals who have an increased risk for pancreatic ductal adenocarcinoma because of genetic predisposition and/or family history of the disease should be offered surveillance if they meet published criteria.
- Current options for surveillance include endoscopic ultrasound and MRI.
- Surveillance should be undertaken in expert centers, ideally in conjunction with research protocols, and only after a thorough discussion of the benefits, limitations, and risks of imaging procedures.
- Data regarding pancreatic ductal adenocarcinoma surveillance outcomes are limited but are beginning to show that high-risk individuals diagnosed with pancreatic ductal adenocarcinoma while undergoing surveillance are more likely to have resectable disease, which should improve survival.
- Research to expand the identification of at-risk individuals and to improve early detection is ongoing and holds promise for the future.

REFERENCES

1. NCI SEER program cancer stat facts: pancreatic cancer. Available at: https://seer.cancer.gov/statfacts/html/pancreas.html. Accessed June 16, 2021.
2. Rulyak SJ, Brentnall TA. Inherited pancreatic cancer: improvements in our understanding of genetics and screening. Int J Biochem Cell Biol 2004;36(8):1386–92.
3. Giardiello FM, Offerhaus GJ, Lee DH, et al. Increased risk of thyroid and pancreatic carcinoma in familial adenomatous polyposis. Gut 1993;34(10):1394–6.
4. Roberts NJ, Jiao Y, Yu J, et al. ATM mutations in patients with hereditary pancreatic cancer. Cancer Discov 2012;2(1):41–6.
5. Thompson D, Easton DF, Breast Cancer Linkage Consortium. Cancer incidence in BRCA1 mutation carriers. J Natl Cancer Inst 2002;94(18):1358–65.
6. Breast Cancer Linkage Consortium. Cancer risks in BRCA2 mutation carriers. J Natl Cancer Inst 1999;91(15):1310–6.
7. Goldstein AM, Fraser MC, Struewing JP, et al. Increased risk of pancreatic cancer in melanoma-prone kindreds with p16INK4 mutations. N Engl J Med 1995;333(15):970–4.
8. Aarnio M, Mecklin JP, Aaltonen LA, et al. Life-time risk of different cancers in hereditary non-polyposis colorectal cancer (HNPCC) syndrome. Int J Cancer 1995;64(6):430–3.
9. Jones S, Hruban RH, Kamiyami M, et al. Exomic sequencing identifies PALB2 as a pancreatic cancer susceptibility gene. Science 2009;324(5924):217.
10. Hearle N, Schumacher V, Menko FH, et al. Frequency and spectrum of cancers in the Peutz-Jeghers syndrome. Clin Cancer Res 2006;12(10):3209–15.
11. Birch JM, Alston RD, McNally RJ, et al. Relative frequency and morphology of cancers in carriers of germline TP53 mutations. Oncogene 2001;20(34):4621–8.
12. Klein AP, Brune KA, Petersen GM, et al. Prospective risk of pancreatic cancer in familial pancreatic cancer kindreds. Cancer Res 2004;64(7):2634–8.
13. Brune KA, Lau B, Palmisano E, et al. Importance of age of onset in pancreatic cancer kindreds. J Natl Cancer Inst 2010;102(2):119–26.
14. Syngal S, Brand RE, Church JM, et al. ACG clinical guideline: genetic testing and management of hereditary gastrointestinal cancer syndromes. Am J Gastroenterol 2015;110(2):223–62.
15. Stoffel EM, McKernin SE, Brand R, et al. Evaluating susceptibility to pancreatic cancer: ASCO provisional clinical opinion. J Clin Oncol 2019;37(2):153–64.
16. Goggins M, Overbeek KA, Brand R, et al. Management of patients with increased risk for familial pancreatic cancer: updated recommendations from the International Cancer of the Pancreas Screening (CAPS) Consortium. Gut 2020;69(1):7–17.
17. NCCN clinical practice guidelines in oncology: genetic/familial high-risk assessment: breast and ovarian. Version 2.2021. 2020. Available at: https://www.nccn.org/login?ReturnURL=https://www.nccn.org/professionals/physician_gls/pdf/genetics_bop.pdf. Accessed June 17, 2021.
18. Hall MJ, Bernhisel R, Hughes E, et al. Germline pathogenic variants in the ataxia telangiectasia mutated (ATM) gene are associated with high and moderate risks for multiple cancers. Cancer Prev Res 2021;14(4):433–40.
19. Yang X, Leslie G, Doroszuk A, et al. Cancer risks associated with germline PALB2 pathogenic variants: an international study of 524 families. J Clin Oncol 2020;38(7):674–85.
20. Brand RE, Lerch MM, Rubinstein WS, et al. Advances in counselling and surveillance of patients at risk for pancreatic cancer. Gut 2007;56(10):1460–9.

21. Roch AM, Schneider J, Carr RA, et al. Are BRCA1 and BRCA2 gene mutation patients underscreened for pancreatic adenocarcinoma? J Surg Oncol 2019;119(6): 777–83.
22. Abe T, Blackford AL, Tamura K, et al. Deleterious germline mutations are a risk factor for neoplastic progression among high-risk individuals undergoing pancreatic surveillance. J Clin Oncol 2019;37(13):1070–80.
23. Bartsch DK, Slater EP, Carrato A, et al. Refinement of screening for familial pancreatic cancer. Gut 2016;65(8):1314–21.
24. Ariyama J, Suyama M, Satoh K, et al. Imaging of small pancreatic ductal adenocarcinoma. Pancreas 1998;16(3):396–401.
25. Hruban RH, Takaori K, Klimstra DS, et al. An illustrated consensus on the classification of pancreatic intraepithelial neoplasia and intraductal papillary mucinous neoplasms. Am J Surg Pathol 2004;28(8):977–87.
26. Tanaka M, Fernandez-del Castillo C, Kamisawa T, et al. Revisions of international consensus Fukuoka guidelines for the management of IPMN of the pancreas. Pancreatology 2017;17(5):738–53.
27. Singhi AD, McGrath K, Brand RE, et al. Preoperative next-generation sequencing of pancreatic cyst fluid is highly accurate in cyst classification and detection of advanced neoplasia. Gut 2018;67(12):2131–41.
28. Canto MI, Hruban RH, Fishman EK, et al. Frequent detection of pancreatic lesions in asymptomatic high-risk individuals. Gastroenterology 2012;142(4):796–804.
29. Harinck F, Konings IC, Klujit I, et al. A multicentre comparative prospective blinded analysis of EUS and MRI for screening of pancreatic cancer in high-risk individuals. Gut 2016;65(9):1503–13.
30. Vasen H, Ibrahim I, Ponce CG, et al. Benefit of surveillance for pancreatic cancer in high-risk individuals: outcome of long-term prospective follow-up studies from three European expert centers. J Clin Oncol 2016;34(17):2010–9.
31. Canto MI, Almario JA, Schulick RD, et al. Risk of neoplastic progression in individuals at high risk for pancreatic cancer undergoing long-term surveillance. Gastroenterol 2018;155(3):740–51.
32. Konings ICAW, Canto MI, Almario JA, et al. Surveillance for pancreatic cancer in high-risk individuals. BJS Open 2019;3(5):656–65.
33. Kogekar N, Diaz KE, Weinberg AD, et al. Surveillance of high-risk individuals for pancreatic cancer with EUS and MRI: a meta-analysis. Pancreatology 2020; 20(8):1739–46.
34. Corral JE, Das A, Bruno MJ, et al. Cost-effectiveness of pancreatic cancer surveillance in high-risk individuals: an economic analysis. Pancreas 2019;48(4): 526–36.
35. Kumar S, Saumoy M, Oh A, et al. Threshold analysis of the cost-effectiveness of endoscopic ultrasound in patients at high risk for pancreatic ductal adenocarcinoma. Pancreas 2021.
36. Canto MI, Kerdsirichairat T, Yeo CJ, et al. Surgical outcomes after pancreatic resection of screening-detected lesions in individuals at high risk for developing pancreatic cancer. J Gastrointest Surg 2020;24(5):1101–10.
37. Overbeek KA, Levink IJM, Koopmann BDM, et al. Long-term yield of pancreatic cancer surveillance in high-risk individuals. Gut 2021.
38. Aslanian HR, Lee JH, Canto MI. AGA clinical practice update on pancreas cancer screening in high-risk individuals: expert review. Gastroenterology 2020; 159(1):358–62.

39. Galeotti AA, Gentiluomo M, Rizzato C, et al. Polygenic and multifactorial scores for pancreatic ductal adenocarcinoma risk prediction. J Med Genet 2021;58(6):369–77.
40. Chari ST, Leibson CL, Rabe KG, et al. Probability of pancreatic cancer following diabetes: a population-based study. Gastroenterol 2005;129(2):504–11.
41. Chen W, Butler RK, Lustigova E, et al. Validation of the enriching new-onset diabetes for pancreatic cancer model in a diverse and integrated healthcare system. Dig Dis Sci 2021;66(1):78–87.
42. Sharma A, Kandlakunta H, Nagpal SJS, et al. Model to determine risk of pancreatic cancer in patients with new-onset diabetes. Gastroenterol 2018;155(3):730–9.
43. A study to establish a new onset hyperglycemia and diabetes cohort. Available at: https://clinicaltrials.gov/ct2/show/NCT03731637. Accessed June 18, 2021.
44. Lowenfels AB, Maisonneuve P, Cavallini G, et al. Pancreatitis and the risk of pancreatic cancer. International Pancreatitis Study Group. N Engl J Med 1993;328(20):1433–7.
45. Malka D, Hammel P, Maire F, et al. Risk of pancreatic adenocarcinoma in chronic pancreatitis. Gut 2002;51(6):849–52.
46. Duell EJ, Lucenteforte E, Olson SH, et al. Pancreatitis and pancreatic cancer risk: a pooled analysis in the International Pancreatic Cancer Case-Control Consortium (PanC4). Ann Oncol 2012;23(11):2964–70.
47. Tong GX, Geng QQ, Chai J, et al. Association between pancreatitis and subsequent risk of pancreatic cancer: a systematic review of epidemiological studies. Asian Pac J Cancer Prev 2014;15(12):5029–34.
48. Greenhalf W, Levy P, Gress T, et al. International consensus guidelines on surveillance for pancreatic cancer in chronic pancreatitis. Recommendations from the Working Group for the International Consensus Guidelines for Chronic Pancreatitis in conjunction with the International Association of Pancreatology, the American Pancreatic Association, the Japan Pancreas Society, and European Pancreatic Club. Pancreatology 2020;20(5):910–8.
49. Liu Y, Kaur S, Huang Y, et al. Biomarkers and strategy to detect preinvasive and early pancreatic cancer: state of the field and impact of the EDRN. Cancer Epidemiol Biomarkers Prev 2020;29(12):2513–23.
50. Goonetilleke KS, Siriwardena AK. Systematic review of carbohydrate antigen (CA19-9) as biochemical marker in the diagnosis of pancreatic cancer. Eur J Surg Oncol 2007;33(3):266–70.
51. Kim J, Bamlet WR, Oberg AL, et al. Detection of early pancreatic ductal adenocarcinoma with thrombospondin-2 and CA19-9 blood markers. Sci Transl Med 2017;9(398):eaah5583.
52. Kaur S, Smith LM, Patel A, et al. A combination of MUC5AC and CA19-9 improves the diagnosis of pancreatic cancer: a multi-center study. Am J Gastroenterol 2017;112(1):172–83.
53. Staal B, Liu Y, Barnett D, et al. The sTRA biomarker: blinded validation of improved accuracy over CA19-9 in pancreatic cancer diagnosis. Clin Cancer Res 2019;25(9):2745–54.
54. Jahan R, Ganguly K, Smith LM, et al. Trefoil factor(s) and CA19-9: a promising panel for early detection of pancreatic cancer. EBioMedicine 2019;42:375–85.
55. A study of IMMRayTM PanCan-d test for early detection of pancreatic cancer in high-risk groups. Available at: https://clinicaltrials.gov/ct2/show/NCT03693378. Accessed June 18, 2021.

56. Mellby LD, Nyberg AP, Johansen JS, et al. Serum biomarker signature-based liquid biopsy for diagnosis of early-stage pancreatic cancer. J Clin Oncol 2018; 36(28):2887–94.
57. Cohen JD, Javed AA, Thoburn C, et al. Combined circulating tumor DNA and protein biomarker-based liquid biopsy for the earlier detection of pancreatic cancers. Proc Natl Acad Sci U S A 2017;114(38):10202–7.
58. Cohen JD, Lu L, Wang Y, et al. Detection and localization of surgically resectable cancers with a multi-analyte blood test. Science 2018;359(6378):926–30.
59. Chu LC, Park S, Kawamoto S, et al. Utility of CT radiomics features in differentiation of pancreatic ductal adenocarcinoma from normal pancreatic tissue. AJR Am J Roentgenol 2019;213(2):349–57.
60. Machicado JD, Koay EJ, Krishna SG. Radiomics for the diagnosis and differentiation of pancreatic cystic lesions. Diagnostics (Basel) 2020;10(7):505.

Genetic Evaluation of Pancreatitis

Yichun Fu, MD[a,b], Aimee L. Lucas, MD, MS[a,b],*

KEYWORDS

- Pancreatitis • Genetics • Hereditary pancreatitis • Familial pancreatitis • *PRSS1*
- *SPINK1* • *CFTR*

KEY POINTS

- Genetic testing is important in evaluating patients with a family history of hereditary pancreatitis (HP), as well as a personal history of unexplained recurrent acute pancreatitis or chronic pancreatitis (CP).
- Certain lifestyle changes are critical for disease modulations, such as tobacco and alcohol cessation. All patients should be counseled, but particularly for carriers of *PRSS1*, *CTRC*, and *CLDN2* mutations.
- Patients with familial pancreatitis should be screened for endocrine and exocrine insufficiency, as well as pancreatic cancer. A multidisciplinary approach including pain management and psychosocial counseling is beneficial.

INTRODUCTION

The initial description of multiple cases of autosomal dominant inherited chronic pancreatitis (CP) in a single family there have been many advances in the understanding of the genetic susceptibility to pancreatitis.[1] Following Since a report on the significant role of serine protease 1 (*PRSS1*) gene in hereditary pancreatitis (HP) in the late 1990s, the cystic fibrosis transmembrane conductance regulator gene (*CFTR*) was also associated with recurrent acute pancreatitis (RAP) and CP.[2–4] In 2000, the serine protease inhibitor gene (*SPINK1*) was also linked to CP.[5] In the next 2 decades, other genes including calcium-sensing receptor (*CASR*),[6–9] chymotrypsin C (*CTRC*),[10] claudin-2 (*CLDN2*),[11] carboxypeptidase A1 (*CPA1*),[12] carboxyl ester lipase (*CEL*),[13] chymotrypsin B1 and B2 (*CTRB1/CTRB2*),[14] and transient receptor cation channel subfamily V member 6 gene (*TRPV6*)[15] have also been associated with RAP and/or CP.

Some patients who present with RAP or CP have a genetic predisposition and the disease may be better characterized as HP or familial pancreatitis.[16] HP has been

Funding sources: None.
[a] Henry D. Janowitz Division of Gastroenterology, One Gustave L. Levy Place, Box 1069, New York, NY 10029, USA; [b] Samuel Bronfman Department of Medicine, Icahn School of Medicine at Mount Sinai, New York, USA
* Corresponding author.
E-mail address: aimee.lucas@mssm.edu

Gastrointest Endoscopy Clin N Am 32 (2022) 27–43
https://doi.org/10.1016/j.giec.2021.08.006
1052-5157/22/© 2021 Elsevier Inc. All rights reserved.

traditionally defined as the presence of ≥2 blood relatives with pancreatitis across ≥2 generations with apparent autosomal dominant inheritance, or pancreatitis in the setting of a pathogenic germline variant in *PRSS1*.[17,18] In comparison, FP is used to describe a broader category of families with higher incidence of pancreatitis than the general population. FP requires ≥2 blood relatives with idiopathic pancreatitis not clearly caused by obstruction or environmental (eg, alcohol) causes, typically in the absence of an identifiable genetic defect.

Patients with genetic predispositions have often been diagnosed initially with RAP and CP, and developed irreversible pancreatic fibrosis, endocrine and exocrine disorders by the time they were diagnosed with HP.[19] Therefore, it is imperative for clinicians to have early suspicion to initiate appropriate management and disease modification. In this review, we summarize the current data on the genetic abnormalities in pancreatitis and discuss the evaluation and clinical management.

OVERALL EPIDEMIOLOGY

The epidemiology of CP and HP is incompletely understood, in part due to challenges with long-term follow-up, variability of disease phenotype, and lack of consistent disease definitions. The estimated prevalence of HP ranges from 0.3 to 0.57 per 100,000, with worldwide variability.[20–22] Most of the data on HP are derived from European cohorts and associated with specific germline variants, as discussed in the following.

GERMLINE VARIANTS
PRSS1

Pathogenic *PRSS1* variants, with penetrance ranging between 40% and 90% in HP families, lead to autosomal dominant expression of pancreatitis.[17] Although more than 40 variants in *PRSS1* have been associated with HP, the most prevalent variants are R122H, N29I, and A16V.[23,24]

Prevalence

As the most recognized genetic variant in HP, the prevalence of *PRSS1* variants has been explored in multiple studies in Europe, Asia, and North America and found in up to 80% of HP worldwide.[23] In 418 individuals from the European Registry of Hereditary Pancreatitis and Pancreatic Cancer (EUROPAC), pathogenic germline variants in *PRSS1* were detected in 327 (78%); 19 (5%) of patients did not pursue testing. Among the pathogenic variants, 58 (52%) of 112 families (222 (53%) of 418 patients) were found to harbor R122H, 24 (21%) families (94 (22%) patients) N29I, and 5 (4%) families (11 (3%) patients) A16V.[18] In a nationwide survey from Japan, 30 (41.1%) of families who underwent genetic testing harbored a *PRSS1* variant: 22 (30.1%) with R122H and 6 (8.2%) N29I. In a study of more than 200 *PRSS1* carriers in the United States, the most common variants were R122H (83.9%) and N29I (11.5).[25] Interestingly, one study found *PRSS1* A16V variants to be present in 0.66% of the general population (4.32% in the African population compared with 0.47% in the European population), suggesting that this variant may have a variable phenotype.[23]

Mechanism of action

The *PRSS1* gene encodes cationic trypsinogen, a zymogen precursor to trypsin. After being secreted by the pancreas into the small intestine, trypsin activates other zymogens in the small intestine. Pancreatic acinar and ductal cells regulate trypsin and prevent premature or excessive trypsin activation, which may lead to an immune response.[2] (**Fig. 1**) Most of the *PRSS1* variants result in single amino acid changes

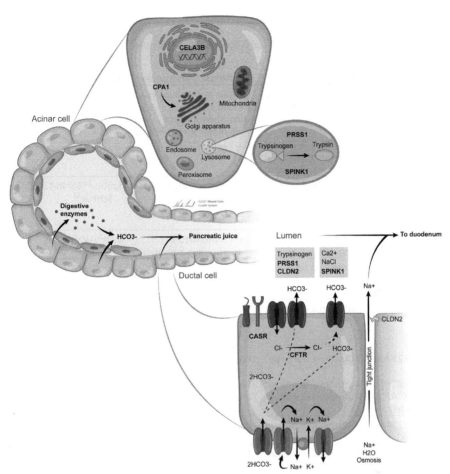

Fig. 1. Genetic variants in chronic pancreatitis. Left panel: several genes affect trypsin activation (*SPINK1*, *PRSS1*, *CELA3B*), secretion (*PRSS1*, *UBR1*, *CEL*), and degradation (*PRSS1*, *CTRC*, *PHLIP*). *CPA1* causes protein misfolding and stress in the endoplasmic reticulum. Right panel: *CFTR* affects duct cell secretion. *CASR* is involved in both calcium regulation and duct cell secretion. *CLDN2* regulates water and sodium transport in the pancreatic duct. (Printed with permission from © Mount Sinai Health System.)

in cationic trypsinogen and some result in an enzyme product that prematurely converts cationic trypsinogen to trypsin within the pancreas, whereas others prevent the degradation of trypsin (**Table 1**). There are 56 known *PRSS1* variants in patients with hereditary, familial, or idiopathic CP, all of which are categorized into copy number variants, gene conversion, and point variants.[23,24] R122H inhibits trypsin autolysis, whereas A16V mutation increases auto-activation and N29I affects both trypsinogen degradation and activation.[26,27] *PRSS1* variants that cause a gain of function of the trypsin TRY-1 proteins have the deleterious effect of promoting increased autoactivation and higher intrapancreatic trypsin activity.[28–30] In addition, less prevalent variants such as R116C, S124F, D100H, C139F, K29N, G208A have been associated with moderate to severe reduction in trypsinogen secretion, which can lead to protein misfolding and endoplasmic reticulum (ER) stress, causing pancreatic injury.[27,31,32]

Table 1
Common pathogenic variants associated with chronic pancreatitis

Gene and Variant	Mode of Inheritance	Functional Consequence	References
PRSS1 (R122H)	Autosomal dominant	Inhibits trypsin autolysis	Whitcomb,[2] Nemoda,[26] Szabo[27]
PRSS1 (N29I)	Autosomal dominant	Inhibits trypsin degradation and increases activation	
PRSS1 (A16V)	Autosomal dominant, low-penetrance pathogenic variant	Increases auto-activation	
PRSS1 (R116C, S124F, D100H, C139F, K29N, G208A)	Autosomal dominant	Causes moderate to severe reduction in trypsinogen secretion	Szabo,[27] Sahin-Toth,[31] Schnur[32]
SPINK1 (N34S)	Autosomal recessive or polygenic	Causes premature trypsinogen activation	Witt,[5] Whitcomb,[28] Muller[38]
CFTR (F508del)	Autosomal recessive or polygenic	Impairs water secretion which causes protein plugs	Rowntree,[41] Cohn,[42] Weiss[43]
CTRC (A73T)	Autosomal dominant	Causes severe reduction in CTRC secretion and decrease in trypsin degradation	Rosendahl,[39] LaRusch[56]
CTRC (R254W)	Autosomal dominant	Promotes CTRC degradation	
CTRC (V235I)	Autosomal dominant	Decreases CTRC activity	
CTRC (K247_R254del)	Autosomal dominant	Produces inactive CTRC	
CPA1 (K374E, N256K)	Autosomal dominant	Causes protein misfolding-induced ER stress	Witt,[12] Nemeth[58]
CASR	Autosomal dominant	Causes hypercalcemia which leads to premature activation of trypsinogen inducing autodigestion	Racz[61]
CLDN2	X chromosome linked	Impairs water and sodium transport in the proximal pancreatic duct	Amasheh,[62] Whitcomb[11]
CEL	Autosomal dominant	Impairs secretion, leading to intracellular accumulation and ER stress	Raeder,[3] Fjeld[13]
CELA3B (R90C)	Autosomal dominant	Enhances the rate of translation, therefore, increasing the total amount of active enzyme	Uhlen,[66] Moore[67]
PHLIP (F300L)	Autosomal recessive	Increases degradation by trypsin and chymotrypsin	Behar[68] Szabo[69]
UBR1	Autosomal recessive	Diminishes response to secretion signals, causing acinar cell stress	Zenker[71]

The pathogenic gene variants with known mechanisms and described in families with chronic and hereditary pancreatitis are summarized later in this article.

Clinical manifestations

Individuals carrying a pathologic *PRSS1* variant can develop symptoms as early as 7 to 13 years, which is significantly earlier than non-*PRSS1* carriers.[18,21,22,25,29] Similar to other forms of pancreatitis, patients present with acute abdominal pain and elevated amylase and lipase. The onset of *PRSS1*-associated pancreatitis is typically before age 20. Howes and colleagues[18] studied 527 individuals from 112 families with HP in 14 countries, demonstrating a median age of pancreatitis onset of 12. In a French study of 200 patients with HP, the onset of pancreatitis was before the age of 10, and morphologic changes such as pancreatic calcification began at 20 to 25 years old.[22] Similar data have been reported from Japan, whereby the mean age of symptom onset was 17.8 years.[21] In the EUROPAC study, patients with R122H had a younger age of onset than other variants and this was not observed in the Japanese study.[18,21]

Signs of CP, such as calcification, may present by the mid-20s.[22] A Japanese study reported exocrine pancreatic insufficiency (EPI) at a median age of 42 years, significantly earlier than HP patients without *PRSS1* or *SPINK1* pathogenic variants.[21] In the European population, the median age to develop EPI in the setting of a pathogenic *PRSS1* variant was 53 years but no differences in age of onset of EPI were noted for those with R122H, N29I, or a different *PRSS1* variant.[18] Additionally, Japanese patients with pathogenic *PRSS1* variants developed diabetes at a median age of 42. Later onset of diabetes was noted in the EUROPAC cohort, with a median age of 58 for R122H carriers and 46 for N29I carriers. Neither study showed a difference in the time to diabetes onset in patients with HP with versus without *PRSS1* variants.[18,21]

SPINK1

The association between *SPINK1* variants and pancreatitis was established in 2000 and more than 30 *SPINK1* variants have been reported.[5]

Prevalence

There is a 2% prevalence of *SPINK1* pathogenic variants (N34S and P55S) among the healthy general population, yet less than 1% of *SPINK1* carriers develop pancreatitis.[33] However, among patients with idiopathic CP, *SPINK1* variants may be seen in up to 23% of cases.[5,34–36] The N34S variant is the most prevalent pathogenic haplotype in the US, Europe, and Japan, and IVS3+2T>C is commonly found in Japan and China.[21,37,38] In a European study, 21.3% and 9.1% of patients with CP exhibited a comutation involving *CFTR* and *CTRC*, respectively, which was higher than 4% in the general population.[38]

Mechanism of action

Located on chromosome 5q32, *SPINK1* encodes a pancreatic secretory trypsin inhibitor. During acute inflammation, this inhibitor is expressed in the pancreatic acinar cells and binds to activated trypsin, and can inhibit 20% of trypsin activity.[5,28] Pathogenic *SPINK1* variants do not lead to pancreatitis in the absence of early or excessive activation of trypsin and inflammation. *SPINK1* may cause CP in the setting of autosomal recessive inheritance; however, most patients with pancreatitis in the setting of *SPINK1* pathogenic variants are heterozygotes with more complex inheritance patterns of pancreatitis including modification by environmental factors. By lowering the threshold for the development of pancreatitis, *SPINK1* variants likely function as a disease modifier because they may not cause pancreatitis in the absence of other supporting factors.[39]

Clinical manifestations

In a histopathologic examination of 28 cases of *SPINK1*-associated CP, there was an increased loss of both acinar cell epithelium and intralobular ducts as the duration of pancreatic symptoms lengthened, as well as intralobular, interlobular, and perilobular fibrosis. Lipomatous atrophy, commonly associated with *PRSS1* and *CFTR* pancreatitis, was not present.[40] Variants in *SPINK1* are associated with a 12-fold increase in pancreatitis; however, controversy exists on whether *SPINK1* is the causative of disease or functions as a disease modifier. For example, in a Japanese study, patients harboring *SPINK1* variants did not develop pancreatitis earlier than controls.[21] In contrast, a large Chinese study of more than 1000 patients with CP and a European study of 209 patients with *SPINK1* mutations did demonstrate a significant difference (27 years and 21 years earlier, respectively) in the age of pancreatitis onset.[37,38] A similar proportion of patients developed diabetes and EPI in the European study, but the *SPINK1* group developed both diabetes and EPI approximately 15 years earlier.[38] Compound heterozygotes, such as those with both *SPINK1* and *CFTR* or *CTR,* exhibit a younger age of disease onset than those with *SPINK1* alone. Additionally, the presence of homozygous N34S did not confer an earlier age of pancreatitis symptom onset, diabetes, or EPI compared with heterozygotes.[38] These observations suggest that compound heterozygosity of *SPINK1,* or other unidentified environmental or genetic factors, rather than *SPINK1* mutation alone enhance the risk for pancreatitis.

Cystic fibrosis transmembrane conductance regulator gene

CFTR variants are associated with pancreatitis, even in the absence of other symptoms of cystic fibrosis (CF). The severity of pancreatitis is related to the specific variant and consequent defects in the CFTR protein, as well as zygosity.[41]

Prevalence

Approximately 1% to 4% of patients with CF will experience an episode of pancreatitis; conversely, approximately 15% of adults with CP carry a *CFTR* variant.[17,42] Incidence of CF varies worldwide and the highest incidence (1/2500) is in Northern Europeans. The most common variant, F508del, can be seen in approximately 70% of those with CF and 40% of those with HP who are found to have a variant in *CFTR.* There are more than 2000 *CFTR* gene variants and they are classified by the primary molecular defect in the protein with Class I–III variants of severe disruptions and Class IV–V of milder dysfunction.[41]

CFTR variants have complex inheritance patterns and heterozygous carriers have a 2-to 5-fold increased risk of pancreatitis.[42,43] In case–control studies from Europe and US, individuals with CP are at least twice more likely to have an aberrant *CFTR* gene than healthy controls.[43–45] In a study of 984 cases from the North America Pancreatitis Study 2 (NAPS2) population of 1000 subjects (460 RAP, 540 CP) and 695 controls, 43 *CFTR* variants were identified and 9 of them were reported in recurrent and CP but not CF. These variants were more prevalent in the pancreatitis cases than controls (14.2% vs 9.8%).[46] In a study of individuals with CP in China, 16 rare *CFTR* variants (allele frequency <1% of the control population) were identified from nearly 1900 individuals, and the aggregated *CFTR* variants confer an odds ratio (OR) of 3.71 for CP.[37]

Mechanism of action

CFTR, an epithelial cell anion channel, regulates chloride and bicarbonate secretion in the ductal cells of the lungs, pancreas, and other organs, thereby affecting the production of sweat, mucus, and digestive fluids.[41] It is theorized that the mutated *CFTR* gene leads to inadequate alkalization of the pancreatic acinar cells and the retained zymogens in the duct digest the surrounding pancreatic tissue, leading to pancreatitis. In fact, electrophysiology studies of the cloned *CFTR* with the 43 variants from the NAPS2 study confirmed diminished bicarbonate conductance.[46] However, some animal model studies suggested that the pathogenesis is more likely linked to the impaired water secretion which causes protein plugs in the pancreatic duct, as well as overexpression of proinflammatory cytokine genes in CFTR knockout and F508del mice.[47,48]

Clinical manifestations

CFTR-associated pancreatitis varies in its manifestations based on the pathogenic variants and other environmental modifiers. The disease patterns and relationship to *CFTR* mutations generally fall into one of the several categories.

Patients with classic CF and abnormal sweat chloride measurement ($\geq$60 mmol/L) have 2 pathogenic *CFTR* alleles (homozygous or compound heterozygous). Pancreatic damage has typically been so severe early in life that their pancreatic acinar reserve is too low to elicit pancreatitis. Freeman and Ooi suggested that a "critical mass" of acinar tissue in the setting of ductal obstruction is required for symptomatic pancreatitis.[49,50] Instead, up to 95% of patients with CF present with severe EPI.[4] In comparison, the risk of developing pancreatitis was 71% higher in patients with a mild genotype than in the moderate–severe group.[50]

Another manifestation of *CFTR* variants is called the *CFTR*-related pancreas-sinus-vas deferens syndrome. There are 9 variants (R117H, R74Q, R75Q, R170H, L967S, L997F, D1152H, S1235R, and D1270N) associated with the development of CP, chronic sinusitis, and male infertility but with minimal lung involvement. Individuals with *CFTR*-related pancreas-sinus-vas deferens syndrome usually have normal or mildly abnormal sweat chloride values, as the variants cause a select deficiency in bicarbonate conductance.[46] Interestingly, patients with less than 2 severe *CFTR* mutations have likely normal sweat chloride values (30–59 mmol/L) and do not meet the criteria for the diagnosis of CF, but still suffer symptoms of CP.[51] For example, one of these variants, R75Q, has deleterious effects on the pancreas but not on the lungs.[52] These patients have *CFTR*-related disorder, typically described as exhibiting one clinical manifestation (eg, pancreatitis or absence of vas deferens) associated with *CFTR* dysfunction.

Patients with *CFTR*-related pancreatitis are typically *CFTR* heterozygotes and have sweat chloride levels less than 30 mmol/L.[42,43,51] This group is generally healthy, but does exhibit a 3- to 4-fold risk of developing CP compared to the general population, especially when there is coexisting *SPINK1*, *CTRC*, or other genotypes.[39,52] Any factors that result in diminished pancreatic juice flow or increased duct resistance can precipitate pancreatitis. Therefore, tobacco use or pancreas divisum in the presence of *CFTR* variants may increase the risk of CP.[53–55]

Chymotrypsin C

CTRC is an enzyme that degrades trypsin in the setting of lower calcium concentrations. Its role in controlling prematurely activated trypsin has sparked interest in its association with pancreatitis.

Prevalence

In a German study, *CTRC* variants were found in 2.9% of patients with CP than 0.7% of controls. *CTRC* variants were also found in 14.1% of Indian patients with tropical pancreatitis than 1.2% of controls.[10] In a North American population, the CTRC R254W variant was found to be equally present in CP, RAP, and controls, whereas the G60G variant, which causes decreased CTRC mRNA, was detected in 16.8% of CP, 11.9% of RAP, and 10.8% of controls. Specifically, there is a high association of G60G variant with CP in people who had a history of smoking than nonsmokers or drinking-only.[56] The evidence is less clear in other populations. In a Chinese study, when all CTRC variants were combined, an OR of 3.58 was found for CP. However, no increased odds of CP were found when individual variants were examined, possibly due to the small sample size of each individual variant.[37] These findings suggest that rather than independently causing CP, CTRC variants may be disease modifiers that exacerbate subclinical pancreatitis in the setting of other inciting factors.[57]

Mechanism of action

The CTRC gene is located on chromosome 19p13 and encodes CTRC. It cleaves trypsin at specific binding sites and its trypsin-regulatory function is affected by calcium concentration. CTRC variants include A73T, which causes a severe reduction in CTRC secretion, R254W which promotes CTRC degradation, V235I which decreases CTRC activity, and K247_R254del which produces inactive CTRC.[39,56]

ADDITIONAL GENES ASSOCIATED WITH PANCREATITIS

Several genes have been implicated in recent studies for the development of CP or HP, including CPA1, CASR, CLDN2, CEL, and others. These genes are considered disease modifying and increase the risk of pancreatitis progression.

Carboxypeptidase A1

The CPA1 gene is located on chromosome 7q32 and encodes CPA1, a pancreatic enzyme that cleaves dietary proteins and involves in zymogen inhibition.[12] Mutations in CPA1, such as K374E and N256K, can cause protein misfolding-induced ER stress, thus increasing risks of pancreatitis.[12,58] N256K is the most frequently described variant. In a large German study, N256K was observed in 0.7% (7/944) of patients with nonalcoholic CP and 0% (0/3938) of controls.[12] Pathogenic variants including V251M, N256K, S282P have also been reported in the US, Poland, and Japan.[21,59,60] CPA1 variants are associated with early-onset pancreatitis, as the risk increasing by 38-fold in patients younger than 20 years and 84-fold in those younger than 10 years.[12]

Calcium-sensing receptor gene CASR

A member of the G protein-coupled receptor family, is expressed in pancreatic acinar and ductal cells. It increases pancreatic ductal fluid secretion in response to high calcium concentrations in the pancreatic juice, thus preventing stone formation and pancreatitis.[61] The initial study that associated CASR with CP included a family of 5 individuals heterozygous for the SPINK1 N34S and only 2 of these individuals developed CP and both were found to have variants in CASR. Several additional studies have further analyzed the relationship between CASR variants and pancreatitis in the setting of SPINK1 mutations and alcohol.[6,8] CASR R990G is associated with the development of CP (OR: 2) and even more in the setting of heavy alcohol consumption (OR: 3.12). In some families, individuals with CP were found to have either CASR variants alone or in combination with SPINK1 mutations, whereas healthy adults and children had SPINK1 alone, suggesting that CASR variants may also function as disease modifiers in the development of CP, particularly in conjunction with pathogenic variants in other genes.[6,8] In a subsequent study of 253 young French idiopathic patients with CP and nearly 500 healthy controls, 10 rare *CASR* coding variants were identified, but only A986 homozygosity was associated with CP. Of note, 3 of the 9 patients with CP with rare *CASR* variants were found to also have variants in *SPINK1* or *CFTR*.[9] Further work is required to better understand the mechanism of *CASR*-associated pancreatitis.

Claudin-2 gene

CLDN2 is expressed along the tight junctions and forms cation-ion and water channels between endothelial cells. It regulates sodium and water movement into the ductal lumen.[62] Interestingly, *CLDN2* has no association with acute pancreatitis. Rather, *CLDN2* variants accelerate the progression from acute pancreatitis to CP. *CLDN2* is located on the X chromosome; therefore, risk CP seems dominant in men and recessive in women. The T allele (rs128688220) is seen in 25.8% of male controls and 6.9% of female controls. However, it has been described in 47.6% men with alcohol-associated CP than 4% of male controls with heavy alcohol use, suggesting an association of the T allele with alcohol-induced CP in male carriers.[11] In subsequent studies in Japan and India, the T allele was associated with significantly increased risk for both alcohol-associated CP and idiopathic CP in male patients.[29,63–65]

Carboxyl ester lipase

CEL is a pancreatic enzyme encoded by the *CEL* gene. Mutations in *CEL* are associated with maturity-onset diabetes of the young type 8 (MODY8) and pancreatic exocrine insufficiency, suggesting the destruction of the islet cells.[3] Another hybrid *CEL* mutation with its adjacent pseudogene, *CELP*, causes a hybrid protein with impaired secretion and intracellular accumulation leading to ER stress. This pathogenic allele was detected in 3.7% (42/1122) of nonalcoholic patients with CP versus 0.7% (30/4152) controls.[13]

Others

Chymotrypsin-like elastase 3B (CELA3B) is a member of 6 elastases, 4 of which are exclusively produced in and secreted by pancreatic acinar cells. CELA3B is cleaved by trypsin on secretion and converted to an active protease.[66] A *CELA3B* R90C variant was recently discovered in a patient with personal and family history of CP.[67] The variant enhances the rate of CELA3B translation, thereby increasing the total amount of active enzyme and risk of pancreatic injury. Subsequent in vitro and murine studies with CRISPR genome editing demonstrated that homozygous *CELA3B* mutant mice only developed pancreatitis after a second insult. Taken together, this illustrates a different pathway from the typical disruption of trypsin regulation or increased ER stress.[67]

The *PNLIP* gene is located on chromosome 10q25. Protease-sensitive pancreatic lipase (PNLIP) is critical for the digestion of dietary triglycerides and is expressed only in the exocrine pancreas.[68,69] In a study of 2 European cohorts of 1052 nonalcoholic CP and 1557 control subjects, missense variants were enriched in 1.7% (18/1061) of patients with CP compared to 0.6% (10/1557) of controls. The most frequent variant was F300L (8/1061), unique to the CP group. Five variants, including F300L, P245A, I265R, S304F, and F314L, showed increased degradation by trypsin and chymotrypsin. These protease-sensitive *PNLIP* variants were found in 1.1% mild RAP pediatric or young adult patients and 0.1% controls (OR: 11.3). These missense variants were subsequently detected in both Japanese patients with CP and controls, but no variants were found in CP cohorts from India and US.[70] Although this study showcased a novel F300L variant associated with potentially early-onset CP, further evidence is needed to characterize its impact on a wider population.

The *UBR1* gene encodes ubiquitin-protein ligase E3, which is expressed in the pancreatic acinar cells and regulates protein degradation. UBR1 deficiency leads to acinar cell destruction that resembles pancreatitis. Homozygous or compound heterozygous mutations in *UBR1* cause Johanson–Blizzard syndrome, characterized by severe EPI and hypoplasia of the nasal alae.[71] In a study of 389 Japanese patients with idiopathic, alcoholic, or hereditary CP, 17 variants were identified in the exons of *UBR1*, albeit in similar frequencies in both cases and controls.[72] In a US study of 100 patients with AP, RAP, or CP, 121 genetic variants in *PRSS1, CFTR, SPINK1, CTRC* as well as *UBR1* were identified by RNA-sequencing. Co-expression analysis revealed the co-occurrence of genes involved in stress response, such as *UBR1* or gamma-glutamyl transferase 1 (*GGT1*), together with at least 1 acinar- or duct-associated gene, such as *CFTR*. Some of the *UBR1* variants were in the noncoding region.[73] This suggested that the generic risk of *UBR1* mutations may not fit a Mendelian model and *UBR1* variants alone may not confer any deleterious effect.

TRPV6 is an active calcium selective ion channel and regulates apical calcium entry in absorptive and secretory tissues. TRPV6 is expressed approximately 6 times higher in pancreatic ductal cells than in acinar cells.[74] In a recent study by Masamune and colleagues,[15] functionally defective *TRPV6* variants caused impaired calcium uptake, and was enriched in both Japanese (4.3%, 13/300) and European patients (2.0%, 18/880) with nonalcoholic CP compared with controls (Japanese: 0.1%, OR: 48.4; European: 0%). It was also correlated with the onset of disease $\leq$20 years of age (OR: 18.8). Notably, 20% of patients with these defective variants also carried *SPINK1* N34S, further highlighting the complexity of genetics in CP.

PANCREATIC CANCER

The etiology of pancreatic cancer in the setting of HP or FP is multifactorial, although the true risk of pancreatic cancer is uncertain because studies are limited by referral, ascertainment, and other biases. CP itself is a strong risk factor for pancreatic cancer due to longstanding inflammation.[75] *PRSS1, SPINK1,* and *CFTR*, which all cause pancreatic cell injury, are known to significantly increase cancer risks.[76,77] For example, a French study found a standardized incidence ratio (SIR) of 87 in HP with *PRSS1* mutations.[76] In a study of symptomatic and asymptomatic white *PRSS1* carriers in the US, the age- and sex-adjusted SIR was 59.[25] In a cohort of patients with *SPINK1* carriers, the cumulative risk of developing pancreatic cancer was significantly higher (HR: 12.0) than in controls. Notably, there is also higher tobacco consumption in the patients who developed pancreatic cancer (15 pack-years) than the entire study population (8 pack-years).[38] *CFTR*-related CP is also associated with increased risk of pancreatic cancer (SIR: 26.5). However, all of the patients with cancer had a smoking history and CP was not more prevalent in the *CFTR* variant carriers than noncarriers.[30,78] In addition, smoking independently doubled the risk of pancreatic cancer in patients with CP, with earlier development of cancer and accounted for 25% to 30% of all pancreatic tumors.[79] More recent data, however, suggest that there may be a lower cumulative risk of pancreatic cancer (7%) reported for patients with CP with *PRSS1* mutations at age 70.[25] It is possible that more stringent regulations leading to decreased tobacco exposure have resulted in a birth cohort effect, resulting in a lower risk of *PRSS1*-associated pancreatic cancer in more recent years.

EVALUATION

Diagnosis of HP requires a comprehensive review of personal and family history, blood tests, and imaging studies, as well as a detailed discussion on the role of genetic testing. Patients with idiopathic pancreatitis, RAP, or CP in the absence of typical inciting factors should undergo evaluation for a hereditary etiology for their pancreatitis. The young age of onset may also prompt genetic risk assessment. For example, one study demonstrated that patients with unexplained first episode of acute pancreatitis less than 35 years are more likely to carry pathogenic mutations when undergoing a four-gene panel test for PRSS1, SPINK1, CFTR, and CRTC than patients with CP without RAP or having later disease onset.[80]

Current guidelines recommend genetic testing for pancreatitis susceptibility genes in patients with pancreatitis and one or more of the following characteristics: an unexplained pancreatitis episode as a child; idiopathic CP with onset before 25 years of age; family history of CP, RAP, or childhood pancreatitis with unknown cause in a first- or second-degree relative; and RAP without an identifiable cause.[81,82]

In children less than the age of 16, genetic testing is recommended for an episode of pancreatitis of unknown etiology and severe enough for hospitalization; 2 or more episodes of pancreatitis of unknown etiology; an episode of pancreatitis in a child with a relative carrying an HP mutation; high suspicion of HP in a child with recurrent abdominal pain; or high suspicion of HP in a child with CP of unknown etiology.[83] The INSPPIRE(International Study Group of Pediatric Pancreatitis: In search for a cuRE) Consortium strongly recommends testing for PRSS1 mutations and for CF in pediatric patients with RAP and CP. If children with RAP and CP have a sweat chloride less than 60 mmol/L, expanded CFTR mutation testing should be performed. Testing for SPINK1 and CTRC may also be considered.[84]

Given the complex, often non–Mendelian, inheritance patterns in patients with HP should undergo pre and posttest genetic counseling.[77,85] Current germline testing often includes PRSS1, SPINK1, CFTR, CEL, CRTC, and CPA1.[86] If a variant has been previously identified in the family, patients may consider testing only for the familial variant or they may choose to interrogate a broader panel of genes associated with HP.

MANAGEMENT

Once a diagnosis of HP has been confirmed, treatment should be initiated to slow disease progression and development of complications. Lifestyle modifications, particularly tobacco and alcohol cessation, are recommended for all patients with RAP, CP, and HP, as they increase risks of symptom progression and cancer. Other factors, such as stress and dehydration, may also exacerbate pancreatitis.[85] Practitioners should be aware of the importance of these and destigmatize patients as alcoholics or substance users.[25,85] Patients at various stages of HP often experience significant pain. A multidisciplinary team should be involved to provide pain management, which may include antioxidant treatment, celiac plexus neurolysis, pancreatic enzyme replacement, counseling on psychosocial well-being, and potential intervention for drug addiction.[87] Families should additionally receive comprehensive counseling and support.[85]

Patients who develop EPI should undergo malnutrition evaluation and evaluation for osteoporosis.[88] Appropriate pancreatic enzyme and fat-soluble vitamin supplementation should be initiated. For patients with endocrine disorder, insulin is the first-line therapy for advanced disease.[88]

Select germline carriers may ultimately consider a total pancreatectomy with islet autotransplantation (TP-IAT) in a high-volume center under multidisciplinary care. Although the primary objective of this procedure is pain relief, it may improve glycemic control and quality of life in selected patients. However, age and prolonged course of pancreatitis adversely affected TP-IAT outcomes, so the patient population needs to be carefully selected.[88,89]

Currently, there have been few therapeutic options targeting specific genetic mutations. The mainstay of treatment focuses on lifestyle modifications based on known risks factors associated with certain mutations. For example, patients with high-risk variants in *PRSS1*, *CLDN2,* or *CTRC* should be counseled for alcohol and tobacco cessation.[11,56] Given several of the HP-causing genes are well characterized, it is to be hoped that new technologies such as preimplantation genetic testing for monogenic disorders (PGT-M) would provide new targeted treatment options in the future.[19,90,91]

SUMMARY

HP and FP highlight a complex multigene, non–Mendelian disorder with environmental interactions. Early identification through genetic evaluation and proper interdisciplinary management may give patients the opportunity to control symptoms and prevent complications.

CLINICS CARE POINTS

- Patients with unexplained RAP or CP should undergo detailed screening for the family history of pancreatic diseases and genetic testing.
- All patients with HP should be counseled on tobacco and alcohol cessation.
- Patients who develop EPI should undergo malnutrition evaluation and evaluation for osteoporosis.
- Total pancreatectomy with islet autotransplantation (TP-IAT) may be indicated to provide pain relief and may improve glycemic control in selected patients.

DISCLOSURES

The authors have nothing to disclose.

REFERENCES

1. Comfort MW, Steinberg AG. Pedigree of a family with hereditary chronic relapsing pancreatitis. Gastroenterology 1952;21(1):54–63.
2. Whitcomb DC, Gorry MC, Preston RA, et al. Hereditary pancreatitis is caused by a mutation in the cationic trypsinogen gene. Nat Genet 1996;14(2):141–5.
3. Raeder H, Johansson S, Holm PI, et al. Mutations in the CEL VNTR cause a syndrome of diabetes and pancreatic exocrine dysfunction. Nat Genet 2006;38(1):54–62.
4. Cohn JA, Friedman KJ, Noone PG, et al. Relation between mutations of the cystic fibrosis gene and idiopathic pancreatitis. N Engl J Med 1998;339(10):653–8.
5. Witt H, Luck W, Hennies HC, et al. Mutations in the gene encoding the serine protease inhibitor, Kazal type 1 are associated with chronic pancreatitis. Nat Genet 2000;25(2):213–6.
6. Muddana V, Lamb J, Greer JB, et al. Association between calcium sensing receptor gene polymorphisms and chronic pancreatitis in a US population: role of serine protease inhibitor Kazal 1type and alcohol. World J Gastroenterol 2008;14(28):4486–91.

7. Felderbauer P, Klein W, Bulut K, et al. Mutations in the calcium-sensing receptor: a new genetic risk factor for chronic pancreatitis? Scand J Gastroenterol 2006; 41(3):343–8.
8. Felderbauer P, Hoffmann P, Einwachter H, et al. A novel mutation of the calcium sensing receptor gene is associated with chronic pancreatitis in a family with heterozygous SPINK1 mutations. BMC Gastroenterol 2003;3:34.
9. Masson E, Chen JM, Ferec C. Overrepresentation of Rare CASR Coding Variants in a Sample of Young French Patients With Idiopathic Chronic Pancreatitis. Pancreas 2015;44(6):996–8.
10. Rosendahl J, Witt H, Szmola R, et al. Chymotrypsin C (CTRC) variants that diminish activity or secretion are associated with chronic pancreatitis. Nat Genet 2008;40(1):78–82.
11. Whitcomb DC, LaRusch J, Krasinskas AM, et al. Common genetic variants in the CLDN2 and PRSS1-PRSS2 loci alter risk for alcohol-related and sporadic pancreatitis. Nat Genet 2012;44(12):1349–54.
12. Witt H, Beer S, Rosendahl J, et al. Variants in CPA1 are strongly associated with early onset chronic pancreatitis. Nat Genet 2013;45(10):1216–20.
13. Fjeld K, Weiss FU, Lasher D, et al. A recombined allele of the lipase gene CEL and its pseudogene CELP confers susceptibility to chronic pancreatitis. Nat Genet 2015;47(5):518–22.
14. Rosendahl J, Kirsten H, Hegyi E, et al. Genome-wide association study identifies inversion in the CTRB1-CTRB2 locus to modify risk for alcoholic and non-alcoholic chronic pancreatitis. Gut 2018;67(10):1855–63.
15. Masamune A, Kotani H, Sorgel FL, et al. Variants That Affect Function of Calcium Channel TRPV6 Are Associated With Early-Onset Chronic Pancreatitis. Gastroenterology 2020;158(6):1626–41.e8.
16. Hasan A, Moscoso DI, Kastrinos F. The Role of Genetics in Pancreatitis. Gastrointest Endosc Clin N Am 2018;28(4):587–603.
17. Shelton C, LaRusch J, Whitcomb DC. Pancreatitis Overview. In: Adam MP, Ardinger HH, Pagon RA, et al, editors. University of Washington: GeneReviews((R)). 1993. Seattle (WA).
18. Howes N, Lerch MM, Greenhalf W, et al. Clinical and genetic characteristics of hereditary pancreatitis in Europe. Clin Gastroenterol Hepatol 2004;2(3):252–61.
19. Whitcomb DC. Barriers and Research Priorities for Implementing Precision Medicine. Pancreas 2019;48(10):1246–9.
20. Joergensen MT, Brusgaard K, Cruger DG, et al. Genetic, epidemiological, and clinical aspects of hereditary pancreatitis: a population-based cohort study in Denmark. Am J Gastroenterol 2010;105(8):1876–83.
21. Masamune A, Kikuta K, Hamada S, et al. Nationwide survey of hereditary pancreatitis in Japan. J Gastroenterol 2018;53(1):152–60.
22. Rebours V, Boutron-Ruault MC, Schnee M, et al. The natural history of hereditary pancreatitis: a national series. Gut 2009;58(1):97–103.
23. Girodon E, Rebours V, Chen JM, et al. Clinical interpretation of PRSS1 variants in patients with pancreatitis. Clin Res Hepatol Gastroenterol 2021;45(1):101497.
24. Nemeth BC, Sahin-Toth M. Human cationic trypsinogen (PRSS1) variants and chronic pancreatitis. Am J Physiol Gastrointest Liver Physiol 2014;306(6): G466–73.
25. Shelton CA, Umapathy C, Stello K, et al. Hereditary Pancreatitis in the United States: Survival and Rates of Pancreatic Cancer. Am J Gastroenterol 2018; 113(9):1376.

26. Nemoda Z, Sahin-Toth M. Chymotrypsin C (caldecrin) stimulates autoactivation of human cationic trypsinogen. J Biol Chem 2006;281(17):11879–86.
27. Szabo A, Sahin-Toth M. Increased activation of hereditary pancreatitis-associated human cationic trypsinogen mutants in presence of chymotrypsin C. J Biol Chem 2012;287(24):20701–10.
28. Whitcomb DC. Genetic aspects of pancreatitis. Annu Rev Med 2010;61:413–24.
29. Whitcomb DC. Genetic risk factors for pancreatic disorders. Gastroenterology 2013;144(6):1292–302.
30. Hegyi E, Sahin-Toth M. Genetic Risk in Chronic Pancreatitis: The Trypsin-Dependent Pathway. Dig Dis Sci 2017;62(7):1692–701.
31. Sahin-Toth M. Genetic risk in chronic pancreatitis: the misfolding-dependent pathway. Curr Opin Gastroenterol 2017;33(5):390–5.
32. Schnur A, Beer S, Witt H, et al. Functional effects of 13 rare PRSS1 variants presumed to cause chronic pancreatitis. Gut 2014;63(2):337–43.
33. Pfutzer RH, Barmada MM, Brunskill AP, et al. SPINK1/PSTI polymorphisms act as disease modifiers in familial and idiopathic chronic pancreatitis. Gastroenterology 2000;119(3):615–23.
34. Abu-El-Haija M, Valencia CA, Hornung L, et al. Genetic variants in acute, acute recurrent and chronic pancreatitis affect the progression of disease in children. Pancreatology 2019;19(4):535–40.
35. Schneider A, Barmada MM, Slivka A, et al. Clinical characterization of patients with idiopathic chronic pancreatitis and SPINK1 Mutations. Scand J Gastroenterol 2004;39(9):903–4.
36. Teich N, Bauer N, Mossner J, et al. Mutational screening of patients with nonalcoholic chronic pancreatitis: identification of further trypsinogen variants. Am J Gastroenterol 2002;97(2):341–6.
37. Zou WB, Tang XY, Zhou DZ, et al. SPINK1, PRSS1, CTRC, and CFTR Genotypes Influence Disease Onset and Clinical Outcomes in Chronic Pancreatitis. Clin Transl Gastroenterol 2018;9(11):204.
38. Muller N, Sarantitis I, Rouanet M, et al. Natural history of SPINK1 germline mutation related-pancreatitis. EBioMedicine 2019;48:581–91.
39. Rosendahl J, Landt O, Bernadova J, et al. CFTR, SPINK1, CTRC and PRSS1 variants in chronic pancreatitis: is the role of mutated CFTR overestimated? Gut 2013;62(4):582–92.
40. Jones TE, Bellin MD, Yadav D, et al. The histopathology of SPINK1-associated chronic pancreatitis. Pancreatology 2020;20(8):1648–55.
41. Rowntree RK, Harris A. The phenotypic consequences of CFTR mutations. Ann Hum Genet 2003;67(Pt 5):471–85.
42. Cohn JA, Neoptolemos JP, Feng J, et al. Increased risk of idiopathic chronic pancreatitis in cystic fibrosis carriers. Hum Mutat 2005;26(4):303–7.
43. Weiss FU, Simon P, Bogdanova N, et al. Complete cystic fibrosis transmembrane conductance regulator gene sequencing in patients with idiopathic chronic pancreatitis and controls. Gut 2005;54(10):1456–60.
44. Choudari CP, Imperiale TF, Sherman S, et al. Risk of pancreatitis with mutation of the cystic fibrosis gene. Am J Gastroenterol 2004;99(7):1358–63.
45. Sharer N, Schwarz M, Malone G, et al. Mutations of the cystic fibrosis gene in patients with chronic pancreatitis. N Engl J Med 1998;339(10):645–52.
46. LaRusch J, Jung J, General IJ, et al. Mechanisms of CFTR functional variants that impair regulated bicarbonate permeation and increase risk for pancreatitis but not for cystic fibrosis. Plos Genet 2014;10(7):e1004376.

47. Lee MG, Ohana E, Park HW, et al. Molecular mechanism of pancreatic and salivary gland fluid and HCO3 secretion. Physiol Rev 2012;92(1):39–74.
48. DiMagno MJ, Lee SH, Owyang C, et al. Inhibition of acinar apoptosis occurs during acute pancreatitis in the human homologue DeltaF508 cystic fibrosis mouse. Am J Physiol Gastrointest Liver Physiol 2010;299(2):G400–12.
49. Freeman AJ, Ooi CY. Pancreatitis and pancreatic cystosis in Cystic Fibrosis. J Cyst Fibros 2017;16(Suppl 2):S79–86.
50. Ooi CY, Durie PR. Cystic fibrosis transmembrane conductance regulator (CFTR) gene mutations in pancreatitis. J Cyst Fibros 2012;11(5):355–62.
51. LaRusch J, Whitcomb DC. Genetics of pancreatitis. Curr Opin Gastroenterol 2011;27(5):467–74.
52. Schneider A, Larusch J, Sun X, et al. Combined bicarbonate conductance-impairing variants in CFTR and SPINK1 variants are associated with chronic pancreatitis in patients without cystic fibrosis. Gastroenterology 2011;140(1):162–71.
53. Bertin C, Pelletier AL, Vullierme MP, et al. Pancreas divisum is not a cause of pancreatitis by itself but acts as a partner of genetic mutations. Am J Gastroenterol 2012;107(2):311–7.
54. Garg PK, Khajuria R, Kabra M, et al. Association of SPINK1 gene mutation and CFTR gene polymorphisms in patients with pancreas divisum presenting with idiopathic pancreatitis. J Clin Gastroenterol 2009;43(9):848–52.
55. Raju SV, Jackson PL, Courville CA, et al. Cigarette smoke induces systemic defects in cystic fibrosis transmembrane conductance regulator function. Am J Respir Crit Care Med 2013;188(11):1321–30.
56. LaRusch J, Lozano-Leon A, Stello K, et al. The Common Chymotrypsinogen C (CTRC) Variant G60G (C.180T) Increases Risk of Chronic Pancreatitis But Not Recurrent Acute Pancreatitis in a North American Population. Clin Transl Gastroenterol 2015;6:e68.
57. Zator Z, Whitcomb DC. Insights into the genetic risk factors for the development of pancreatic disease. Therap Adv Gastroenterol 2017;10(3):323–36.
58. Nemeth BC, Orekhova A, Zhang W, et al. Novel p.K374E variant of CPA1 causes misfolding-induced hereditary pancreatitis with autosomal dominant inheritance. Gut 2020;69(4):790–2.
59. Hegyi E, Sahin-Toth M. Human CPA1 mutation causes digestive enzyme misfolding and chronic pancreatitis in mice. Gut 2019;68(2):301–12.
60. Kujko AA, Berki DM, Oracz G, et al. A novel p.Ser282Pro CPA1 variant is associated with autosomal dominant hereditary pancreatitis. Gut 2017;66(9):1728–30.
61. Racz GZ, Kittel A, Riccardi D, et al. Extracellular calcium sensing receptor in human pancreatic cells. Gut 2002;51(5):705–11.
62. Amasheh S, Meiri N, Gitter AH, et al. Claudin-2 expression induces cation-selective channels in tight junctions of epithelial cells. J Cell Sci 2002;115(Pt 24):4969–76.
63. Giri AK, Midha S, Banerjee P, et al. Common Variants in CLDN2 and MORC4 Genes Confer Disease Susceptibility in Patients with Chronic Pancreatitis. PLoS One 2016;11(1):e0147345.
64. Masamune A, Nakano E, Hamada S, et al. Common variants at PRSS1-PRSS2 and CLDN2-MORC4 loci associate with chronic pancreatitis in Japan. Gut 2015;64(8):1345–6.
65. Derikx MH, Kovacs P, Scholz M, et al. Polymorphisms at PRSS1-PRSS2 and CLDN2-MORC4 loci associate with alcoholic and non-alcoholic chronic pancreatitis in a European replication study. Gut 2015;64(9):1426–33.

66. Uhlen M, Fagerberg L, Hallstrom BM, et al. Proteomics. Tissue-based map of the human proteome. Science 2015;347(6220):1260419.
67. Moore PC, Cortez JT, Chamberlain CE, et al. Elastase 3B mutation links to familial pancreatitis with diabetes and pancreatic adenocarcinoma. J Clin Invest 2019; 129(11):4676–81.
68. Behar DM, Basel-Vanagaite L, Glaser F, et al. Identification of a novel mutation in the PNLIP gene in two brothers with congenital pancreatic lipase deficiency. J Lipid Res 2014;55(2):307–12.
69. Szabo A, Xiao X, Haughney M, et al. A novel mutation in PNLIP causes pancreatic triglyceride lipase deficiency through protein misfolding. Biochim Biophys Acta 2015;1852(7):1372–9.
70. Lasher D, Szabo A, Masamune A, et al. Protease-Sensitive Pancreatic Lipase Variants Are Associated With Early Onset Chronic Pancreatitis. Am J Gastroenterol 2019;114(6):974–83.
71. Zenker M, Mayerle J, Reis A, et al. Genetic basis and pancreatic biology of Johanson-Blizzard syndrome. Endocrinol Metab Clin North Am 2006;35(2): 243–253, vii-viii.
72. Masamune A, Nakano E, Niihori T, et al. Variants in the UBR1 gene are not associated with chronic pancreatitis in Japan. Pancreatology 2016;16(5):814–8.
73. Ellison MA, Spagnolo DM, Shelton C, et al. Complex Genetics in Pancreatitis: Insights Gained From a New Candidate Locus Panel. Pancreas 2020;49(7):983–98.
74. Fecher-Trost C, Wissenbach U, Weissgerber P. TRPV6: From identification to function. Cell Calcium 2017;67:116–22.
75. Raimondi S, Lowenfels AB, Morselli-Labate AM, et al. Pancreatic cancer in chronic pancreatitis; aetiology, incidence, and early detection. Best Pract Res Clin Gastroenterol 2010;24(3):349–58.
76. Rebours V, Boutron-Ruault MC, Schnee M, et al. Risk of pancreatic adenocarcinoma in patients with hereditary pancreatitis: a national exhaustive series. Am J Gastroenterol 2008;103(1):111–9.
77. Whitcomb DC, Shelton CA, Brand RE. Genetics and Genetic Testing in Pancreatic Cancer. Gastroenterology 2015;149(5):1252–64.e4.
78. McWilliams RR, Petersen GM, Rabe KG, et al. Cystic fibrosis transmembrane conductance regulator (CFTR) gene mutations and risk for pancreatic adenocarcinoma. Cancer 2010;116(1):203–9.
79. Lowenfels AB, Maisonneuve P, Whitcomb DC, et al. Cigarette smoking as a risk factor for pancreatic cancer in patients with hereditary pancreatitis. JAMA 2001;286(2):169–70.
80. Jalaly NY, Moran RA, Fargahi F, et al. An Evaluation of Factors Associated With Pathogenic PRSS1, SPINK1, CTFR, and/or CTRC Genetic Variants in Patients With Idiopathic Pancreatitis. Am J Gastroenterol 2017;112(8):1320–9.
81. Fink EN, Kant JA, Whitcomb DC. Genetic counseling for nonsyndromic pancreatitis. Gastroenterol Clin North Am 2007;36(2):325–333, ix.
82. Solomon S, Whitcomb DC. Genetics of pancreatitis: an update for clinicians and genetic counselors. Curr Gastroenterol Rep 2012;14(2):112–7.
83. Whitcomb DC. Value of genetic testing in the management of pancreatitis. Gut 2004;53(11):1710–7.
84. Gariepy CE, Heyman MB, Lowe ME, et al. Causal Evaluation of Acute Recurrent and Chronic Pancreatitis in Children: Consensus From the INSPPIRE Group. J Pediatr Gastroenterol Nutr 2017;64(1):95–103.
85. Shelton CA, Grubs RE, Umapathy C, et al. Impact of hereditary pancreatitis on patients and their families. J Genet Couns 2020;29(6):971–82.

86. Hegyi P, Parniczky A, Lerch MM, et al. International Consensus Guidelines for Risk Factors in Chronic Pancreatitis. Recommendations from the working group for the international consensus guidelines for chronic pancreatitis in collaboration with the International Association of Pancreatology, the American Pancreatic Association, the Japan Pancreas Society, and European Pancreatic Club. Pancreatology 2020;20(4):579–85.

87. Gardner TB, Adler DG, Forsmark CE, et al. ACG Clinical Guideline: Chronic Pancreatitis. Am J Gastroenterol 2020;115(3):322–39.

88. Ramalho GX, Dytz MG. Diabetes of the Exocrine Pancreas Related to Hereditary Pancreatitis, an Update. Curr Diab Rep 2020;20(6):16.

89. Bellin MD, Prokhoda P, Hodges JS, et al. Age and Disease Duration Impact Outcomes of Total Pancreatectomy and Islet Autotransplant for PRSS1 Hereditary Pancreatitis. Pancreas 2018;47(4):466–70.

90. Girardet A, Viart V, Plaza S, et al. The improvement of the best practice guidelines for preimplantation genetic diagnosis of cystic fibrosis: toward an international consensus. Eur J Hum Genet 2016;24(4):469–78.

91. Group EP-MW, Carvalho F, Moutou C, et al. ESHRE PGT Consortium good practice recommendations for the detection of monogenic disorders. Hum Reprod Open 2020;2020(3):hoaa018.

Identification of Lynch Syndrome

Jennifer K. Maratt, MD, MS[a,b,c,*], Elena Stoffel, MD, MPH[d,e]

KEYWORDS

- Lynch syndrome • Hereditary colorectal cancer syndrome • Mismatch repair
- Hereditary nonpolyposis colorectal cancer

KEY POINTS

- Lynch syndrome (LS) is caused by pathogenic germline variants (PGV) in DNA mismatch repair (MMR) genes, inherited in an autosomal dominant pattern.
- Individuals at risk for LS can be identified through the use of clinical diagnostic criteria, prediction models, and universal tumor screening.
- Universal screening of all colorectal and endometrial cancers for Lynch syndrome involves evaluation for DNA mismatch repair deficiency (MMRd) and includes microsatellite instability and immunohistochemical testing for the protein expression of MMR genes related to LS.
- Individuals suspected to have LS should receive genetic counseling and undergo germline genetic testing to confirm the diagnosis.

INTRODUCTION

Lynch syndrome (LS) is the most common hereditary colorectal cancer (CRC) syndrome, with a prevalence of 1 in 279 (0.36%) individuals in the general population.[1] Previously referred to as hereditary nonpolyposis colorectal cancer (HNPCC) syndrome, LS was one of the earliest recognized familial cancer syndromes.[2] Individuals with LS are at risk for CRC and various types of extracolonic cancers, including endometrial, ovarian, urinary tract (ureters, renal, bladder), gastric, small intestine cancers along with brain tumors, and sebaceous neoplasms. Fortunately, the implementation of specialized surveillance has been shown to be effective in reducing morbidity from LS-associated cancers and improving clinical outcomes. In this review, we highlight

[a] Division of Gastroenterology and Hepatology, Indiana University School of Medicine, 1101 West Tenth Street, Indianapolis, IN 46202, USA; [b] Richard L. Roudebush Veterans Affairs Medical Center, Indianapolis, IN, USA; [c] Regenstrief Institute, Inc, Indianapolis, IN, USA; [d] Division of Gastroenterology, Department of Internal Medicine, University of Michigan, 1500 East Medical Center Drive, Ann Arbor, MI 48109, USA; [e] Rogel Cancer Center, Ann Arbor, MI, USA
* Corresponding author. 1101 West Tenth Street, Indianapolis, IN 46032.
E-mail address: jmaratt@iu.edu

Gastrointest Endoscopy Clin N Am 32 (2022) 45–58
https://doi.org/10.1016/j.giec.2021.09.002
1052-5157/22/Published by Elsevier Inc.
giendo.theclinics.com

the history and pathogenesis of LS, and discuss strategies that are available to effectively identify individuals with LS, which include clinical diagnostic criteria based on personal and family cancer history, risk prediction models, universal tumor screening, and next-generation DNA sequencing.

HISTORY OF LYNCH SYNDROME

The groundwork for establishing what we know as LS today dates back to 1895, when Aldred S. Warthin, MD, PhD, a pathologist at the University of Michigan, studied relatives of a family who had been afflicted with multiple cancers including those of the colon, stomach, and uterus. Dr. Warthin's study of 'Family G' led to the notion that the observed cancers may be related to an autosomal dominant pattern of inheritance.[2] In 1962, Dr. Henry T. Lynch studied relatives of "Family N" in Nebraska, who had been afflicted with CRCs across multiple generations. Along with colleague Dr. Marjorie Shaw, who was simultaneously studying another family ("Family M") affected by multiple similar cancers at the University of Michigan, Dr. Lynch coined the term "cancer family syndrome" in 1971 to reflect a suspected genetic basis for the cancer trends and burden in these families. In 1984, Cancer Family Syndrome was renamed Hereditary Nonpolyposis Colorectal Cancer (HNPCC) to distinguish it from familial adenomatous polyposis (FAP), but HNPCC was not widely accepted as a cancer predisposition syndrome until the early 1990s when a genetic basis of the disease was identified and clinical criteria established.[3] Eventually, the term HNPCC was replaced by Lynch Syndrome, acknowledging Dr. Lynch's contribution in characterizing the condition as well as the fact that the cancer spectrum encompasses various tumor types beyond CRC.

PATHOGENESIS

LS is an autosomal dominant hereditary cancer syndrome caused by pathogenic germline variants (PGV) in any of 4 DNA mismatch repair (MMR) genes, *MLH1*, *MSH2*, *MSH6*, or *PMS2*. In addition, deletions in epithelial cell adhesion molecule (*EPCAM*) can also lead to the silencing of *MSH2*, with similar clinical phenotype.[4]

The genetic basis of LS was elucidated through linkage analysis and informed by the unusual molecular phenotype of the associated tumors, which exhibit high rates of somatic mutations at specific genomic regions known as DNA microsatellites. Clues regarding the pathogenesis of LS were garnered through the study of familial clusters of CRC in patients without colorectal polyposis.[3] International collaborative groups of investigators initiated the search for candidate genes using DNA linkage analysis in families with nonpolyposis CRC, which identified a region of interest in chromosome 2p.[5,6] CRC tumors from these cases exhibited high levels of instability at specific DNA microsatellites (MSI-H), caused by errors in the replication of repetitive DNA nucleotide sequences.[7] At the time, studies in bacteria and yeast had already identified pathogenic variants in MMR genes as a cause of MSI. Dr. Richard Kolodner's identification of the *MSH2* gene in yeast enabled his team to clone the human *MSH2* gene, which led to the discovery of a PGV in *MSH2* in individuals from a family affected with nonpolyposis CRC. This was followed by the characterization of a separate family with LS in whom genetic linkage identified a locus on chromosome 3p, leading to the identification of PGVs in *MLH1*. Soon thereafter, *PMS2* and *MSH6* were also identified as MMR genes implicated in risk for familial nonpolyposis CRC.

Once the molecular basis for LS was established, studies of affected families yielded information about the phenotypic variability, with regard to risk for colorectal and extracolonic neoplasms. Universal screening of CRC tumors for MMR deficiency confirmed that approximately 3% of all CRCs are attributable to LS.[8] Of the 4 MMR genes, PGVs in *PMS2 and MSH6* seem to have the highest population prevalence (0.14% and 0.13%, respectively), followed by *MLH1* (0.05%) and *MSH2* (0.04%).[1] However, the lifetime risk for CRC is higher for *MLH1* and *MSH2* PGV carriers, with tumors diagnosed at earlier ages when compared with *PMS2* and *MSH6* PGV carriers.[1] The prevalence of LS in endometrial cancers is similar to CRC, with PGVs identified in 3% of women diagnosed with endometrial cancers.[9,10]

DIAGNOSIS OF LYNCH SYNDROME
Evolution of Clinical Criteria

The first clinical criteria used to identify individuals at risk for LS were proposed at the International Collaborative Group on HNPCC (ICG-HNPCC) meeting in Amsterdam in 1990.[11] These original Amsterdam criteria (also referred to as Amsterdam I) were created to help identify patients meeting criteria for familial CRC (without a polyposis phenotype), to facilitate their inclusion in collaborative studies seeking to better characterize this condition. The Amsterdam I clinical criteria required that all of the following 3 criteria be met: (1) at least 3 relatives with histologically confirmed CRC, one of whom is a first degree relative (FDR) of the other 2; (2) at least 2 generations affected by CRC; and (3) at least 1 relative diagnosed with CRC under the age of 50 years. As analyses of these families revealed that risks for other cancers beyond CRC were also increased, the ICG-HNPCC revised the criteria in 1999, such that Amsterdam II included additional LS-associated cancers (endometrial, small bowel, ureter, and renal pelvis) in addition to CRC (**Table 1**).[12]

Recognizing the association between the clinicopathologic tumor phenotype of MMRd and PGVs in DNA MMR genes, the 1996 National Cancer Institute International Workshop on HNPCC drafted the Bethesda Guidelines to help identify which patients with CRC or HNPCC-associated cancers should undergo tumor testing for MSI as a screen for LS.[13] The poor performance of some of the histologic features included in the original Bethesda Guidelines led to their revision in 2002 (see **Table 1**).[14]

Importantly, the discussions about clinical diagnostic criteria for HNPCC revealed some key concepts for the effective identification of patients at-risk for LS. First, that screening tumor specimens for mismatch repair deficiency (through MSI or immunohistochemistry (IHC) for proteins MLH1, MSH2, MSH6, or PMS2 corresponding to the MMR genes) was an effective way to identify patients with cancer who would benefit from germline genetic testing for Lynch syndrome, which formed the basis for implementing "universal tumor screening" for all colorectal and endometrial cancers. Next, was that the term HNPCC was a misnomer, as some affected families manifested an excess of extracolonic cancers, particularly endometrial cancer. The observation that 3% of endometrial cancers and 3% of CRCs were associated with PGVs in mismatch repair genes was one of the several factors prompting the transition away from the term HNPCC and in favor of the term LS. Finally, despite revisions to the Amsterdam criteria and Bethesda Guidelines, identification of patients with LS continued to present challenges, as the various clinical criteria were not only difficult to remember, but also demonstrated suboptimal performance with limited sensitivity and specificity.[15,16]

Prediction Models

Prediction models were developed as an additional means to identify individuals at risk for LS who would benefit from germline testing—unlike the Amsterdam criteria and Bethesda guidelines, risk models offered the ability to quantify the probability

Table 1
Clinical criteria to identify individuals at-risk for lynch syndrome

Criteria	Details	Performance Characteristics[15]
Amsterdam I[11]	Individuals who meet all of the following criteria: • ≥3 relatives with histologically-confirmed CRC, 1 of whom is an FDR of the other 2 • ≥2 generations affected by CRC • ≥1 relative diagnosed with CRC under the age of 50 y	Sensitivity 61% (95% CI: 43%–79%) Specificity 67% (95% CI: 50%–85%)
Amsterdam II[12]	Individuals who meet all of the following criteria: • ≥3 relatives with histologically-confirmed LS-associated[a] cancer, 1 of whom is an FDR of the other 2 • ≥2 generations affected by LS-associated cancer • ≥1 relative diagnosed with LS-associated under the age of 50 y	Sensitivity 78% (95% CI: 64%–92%) Specificity 61% (95% CI: 45%–78%)
Bethesda Guidelines[13]	Test colorectal tumors for MSI in individuals who meet any of the following criteria: • Amsterdam criteria met • Presence of 2 or more LS-associated cancers including synchronous and metachronous CRC • Presence of CRC and an FDR with CRC or LS-associated extracolonic cancer with ≥1 cancer diagnosed at age <45 y and/or colorectal adenoma at age <40 y • CRC or EC diagnosed at age <45 y • Presence of right-sided CRC with an undifferentiated pattern (solid/cribriform), diagnosed at age <45 y • Presence of signet-ring cell type CRC diagnosed at age <45 y • Presence of adenomas diagnosed at age <40 y	Sensitivity 94% (95% CI: 88%–100%) Specificity 25% (95% CI: 14%–36%)
Revised Bethesda Guidelines[14]	Test colorectal tumors for MSI in individuals who meet any of the following criteria: • CRC diagnosed at age <50 y • Presence of synchronous or metachronous CRC, or other LS-associated cancers, regardless of age of diagnosis • CRC with MSI-high histology (tumor-infiltrating lymphocytes, Crohn's-like lymphocytic reaction, mucinous/signet-ring differentiation, or medullary growth pattern) diagnosed at age <60 y • CRC diagnosed in 1 or more FDR with an LS-associated tumor, with 1 of the cancers diagnosed at age <50 y • CRC diagnosed in 2 or more FDR or SDR with LS-associated cancers, regardless of the age	Sensitivity 94% (95% CI: 88%–100%) Specificity 49% (95% CI: 34%–64%)

Abbreviations: CI, confidence interval; CRC, colorectal cancer; EC, endometrial cancer; FDR, first degree relatives; LS, lynch syndrome; MSI, microsatellite instability; SDR, second-degree relatives.
[a] Lynch syndrome-associated cancers in the revised Bethesda guidelines are listed as those that include colorectal, endometrial, small bowel, ureter, and renal pelvis cancers.

of MMR PGV and do not require that clinicians remember complex lists of criteria. Although several models have been developed,[17] here we will highlight the 3 best-studied models: MMRPredict, MMRpro, and Prediction of MMR Gene Mutations (PREMM), which are also summarized in **Table 2**.

MMRPredict was developed using a cohort of 870 patients with CRC who were 55 years of age or younger[18] and has been externally validated in a diverse patient population, demonstrating modest discrimination (area under the receiver operating characteristic curve, AUC: 0.77 (95% confidence interval (CI): 0.73–0.82)) and poor calibration with observed to an expected ratio (O/E) 0.31 (95% CI: 0.24–0.39).[19] MMRPredict incorporates age, sex, personal history of CRC, along with family history of CRC, and/or endometrial cancer in FDRs to provide an overall probability of carrying PGVs of any MMR gene (*MLH1, MSH2, MSH6*). Limitations of MMRPredict include the lack of incorporation of tumor MSI or IHC results, lack of gene-specific risk estimates, and the need to apply to probands who have already been diagnosed with CRC. Additional limitations to this model include the lack of inclusion of extracolonic cancers (aside from endometrial cancer), family history beyond FDRs,[17] and online accessibility for clinical use.

MMRpro was developed and validated using a cohort of 279 individuals from 226 families identified to be at risk for LS through familial cancer registries in the United States, Canada, and Australia.[20] It uses a Bayesian approach and incorporates results from tumor MSI and IHC testing to calculate the risk of carrying PGVs of *MLH1, MSH2,*

Table 2
Risk prediction models for Lynch syndrome[a]

Model	Inputs	Output	Performance Characteristics[19]
MMRpro[20]	• Family history of CRC and/or EC in FDR or SDR • Tumor MSI and IHC results • Result of previous germline testing of *MLH1, MSH2,* or *MSH6* (positive or not found)	Gene-specific probabilities of having PGV in one of the following MMR genes: *MLH1, MSH2, MSH6*	AUC: 0.85 (95% CI: 0.81–0.88) O/E 0.36 (95% CI: 0.27–0.47)
PREMM₅[b,22]	• Age • Sex • Personal history of LS-associated cancer(s)[c] • Family history of LS-associated cancers in FDR and SDR	Gene-specific probabilities of having PGV in one of the following MMR genes: *MLH1, MSH2, MSH6, PMS2,* or deletions in *EPCAM*	AUC: 0.83 (95% CI: 0.75–0.92) *for any MMR gene*

Abbreviations: AUC, area under the receiver operator characteristic curve; CRC, colorectal cancer; EC, endometrial cancer; FDR, first-degree relatives; IHC, immunohistochemistry; LS, Lynch syndrome; MMR, mismatch repair; MSI, microsatellite instability; O/E, observed to expected ratio; PGV, pathogenic germline variants; SDR, second-degree relatives.
  [a] MMRPredict has not been included as it is unavailable for clinical use.
  [b] PREMM model includes PREMM₁,₂, PREMM₁,₂,₆, and PREMM₅, the latter of which is the most recent version.
  [c] Lynch syndrome-associated cancers in the PREMM model are defined as cancers of the ovaries, stomach, small intestine, urinary tract/bladder/kidney, bile ducts, brain, pancreas, and sebaceous gland skin tumors.

and *MSH6* for individuals who are affected or unaffected by CRC and/or endometrial cancer. When externally validated, MMRpro showed good discrimination (AUC: 0.85; 95% CI: 0.81–0.88), but poor calibration with O/E ratio 0.36 (95% CI: 0.27–0.47).[19] Similar to MMRPredict, MMRpro also includes personal CRC and endometrial cancer history, but does not consider other LS-associated cancers. Although MMRpro can provide outputs for gene-specific (*MLH1*, *MSH2*, *MSH6*) probabilities of having LS, the main limitation of this model is that it requires the input of age and cancer history for all relatives, including both cancer-affected and unaffected relatives across the 3 generation pedigree.

PREMM$_{1,2}$ was the first of the PREMM models, developed and validated using a cohort of 1914 (898 for development; 1016 for validation) unrelated probands who had submitted blood samples for clinical testing for *MLH1* and *MSH2* at a commercial genetic testing laboratory.[21] This model includes the following variables: age, sex, personal history of CRC, or other LS-associated cancers, family history of FDRs and SDRs with CRC or any other LS-associated cancer to calculate the probability of having a PGV in an MMR gene. Similar to MMRPredict and MMRpro, PREMM$_{1,2}$ initially included only *MLH1* and *MSH2*. However, it was later expanded to include *MSH6* (PREMM$_{1,2,6}$) and revised to include *PMS2* such that probabilities for mutation in any of the 5 MMR genes associated with LS were calculated (PREMM$_5$).[22] Compared with MMRpro and MMRPredict, PREMM$_5$ has good discrimination to identify the risk of PGV in any of the LS-associated MMR genes (AUC: 0.83; 95% CI: 0.75–0.92). Other advantages to the PREMM$_5$ model are that it can also be applied to healthy individuals who have not had CRC, are user-friendly and easily-accessible online (https://premm.dfci.harvard.edu).[23] With a median PREMM$_5$ estimate of 9.8% for carriers of an MMR PGV and 2.6% for noncarriers, Kastrinos and colleagues found that risk estimates of 2.5% to 10% using PREMM$_5$ achieved a negative predictive value (to identify individuals with negative genetic testing) of 97% to 99%.[22] Therefore, PREMM$_5$ score $\geq$2.5% has been proposed as the threshold above which an individual should be offered genetic counseling and germline genetic testing. Although there have been data to suggest that PREMM$_5$ may be less sensitive for identifying individuals with the PGV in *PMS2* (AUC: 0.51; 95% CI: 0.35–0.66), adding CRC location improved the discriminatory power for *PMS2* carriers (AUC: 0.77; 95% CI: 0.63–0.90).[24] Studies support the feasibility of integrating the PREMM model into clinical practice settings to systematically, and accurately, identify patients at high risk for LS.[25,26]

Universal Tumor Screening

Clinical criteria and risk prediction models for LS rely heavily on having detailed information available about a patient's family history of cancer (including types of cancer and ages of diagnosis). Since this information is often lacking in the medical record, alternative strategies have focused on implementing universal testing of all CRC tumors for mismatch repair deficiency using MSI and/or IHC for MMR proteins. The prevalence of MSI-H among CRC tumors has been estimated as 22%, with most of these (approximately 15%) demonstrating somatic mutations in *BRAF* and/or hypermethylation of the *MLH1* promoter (ie, sporadic CRCs).[27] Patients whose CRC tumors are MSI-H without somatic BRAF mutation or MLH1 promoter hypermethylation should be referred for germline sequencing for PGVs associated with LS.

Routine molecular screening of tumors from patients diagnosed with colorectal adenocarcinoma has been shown to be effective for identifying individuals with PGVs in LS genes who would not have been diagnosed with LS from clinical criteria.[28]

This led to the recommendation from the Evaluation of Genomic Applications in Practice and Prevention (EGAPP) 2009 working group to implement MMR testing for all individuals with newly diagnosed CRC[29] which is now widely accepted as a cost-effective strategy to screen all CRC patients for risk for LS.[30] It is worthy of mention that this recommendation came nearly 25 years after the essential role of MSI as a tumor molecular phenotype indicating risk for LS was first reported.

Similarly, universal testing of endometrial cancers has also been shown to improve identification of individuals with LS who would have otherwise been missed if germline testing was only offered based on clinical criteria and/or prediction models alone.[31] In a large systematic review and meta-analysis, Kahn and colleagues pooled data from 29 studies comprising 6649 patients with endometrial cancer.[10] They found that among those who had testing that was positive for an MMR PGV, 19% had tumors that were MSI-H, and 15% had loss of MMR protein expression on IHC. Therefore, as of 2014, the American College of Obstetricians and Gynecologists also recommend testing all endometrial cancers for MMRd to identify individuals at-risk for LS.[32]

Universal tumor screening refers to testing for DNA mismatch repair deficiency through either MSI by polymerase chain reaction or IHC analysis to detect the loss of MMR proteins. For CRC specimens, MSI testing has a sensitivity of 85% and specificity of 90% for the diagnosis of LS and IHC has a sensitivity of 83% and specificity of 89%.[33] Tumors that are determined to be microsatellite stable and/or have intact MMR proteins are considered to be sporadic. For individuals who are found to have tumors that are MSI-H and/or have a loss of MMR protein expression further testing is required (**Fig. 1**). Tumors that are MSI-high with the loss of *MLH1* and *PMS2* protein expression should undergo additional somatic testing for *MLH1* promoter hypermethylation or *BRAF* V600E mutation, which, if found, are suggestive of a sporadic cancer.[34,35] If *MLH1* promoter hypermethylation and *BRAF* V600 E are not identified, then germline testing for LS should be offered. If tumors show loss of *MSH2*, *MSH6*, or *PMS2* proteins only, then germline testing for LS should be performed. Given the 5% to 10% of false-negative results with tumor screening with MSI and/or IHC, the presence of a strong family history of cancer may still justify germline testing.[36] **Fig. 2** presents an algorithm for universal tumor testing.

Next-Generation DNA Sequencing

Next-generation sequencing (NGS) technologies make it possible to sequence dozens of genes simultaneously and have revolutionized genetic testing for hereditary CRC. NGS can be applied to sequence germline and tumor DNA samples, and has been validated as an approach to identify MMRd in tumors.[37,38] Increased availability of DNA sequencing (at reduced cost) offers opportunities for sequencing tumor and germline DNA samples collected from population-based cohorts. Using WGS, Haraldsdottir and colleagues conducted a population-wide analysis to screen for LS in Iceland.[39] Sequencing of 1208 patients diagnosed with CRC and cancer-free controls found that 2.3% of all CRCs could be attributed to Lynch syndrome, with population prevalence of PGV in LS genes of 0.442%, or 1 in 226.

Strategies that incorporate NGS for tumor testing (with or without germline sequencing) offer the potential to overcome the limited sensitivity of MSI and/or IHC for MMRd while also testing for somatic BRAF mutations, as well as somatic mutations in DNA MMR genes. In fact, tumor sequencing has been shown to have improved sensitivity (100%; 95% CI: 94%–100%) than universal tumor testing with IHC *and BRAF* (90%; 95% CI: 79%–96%) or MSI *and BRAF* (91%; 95% CI: 81%–97%) with equal specificity.[40]

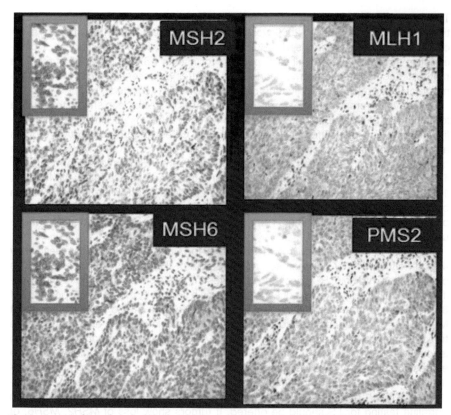

Fig. 1. Immunohistochemical testing of a colorectal cancer tumor for the protein expression of mismatch repair genes associated with Lynch syndrome. Protein expression is preserved for MSH2 and MSH6 (inset) and absent for MLH1 and PMS2 (inset). The absence of MMR protein expression is suggestive of Lynch syndrome and warrants additional evaluation. (*From* PDQ Cancer Genetics Editorial Board. PDQ Genetics of Colorectal Cancer. Bethesda, MD: National Cancer Institute. Available at: https://www.cancer.gov/types/colorectal/hp/colorectal-genetics-pdq. Accessed September 1, 2021.)

LYNCH SYNDROME MIMICS

A discussion about screening for LS would not be complete without mentioning LS mimics.[41] LS mimics are broadly defined as cases with clinical features suggestive of LS in which germline sequencing does not identify a PGV in an LS gene. These include:

Tumor Lynch or Lynch-like syndrome

Defined as individuals with tumors that exhibit mismatch repair-deficient phenotypes, without somatic *BRAF* mutation or *MLH1* promoter hypermethylation who have no identifiable PGV in the LS genes. Although these LLS cases initially raised concern for an unidentified PGV, recent studies suggest that most of these tumors develop in the setting of double somatic mutations in MMR genes which seem to be sporadic..[41,42] Studies of LLS cases suggest the risk of CRC is lower in families of individuals with LLS than LS with one population-based study showing standardized incidence ratios of 2.12 (95% CI: 1.16–3.56) and 6.04 (95% CI: 3.58–9.54) for LLS

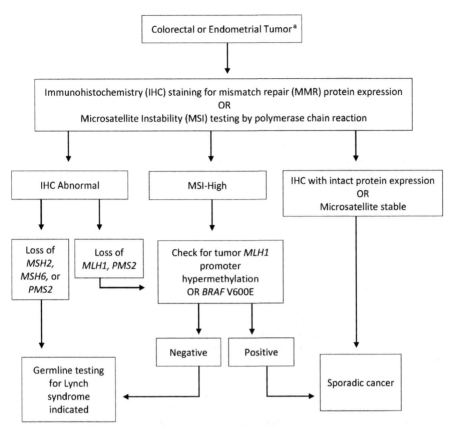

Fig. 2. Algorithm for universal tumor testing. [a] For any individual with highly suspicious family history, germline genetic testing should be performed regardless of the above results.

and LS, respectively.[43] Although CRCs associated with LLS are diagnosed at early ages than sporadic CRC, extracolonic cancers are rare.[43,44]

Amsterdam + Family History with Mismatch Repair Proficient Colorectal Cancers

Individuals with a family history of CRC affecting 3 generations with 1 or more diagnoses age less than 50, but whose colorectal tumors do not exhibit MSI and have germline testing that rules out PGV in MMR genes are generally classified as familial colorectal cancer type X (FCCTX). CRC is predominant cancer in FCCTX, and whereas the mean age of CRC onset is earlier when compared with sporadic CRC, it is higher in FCCTX than LS (54 years vs 44 years of age; $P<.001$).[45] Fortunately, extracolonic cancers do not seem to feature in FCCTX, and the lifetime risk of CRC is lower when compared with LS, justifying every 3-year colonoscopy surveillance intervals. To date, no PGV have been consistently associated with FCCTX.

Finally, a discussion of LS would not be complete without the mention of constitutional mismatch repair deficiency syndrome (CMMRD). This entity is caused by biallelic, rather than monoallelic, PGVs in the MMR genes, most commonly *PMS2* or *MSH6*.[41,46] Individuals with CMMRD often develop LS-associated malignancies (such as brain tumors, hematologic, gynecologic, and gastrointestinal cancers) during childhood or adolescence and can present with features similar to neurofibromatosis type 1. The phenotype can be quite variable, and the European Consortium for CMMRD has developed a scoring system to help identify patients who may be eligible for germline testing.[47]

FUTURE DIRECTIONS

Identification of LS using the currently available clinical criteria and prediction models inherently starts with identifying patterns of LS-associated cancers across multiple generations. Universal testing of all colorectal and endometrial cancers for MSI or loss of MMR protein expression increases the potential to identify individuals with LS, but given their limited sensitivities, perhaps an even more broad approach to identify at-risk individuals may be warranted. One such approach would be to test tumors beyond colorectal or endometrial origin for MMRd. With the U.S. Food and Drug Administration's approval of pembrolizumab, a monoclonal antibody that targets programmed death receptor-1 (PD-1) or programmed death ligand-1 (PD-L1), for treatment of advanced solid tumors with MMRd,[48] testing for MSI has increased. In 2018, Latham and colleagues sought to determine the LS prevalence using a cohort of 15,045 individuals with more than 50 types of solid tumors.[49] They identified LS in the setting of MSI-H in 16% (53/326), MSI-indeterminate in 2% (13/699), and microsatellite stable in another 0.3%. Of the MSI-H and MSI-indeterminate cohorts, 50% (33/66) had tumors other than CRC or endometrial cancer and of these, 45% (15/33) would not have met eligibility for LS testing based on personal and/or family history. This study highlights the heterogeneity of LS, recognizing the limitations of our current clinical criteria, and underscores the importance of germline testing for MMR PGV when MSI-H tumors are identified.

Another approach for the early identification of individuals at-risk for Lynch syndrome is the consideration of genetic risk assessment in the general population and in the absence of a colorectal cancer diagnosis. Using a simulation framework, Dinh and colleagues[50] integrated models of colorectal and endometrial cancers with a 5-generation family history to determine whether primary genetic screening for LS in the general population is a cost-effective approach. They tested 20 screening strategies for individuals starting at the age of 20 years who met thresholds of 0%, 2.5%, 5%, or 10% risk for carrying an LS-associated PGV using the $PREMM_{126}$ model. Risk assessment starting at the ages of 25, 30, or 35 with germline testing for those who exceeded a risk threshold of 5% reduced the incidence of colorectal and endometrial cancers by 12% and 9%, respectively, and was the most cost-effective approach with 135 quality-adjusted life-years (QALYs) gained at a cost of $26,000 per QALY. Universal primary genetic screening (ie, testing when risk was estimated as 0%) starting at the age of 20 years led to the greatest reduction in colorectal and endometrial cancers, 44% and 40%, respectively, with a gain of 933 QALYs, but at the cost of $401,019 per QALY.

SUMMARY

LS is the most common hereditary CRC syndrome. The use of clinical criteria, prediction models, and universal tumor testing strategies, provides ample opportunities to identify LS carriers and apply risk-reducing interventions to decrease cancer-related morbidity and mortality. Advances in NGS allow for the testing of tumors and germline DNA samples at a large scale. Ultimately, screening approaches that are cost-effective and can be easily integrated into clinical practice, coupled with strategies to improve the uptake of genetic counseling and testing, are all necessary to optimize the identification and management of individuals at risk for LS.

CLINICS CARE POINTS

- Colorectal and endometrial tumors that are microsatellite stable and/or have intact mismatch repair (MMR) proteins are considered to be sporadic. Those that are microsatellite instability-high (MSI-H) with the loss of *MLH1* and *PMS2* should undergo somatic testing for *MLH1* promoter hypermethylation or *BRAF V600 E* mutation, which, if present, also suggests sporadic cancer.
- If tumor testing does not reveal MMR deficiency (microsatellite stable and/or immunohistochemistry shows intact MMR protein expression), but there is a strong family history of Lynch syndrome-associated cancers, referral for genetic counseling and germline testing for pathogenic variants (PGVs) of MMR genes should still be considered.
- Individuals who clinically meet criteria for Lynch syndrome, but do not have PGVs of MMR genes should be further evaluated for LS mimics.

DISCLOSURE

Dr. Maratt receives support from Grant Number UL1TR002529 from the National Institutes of Health (NIH), National Center for Advancing Translational Sciences, Clinical and Translational Sciences Award. The views expressed in this manuscript do not reflect views of the NIH.

REFERENCES

1. Win AK, Jenkins MA, Dowty JG, et al. Prevalence and penetrance of major genes and polygenes for colorectal cancer. Cancer Epidemiol Biomarkers Prev 2017; 26(3):404–12.
2. Lynch HT, Snyder CL, Shaw TG, et al. Milestones of Lynch syndrome: 1895-2015. Nat Rev Cancer 2015;15(3):181–94.
3. Boland CR, Lynch HT. The history of Lynch syndrome. Fam Cancer 2013;12(2): 145–57.
4. Ligtenberg MJL, Kuiper RP, Chan TL, et al. Heritable somatic methylation and inactivation of MSH2 in families with Lynch syndrome due to deletion of the 3' exons of TACSTD1. Nat Genet 2009;41(1):112–7.
5. Aaltonen LA, Peltomäki P, Leach FS, et al. Clues to the pathogenesis of familial colorectal cancer. Science 1993;260:812–6.
6. Ionov Y, Peinado MA, Malkhosyan S, et al. Ubiquitous somatic mutations in simple repeated sequences reveal a new mechanism for colonic carcinogenesis. Nature 1993;363(6429):558–61.
7. Grady WM, Carethers JM. Genomic and epigenetic instability in colorectal cancer pathogenesis. Gastroenterology 2008;135(4):1079–99.
8. Boland PM, Yurgelun MB, Boland CR. Recent progress in Lynch syndrome and other familial colorectal cancer syndromes. CA Cancer J Clin 2018;68(3): 217–31.
9. Watkins JC, Yang EJ, Muto MG, et al. Universal screening for mismatch-repair deficiency in endometrial cancers to identify patients with lynch syndrome and lynch-like syndrome. Int J Gynecol Pathol 2017;36(2):115–27.
10. Kahn RM, Gordhandas S, Maddy BP, et al. Universal endometrial cancer tumor typing: How much has immunohistochemistry, microsatellite instability, and MLH1 methylation improved the diagnosis of Lynch syndrome across the population? Cancer 2019;125(18):3172–83.

11. Vasen HFA, Mecklin JP, Meera Khan P, et al. The International Collaborative Group on hereditary non-polyposis colorectal cancer (ICG-HNPCC). Dis Colon Rectum 1991;34(5):424–5.

12. Vasen HFA, Watson P, Mecklin JP, et al. New clinical criteria for hereditary nonpolyposis colorectal definition of HNPCC. Gastroenterology 1999;116:1453–6.

13. Rodriguez-Bigas MA, Boland CR, Hamilton SR, et al. A National Cancer Institute Workshop on hereditary nonpolyposis colorectal cancer syndrome: meeting highlights and Bethesda guidelines. J Natl Cancer Inst 1997;89(23):1758–62.

14. Umar A, Boland CR, Terdiman JP, et al. Revised Bethesda guidelines for hereditary nonpolyposis colorectal cancer (Lynch syndrome) and microsatellite instability. J Natl Cancer Inst 2004;96(4):261–8.

15. Syngal S, Fox EA, Eng C, et al. Sensitivity and specificity of clinical criteria for hereditary non-polyposis colorectal cancer associated mutations in MSH2 and MLH1. J Med Genet 2000;37(9):641–5.

16. Sjursen W, Haukanes BI, Grindedal EM, et al. Current clinical criteria for Lynch syndrome are not sensitive enough to identify MSH6 mutation carriers. J Med Genet 2010;47(9):579–85.

17. Kastrinos F, Balmaña J, Syngal S. Prediction models in Lynch syndrome. Fam Cancer 2013;12(2):217–28.

18. Barnetson RA, Tenesa A, Farrington SM, et al. Identification and survival of carriers of mutations in DNA mismatch-repair genes in colon cancer. N Engl J Med 2006;354(26):2751–63.

19. Kastrinos F, Ojha RP, Leenen C, et al. Comparison of prediction models for Lynch syndrome among individuals with colorectal cancer. J Natl Cancer Inst 2016; 108(2):1–9.

20. Chen S, Wang W, Lee S, et al. Prediction of germline mutations and cancer risk in the Lynch syndrome. JAMA 2006;296(12):1479–87.

21. Balmaña J, Stockwell DH, Steyerberg EW, et al. Prediction of MLH1 and MSH2 mutations in Lynch syndrome. JAMA 2006;296(12):1469–78.

22. Kastrinos F, Uno H, Ukaegbu C, et al. Development & validation of the PREMM5 model for comprehensive risk assessment of lynch syndrome. J Clin Oncol 2017; 35(19):2165–72.

23. Pouchet CJ, Wong N, Chong G, et al. A comparison of models used to predict MLH1, MSH2 and MSH6 mutation carriers. Ann Oncol 2009;20(4):681–8.

24. Goverde A, Spaander MCW, Nieboer D, et al. Evaluation of current prediction models for Lynch syndrome: updating the PREMM5 model to identify PMS2 mutation carriers. Fam Cancer 2018;17(3):361–70.

25. Guivatchian T, Koeppe ES, Baker JR, et al. Family history in colonoscopy patients: feasibility and performance of electronic and paper-based surveys for colorectal cancer risk assessment in the outpatient setting. Gastrointest Endosc 2017;86(4):684–91.

26. Luba DG, DiSario JA, Rock C, et al. Community practice implementation of a self-administered version of PREMM1,2,6 to assess risk for Lynch syndrome. Clin Gastroenterol Hepatol 2018;16(1):49–58.

27. Karlitz JJ, Hsieh MC, Liu Y, et al. Population-based lynch syndrome screening by microsatellite instability in patients ≤50: prevalence, testing determinants, and result availability prior to colon surgery. Am J Gastroenterol 2015;110(7):948–55.

28. Hampel H, Frankel WL, Martin E, et al. Screening for the Lynch Syndrome (Hereditary Nonpolyposis Colorectal Cancer). N Engl J Med 2005;352(18):1851–60.

29. Berg AO, Armstrong K, Botkin J, et al. Recommendations from the EGAPP Working Group: genetic testing strategies in newly diagnosed individuals with

colorectal cancer aimed at reducing morbidity and mortality from Lynch syndrome in relatives. Genet Med 2009;11(1):35–41.

30. Giardiello FM, Allen JI, Axilbund JE, et al. Guidelines on genetic evaluation and management of lynch syndrome: a consensus statement by the US multisociety task force on colorectal cancer. Gastroenterology 2014;147(2):502–26.

31. Adar T, Rodgers LH, Shannon KM, et al. Universal screening of both endometrial and colon cancers increases the detection of Lynch syndrome. Cancer 2018; 124(15):3145–53.

32. ACOG practice bulletin no. 147: Lynch syndrome. Obstet Gynecol 2014;124(5): 1042–54.

33. Palomaki GE, McClain MR, Melillo S, et al. EGAPP supplementary evidence review: DNA testing strategies aimed at reducing morbidity and mortality from Lynch syndrome. Genet Med 2009;11(1):42–65.

34. Jin M, Hampel H, Zhou X, et al. BRAF V600E mutation analysis simplifies the testing algorithm for lynch syndrome. Am J Clin Pathol 2013;140(2):177–83.

35. McGivern A, Wynter CVA, Whitehall VLJ, et al. Promoter hypermethylation frequency and BRAF mutations distinguish hereditary non-polyposis colon cancer from sporadic MSI-H colon cancer. Fam Cancer 2004;3(2):101–7.

36. National Comprehensive Cancer Network (NCCN) Clinical Practice Guidelines in Oncology. Genetic/familial high-risk assessment: colorectal. 2020. Available at: nccn.org. Accessed April 22, 2021.

37. Papke DJ, Nowak JA, Yurgelun MB, et al. Validation of a targeted next-generation sequencing approach to detect mismatch repair deficiency in colorectal adenocarcinoma. Mod Pathol 2018;31(12):1882–90.

38. Nowak JA, Yurgelun MB, Bruce JL, et al. Detection of mismatch repair deficiency and microsatellite instability in colorectal adenocarcinoma by targeted next-generation sequencing. J Mol Diagn 2017;19(1):84–91.

39. Haraldsdottir S, Rafnar T, Frankel WL, et al. Comprehensive population-wide analysis of Lynch syndrome in Iceland reveals founder mutations in MSH6 and PMS2. Nat Commun 2017;8:1–11.

40. Hampel H, Pearlman R, Beightol M, et al. Assessment of tumor sequencing as a replacement for lynch syndrome screening and current molecular tests for patients with colorectal cancer. JAMA Oncol 2018;4(6):806–13.

41. Carethers JM, Stoffel EM. Lynch syndrome and Lynch syndrome mimics: the growing complex landscape of hereditary colon cancer. World J Gastroenterol 2015;21(31):9253–61.

42. Pearlman R, Haraldsdottir S, De La Chapelle A, et al. Clinical characteristics of patients with colorectal cancer with double somatic mismatch repair mutations compared with Lynch syndrome. J Med Genet 2019;56(7):462–70.

43. Rodríguez-Soler M, Pérez-Carbonell L, Guarinos C, et al. Risk of cancer in cases of suspected lynch syndrome without germline mutation. Gastroenterology 2013; 144(5):926–32.e1.

44. Xicola RM, Clark JR, Carroll T, et al. Implication of DNA repair genes in Lynch-like syndrome. Fam Cancer 2019;18(3):331–42.

45. Xu Y, Li C, Zhang Y, et al. Comparison between familial colorectal cancer type X and Lynch syndrome: molecular, clinical, and pathological characteristics and pedigrees. Front Oncol 2020;10:1–11.

46. Aronson M, Colas C, Shuen A, et al. Diagnostic criteria for constitutional mismatch repair deficiency (CMMRD): recommendations from the international consensus working group. J Med Genet 2021;1–10.

47. Katharina W, Kratz CP, Vasen HFA, et al. Diagnostic criteria for constitutional mismatch repair deficiency syndrome: suggestions of the European consortium "Care for CMMRD" (C4CMMRD). J Med Genet 2014;51(6):355–65.
48. Boyiadzis MM, Kirkwood JM, Marshall JL, et al. Significance and implications of FDA approval of pembrolizumab for biomarker-defined disease. J Immunother Cancer 2018;6(1):1–7.
49. Latham A, Srinivasan P, Kemel Y, et al. Microsatellite instability is associated with the presence of Lynch syndrome pan-cancer. J Clin Oncol 2019;37(4):286–95.
50. Dinh TA, Rosner BI, Boland CR, et al. Screening for lynch syndrome in the general population - Response. Cancer Prev Res 2011;4(3):472.

Colorectal Cancer Screening Recommendations and Outcomes in Lynch Syndrome

Christine Drogan, MS, CGC, Sonia S. Kupfer, MD*

KEYWORDS

- Lynch syndrome • Colorectal cancer • Screening • Chromoendoscopy
- Artificial intelligence • Quality

KEY POINTS

- Colorectal cancer (CRC) screening guidelines in Lynch syndrome have evolved from universal to gene-specific recommendations based on differences in lifetime neoplasia risks.
- CRC screening reduces cancer incidence and overall mortality in Lynch syndrome.
- High CRC incidence with regular colonoscopy screening intervals suggests the possibility of accelerated, nonpolypoid, or missed lesions.
- Adjunctive tools such as chromoendoscopy have not been shown to enhance high-definition white-light examination in Lynch syndrome.
- Optimal screening approaches in Lynch syndrome are needed and should include systemic and coordinated care.

INTRODUCTION

Screening for colorectal cancer (CRC) in Lynch syndrome enables early detection and likely also cancer prevention. In this review, the term "screening" (also referred to as surveillance) is used to describe regular tests performed in asymptomatic individuals with Lynch syndrome for the purpose of detection of cancers or precancerous polyps. CRC screening guidelines in Lynch syndrome have evolved from universal recommendations common to all carriers of mismatch repair gene pathogenic and likely pathogenic (P/LP) variants to gene-specific recommendations based on differences in lifetime neoplasia risks. Regular screening for Lynch syndrome reduces CRC-related mortality likely due to early CRC detection and surgery as well as polypectomy. Elevated CRC incidence in individuals undergoing regular colonoscopy screening

Grant support: R01 CA220329 to S.S. Kupfer.

Section of Gastroenterology, Hepatology and Nutrition, Department of Medicine, University of Chicago, Chicago, IL, USA

* Corresponding author. Section of Gastroenterology, Hepatology and Nutrition, Department of Medicine, University of Chicago, 900 East 57th Street, #9120, Chicago, IL 60637.

E-mail address: skupfer@medicine.bsd.uchicago.edu

Gastrointest Endoscopy Clin N Am 32 (2022) 59–74
https://doi.org/10.1016/j.giec.2021.08.001

suggests the possibility of a nonadenomatous carcinogenesis pathway that might vary by mismatch repair gene. Colonoscopy is the primary modality for screening for Lynch syndrome with mixed and emerging data on the benefit of quality metrics, chromoendoscopy, artificial intelligence, and nonendoscopic modalities. The success of screening depends on adherence which varies across studies in different health care systems and countries. The current state of CRC screening recommendations, outcomes, and modalities in Lynch syndrome with emphasis on new and emerging studies in the field is reviewed here.

COLORECTAL CANCER SCREENING GUIDELINES IN LYNCH SYNDROME

Management recommendations for CRC and other cancer screening for Lynch syndrome are consistently reviewed and revised as additional data are published on the efficacy of current modalities, age to initiate screening, and surveillance intervals. Professional organizations, in the United States and worldwide, have published guidelines with differing recommendations for Lynch syndrome over time. In 2018, the International Mismatch Repair Consortium conducted a survey of clinical centers that care for patients with Lynch syndrome and demonstrated little consensus among centers, with most respondents indicating that they perform colonoscopy every year or every 1 to 2 years.[1] The lack of expert consensus in professional guidelines leads to some confusion, especially in regards to the appropriate management of individuals with P/LP variants in less penetrant genes such as *MSH6* or *PMS2*. Current CRC screening recommendations in Lynch syndrome from various professional groups are summarized in **Table 1**.

The National Comprehensive Cancer Network (NCCN) consistently updates screening recommendations for Lynch syndrome and is among the most widely referenced guidelines in the United States. In the 2020 version, recommendations for Lynch syndrome screening were separated by the gene for the first time, based on gene-specific risks.[2] For individuals with an *MLH1* or *MSH2* P/LP variant, CRC screening with colonoscopy is recommended to begin between ages 20 and 25 or 2 and 5 years before the earliest age of diagnosis of CRC in the family if it is before age 25, whichever comes first. In individuals with an *MSH6* or *PMS2* P/LP variant, colonoscopy can start at a later age, between ages 30 and 35 or 2 and 5 years earlier than the youngest diagnosis in the family. Regardless of the gene that is mutated, the NCCN recommends that individuals with Lynch syndrome should have a colonoscopy every 1 to 2 years. Recommendations for colonoscopy do not vary by gender.

Similar to the NCCN, the 2017 American Society of Colon and Rectal Surgeons (ASCRS) guidelines include gene-specific recommendations.[3] Colonoscopy should be considered annually starting at age 20 to 25 for *MLH1/MSH2* carriers or 2–5 years before the youngest age of CRC if younger than 25. For first-degree relatives (FDRs) of an individual who is a known carrier of a Lynch syndrome-associated P/LP variant (sibling, parent, or child), colonoscopy is recommended to commence at age 20 to 25 until they have genetic testing to confirm their carrier or true negative status. Individuals with *MSH6* and *PMS2* P/LP variants are recommended to start colonoscopy at age 30 and 35, respectively, unless there is an earlier onset of CRC in the family.

The American Gastrointestinal Association (AGA) published guidelines for Lynch syndrome in 2015 and recommendations are consistent for all individuals who have Lynch syndrome, regardless of the gene that is mutated.[4] The AGA recommends that all individuals with Lynch syndrome have a colonoscopy starting at age 20 to 25 or 5 years before the youngest diagnosis of CRC in the family and repeating every 1 to 2 years. The American College of Gastroenterology (ACG) also published

Table 1
CRC screening recommendations in Lynch syndrome by professional organizations

Organization (year)	Age/frequency	MLH1	MSH2	MSH6	PMS2
NCCN (2020)	Age		20-25yª		30-35yª
	Frequency		1-2y		1-2y
ASCRS (2017)	Age		20-25yª	30yª	35yª
	Frequency		1y		1y
AGA (2015)	Age			20-25yᵇ	
	Frequency			1-2y	
ACG (2015)	Age			20-25y	
	Frequency			1-2y (1y for confirmed carriers)	
USMSTF (2014)	Age		20-25yª	30yª	35yª
	Frequency			1 y	
ASCO/ESMO (2015)	Age			20-25yᵇ	
	Frequency			1-2y	
EHTG/ESCP (2020)	Age		25y		35y
	Frequency			2-3yᶜ	Consider 5y
BSG/ACPGBI/UKCGG (2020)	Age		25y		35y
	Frequency		2y		2 y
CGN Australia (2017)	Age		25yᵇ		30yᵇ
	Frequency			1-2y	
JSCCR (2018)	Age			20-25y	
	Frequency			1-2y	

Abbreviations: ACPGBI, Association of Coloproctology of Great Britain and Ireland; AGA, American Gastroenterology Association; ASCO, American Society of Clinical Oncology; ASCRS, American Society of Colon and Rectal Surgeons; BSG, British Society of Gastroenterology; CGN, Clinical Guidelines Network Australia; EHTG, European Hereditary Tumour Group; ESCP, European Society of Coloproctology; ESMO, European Society of Medical Oncology; JSCCR, Japanese Society of Cancer of the Colon and Rectum; NCCN, National Comprehensive Cancer Network; UKCGG, United Kingdom Cancer Genetics Group; USMSTF, United States Multi-Society Task Force.
  ª 2–5y younger than the earliest diagnosis in the family.
  ᵇ 5y younger than the earliest diagnosis in the family.
  ᶜ Unless prior history of CRC then every 2y.

guidelines in 2015 to start screening with colonoscopy starting at age 20 to 25 and repeating at least every 2 years and annually for confirmed P/LP variant carriers.[5]

In 2014, the United States Multi-Society Task Force (USMSTF) published a position statement that individuals with an *MLH1* of *MSH2* P/LP variant and FDR of a P/LP variant carrier in these 2 genes undergo colonoscopy every 1 to 2 years, starting between ages 20 and 25, or 2 to 5 years before the youngest diagnosis in the family if that diagnosis is under 25 years of age.[6] Carriers of an *MSH6* or *PMS2* P/LP variant can consider starting screening at 30 and 35, respectively, unless there is an earlier CRC diagnosis in the family. Colonoscopy can be considered on an annual basis for those with a confirmed germline P/LP variant.

The American Society of Clinical Oncology (ASCO) published clinical guidelines in 2015 endorsing those previously established by the European Society for Medical Oncology (ESMO).[7,8] They agree that for individuals with Lynch syndrome, colonoscopy every 1 to 2 years should be performed starting between ages 20 and 25, or 5 years younger than the earliest diagnosis of CRC in the family. No upper age limit is suggested; however, ESMO notes that the decision to continue with colonoscopy should be based on the individual's other health problems.

Additional organizations around the world have also published guidelines on CRC screening for Lynch syndrome. In 2020, the European Hereditary Tumor Group (EHTG) and European Society of Coloproctology (ESCP) published guidelines that also provide gene-specific screening recommendations.[9] Individuals with an *MLH1* or *MSH2* P/LP variant should begin colonoscopy at 25, whereas people with an *MSH6* or *PMS2* gene P/LP variant should start at age 35. Colonoscopy for carriers of an *MLH1*, *MSH2,* or *MSH6* P/LP variant should undergo colonoscopy every 2 to 3 years, unless they have a prior history of CRC, in which case colonoscopy should be conducted every 2 years. Colonoscopy can be considered every 5 years for *PMS2* carriers. These guidelines also note that CRC screening recommendations should not differ between genders.

The British Society of Gastroenterology (BSG), Association of Coloproctology of Great Britain and Ireland (ACPGBI), and United Kingdom Cancer Genetics Group (UKCGG) published joint guidelines, also in 2020, that recommend individuals with an *MLH1* or *MSH2* P/LP variant variants begin colonoscopy at 25 and repeating every 2 years.[10] Individuals with an *MSH6* or *PMS2* P/LP variant should begin colonoscopy at 35 and repeat every 2 years. These guidelines also propose an upper age limit to screening at the age of 75. Similar to the European publication, these guidelines note that there is insufficient evidence to support risk stratification by gender at this time.

Clinical Guidelines Network in Australia's most recent Lynch syndrome management guidelines was published in 2017.[11] This group recommends colonoscopy every 1 to 2 years, for known carriers and individuals at risk of carrying a P/LP variant in which definitive testing is not available, like in a family without an identifiable P/LP variant or no informative relatives available to test. Known carriers should ideally have a colonoscopy annually, beginning at 25 for individuals with an *MLH1* or *MSH2* P/LP variant and consider starting at age 30 for carriers of an *MSH6* or *PMS2* P/LP variant. If there is an earlier diagnosis in the family, colonoscopy should begin 5 years younger than that diagnosis.

The Japanese Society for Cancer of the Colon and Rectum (JSCCR) guidelines do not delineate by gene P/LP variant.[12] All carriers of a P/LP variant in any Lynch syndrome gene are recommended to begin colonoscopy between 20 and 25 years and repeat every 1 to 2 years.

OUTCOMES OF COLORECTAL CANCER SCREENING FOR LYNCH SYNDROME

The increased risk of CRC in Lynch syndrome has long been appreciated with carriers of P/LP variants in *MLH1*, *MSH2 (EPCAM)*, *MSH6* or *PMS2* being recommended to undergo colonoscopies earlier and more often than those at average risk as summarized in **Table 1**. Multiple prospective studies have been published outlining the outcomes of colonoscopy screening for Lynch syndrome, supporting the efficacy of this screening modality, though recent studies highlight potential limitations of colonoscopy for CRC prevention.

The first and longest controlled studies of CRC screening for Lynch syndrome were performed in Finland beginning in the early 1980s, in which individuals from 22 families with Lynch syndrome (initially defined clinically and over time by genetic testing) who choose to undergo CRC screening (initially by colonoscopy or barium enema with flexible sigmoidoscopy and over time predominantly by colonoscopy) every 3 years were compared with individuals with Lynch syndrome who did not choose to undergo CRC screening.[13] Although the study design was complicated because of the introduction of genetic testing and lack of randomization, this study showed a 62% reduction in CRC incidence and, importantly, a 65% reduction in overall mortality with CRC screening for Lynch syndrome over the 15-year time period. These landmark findings solidified regular colonoscopy screening as the preferred strategy in Lynch syndrome carriers.

A prospective study in England followed individuals with a family history of CRC for 16 years with colonoscopy.[14] The most advanced lesion for each individual was recorded. The study reported that individuals who met Amsterdam criteria were more likely to develop CRC or a high-risk adenoma than those with a family history that did not meet Amsterdam criteria. On follow-up colonoscopies, individuals who met Amsterdam criteria were more likely to have high-risk findings than individuals at moderate risk. On average, the subsequent colonoscopies occurred in shorter intervals for individuals at high risk. Additionally, high-risk lesions were identified in all age groups examined in this study, supporting high-risk individuals initiating colonoscopy between ages 20 and 25 years. The study was limited by the lack of a control group but provides additional support for regular colonoscopy screening for Lynch syndrome.

Recently, the Prospective Lynch Syndrome Database (PLSD), a multi-center European prospective study, published cancer incidence among Lynch syndrome carriers engaged in screening programs (screening intervals varied across countries).[15] Prospectively acquired data from several European registries were combined to determine CRC incidence in Lynch syndrome P/LP variant carriers. The original PLSD reported incidence of first CRC by age 70 for *MLH1, MSH2, MSH6,* and *PMS2* of 46%, 35%, 20%, and 0%, respectively, which were similar in an expanded dataset.[16] The cumulative number of CRC cases within 2 years since the last colonoscopy was 31%. CRC incidence by age 70 could not be accurately calculated in *PMS2* variant carriers due to low case numbers supporting less intensive surveillance in this group.[16] Data from 3 countries included in the PLSD that perform colonoscopy at different intervals for Lynch syndrome, with Germany screening annually, the Netherlands every 1 to 2 years, and Finland every 2 to 3 years[17] did not find differences in the incidence of CRC by country, or differences in stage at diagnosis, indicating that shorter interval of colonoscopy was not necessarily beneficial. This study did not include the analysis of CRC risk in *PMS2* carriers.

Based on results from PLSD and other prospective and retrospective studies, it is clear that regular colonoscopy screening does not entirely prevent CRC. There are several possible explanations for these observations including that precursor lesions are missed, fast-growing, nonpolypoid, disappearing or, less likely, induced.[18] Seminal work from the group in Heidelberg, Germany has shown the presence of mismatch repair-deficient crypts that could lead to CRC without adenoma formation[19,20] and are hypothesized to contribute to the high incidence of CRC despite regular colonoscopy screening.

Precursor lesions and somatic profiles differ by affected mismatch repair gene. The risk of adenomas was reported to be higher in individuals with *MSH2* P/LP variants (17.8% 10-year risk) than *MLH1* P/LP variant carriers (7.7% 10-year risk), though overall CRC rates were similar.[21,22] *MSH6* carriers had a similar rate of adenomas as *MSH2;* however, the CRC risk associated with *MSH6* P/LP variants was significantly lower than P/LP variants in *MSH2.*[22] *MSH2* and *MSH6* carriers were more likely to have somatic *APC* P/LP variants, whereas *MLH1* carriers were more likely to have somatic *CTNNB1* P/LP variants. Thus, it is likely that some *MLH1*-related tumors develop through a nonadenoma pathway that might not be readily detectable by colonoscopy, whereas *MSH2* and *MSH6* tumors follow a more conventional adenoma to carcinoma pathway with advanced neoplasia progression being slower in *MSH6* carriers.[23]

These results provide further evidence of unique carcinogenic pathways for each mismatch repair gene that could inform a more specific initiation age for screening, intervals, and possibly modalities. A recent Markov modeling study of colonoscopy screening intervals based on mismatch repair genes supported this approach.[24] Initiation of colonoscopy screening at age 25 and repeating every 1 to 2 years in *MLH1/MSH2* carriers was cost-effective, whereas delaying the start of screening for *MSH6* and *PMS2* carriers to ages 35 and 40, respectively, and repeating every 3 years was also found to be cost-effective.

Several illustrative examples of CRC screening findings in patients with Lynch syndrome are shown in **Figs. 1–3**. The first patient is a 49-year-old woman with personal history of endometrial cancer at age 48 and family history of early-onset CRC in multiple paternal relatives. A pathogenic *MSH2* variant was identified. The patient underwent colonoscopy 16 months after her last screening examination at another hospital. An 18 mm mass was identified in the transverse colon (see **Fig. 1**). Biopsies confirmed a poorly differentiated mucinous adenocarcinoma with signet ring cells. After the discussion of surgical options including total colectomy, the patient opted for subtotal colectomy with ileosigmoid anastomosis.

The second patient is a 45-year-old woman with multiple maternal relatives with CRC including her mother at age 37. A pathogenic variant was found in *MLH1*. She had a colonoscopy 4 years ago that was normal including retroflexion in the right colon (see **Fig. 2**A, B). She returned 4 years later for her next colonoscopy and was noted to have a 20 mm polyp near the ileocecal valve (see **Fig. 2**C), biopsies of which showed tubular adenoma. Endoscopic resection was performed (see **Fig. 2**D); pathologic condition showed a focus of invasive moderately differentiated adenocarcinoma within a tubular adenoma. The patient then underwent right hemicolectomy with no evidence of residual cancer.

Fig. 3 shows findings from 2 patients with *MSH6* pathogenic variants. The first patient is a 59-year-old woman with a history of a tubular adenoma 5 years prior who underwent colonoscopy for a change in bowel habits and hematochezia that showed an

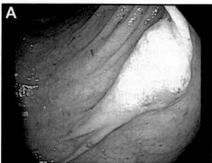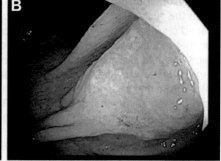

Fig. 1. Colonoscopy screening in an *MSH2* carrier. The patient is a 49-year-old woman with personal history of endometrial cancer at age 48 and family history of early-onset CRC in multiple paternal relatives. A pathogenic *MSH2* variant was identified. The patient underwent colonoscopy 16 months after her last screening examination at another hospital. An 18 mm mass was identified in the transverse colon (*A, B*). Biopsies confirmed a poorly differentiated mucinous adenocarcinoma with signet ring cells. After the discussion of surgical options including total colectomy, the patient opted for subtotal colectomy with ileosigmoid anastomosis.

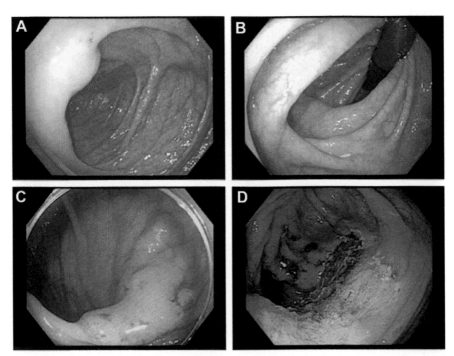

Fig. 2. Colonoscopy screening in an *MLH1* carrier. The patient is a 45-year-old woman with multiple maternal relatives with CRC including her mother at age 37. A pathogenic variant was found in *MLH1*. She had a colonoscopy 4 years ago that was normal including retroflexion in the right colon (*A, B*). She returned 4 years later for her next colonoscopy and was noted to have a 20 mm polyp near the ileocecal valve (*C*), biopsies of which showed tubular adenoma. Endoscopic resection was performed (*D*); pathologic condition showed a focus of invasive moderately differentiated adenocarcinoma within a tubular adenoma. The patient then underwent right hemicolectomy with no evidence of residual cancer.

ulcerated polypoid lesion in the cecum and 3 smaller polyps (see **Fig. 3**A, B). Pathologic condition showed a well-differentiated adenocarcinoma with loss of *MSH6* protein expression on immunohistochemistry and tubular adenomas. A germline pathogenic *MSH6* variant was confirmed. The second patient is a 74-year-old woman with a personal history of uterine cancer at age 56 treated with hysterectomy, oophorectomy, and radiation. Three sisters also had endometrial cancer and a nephew was diagnosed with colon cancer at age 24. A pathogenic variant in *MSH6* was identified in the family. Screening colonoscopy was difficult due to restricted mobility from previous radiation but was complete to the cecum. A 20 mm polyp was identified at the hepatic flexure and removed by endoscopic mucosal resection (see **Fig. 3**C, D). Pathologic condition showed complete resection of a tubular adenoma. The patient continued annual surveillance but, unfortunately, had a perforation during a colonoscopy at age 78 that was successfully treated endoscopically. Discussions about ongoing screening continue on a yearly basis now that the patient is 80 years old and history of difficult colonoscopies.

COLORECTAL CANCER SCREENING MODALITIES IN LYNCH SYNDROME

Colonoscopy is the primary screening modality in Lynch syndrome. A complete examination of the colon and rectum enables evaluation, sampling, and/or complete

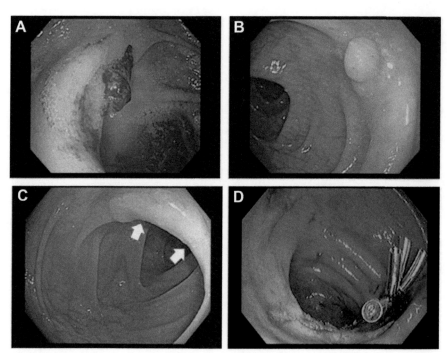

Fig. 3. Colonoscopy screening in 2 *MSH6* carriers. The first patient is a 59-year-old woman with history of a tubular adenoma at age 49 who underwent colonoscopy for a change in bowel habits and hematochezia that showed an ulcerated polypoid lesion in the cecum and 3 smaller polyps (*A, B*). Pathologic condition showed a well-differentiated adenocarcinoma with loss of *MSH6* protein expression on immunohistochemistry and tubular adenomas. A germline pathogenic *MSH6* variant was confirmed. The second patient is a 74-year-old woman with personal history of uterine cancer at age 56 treated with hysterectomy, oophorectomy, and radiation. Three sisters also had endometrial cancer and a nephew was diagnosed with colon cancer at age 24. A pathogenic variant in *MSH6* was identified in the family. Screening colonoscopy was difficult due to restricted mobility from previous radiation but was complete to the cecum. A 20 mm polyp was identified at the hepatic flexure and removed by endoscopic mucosal resection (*C, D*). Arrows are pointing to the polyp. Pathologic condition showed complete resection of a tubular adenoma. The patient continued annual surveillance but, unfortunately, had a perforation during a colonoscopy at age 78 that was successfully treated endoscopically. Discussions about ongoing screening continue on a yearly basis now that the patient is 80 years old and history of difficult colonoscopies.

removal of polyps and cancers. Several quality metrics have been established for average-risk CRC screening; however, the impact of these quality metrics on Lynch syndrome screening is not well established. Moreover, the added benefit of chromoendoscopy in Lynch syndrome is debated, whereas computer-assisted colonoscopy has yet to be studied in Lynch syndrome specifically. Finally, whether nonendoscopic screening modalities could augment current colonoscopy CRC screening for Lynch syndrome remains an open question.

In average-risk CRC screening, the quality of colonoscopy and polypectomy (or surgery for cancers) reduces CRC incidence and mortality.[25] Documentation and adherence to quality metrics such as adenoma detection rate, cecal intubation, withdrawal time, and adequacy of bowel preparation are recommended.[26] The use of high-definition colonoscopes is standard-of-care. However, quality measures and their impact in Lynch syndrome CRC screening are not well established and debated. As discussed previously, the finding of high incidence of CRC among Lynch syndrome carriers despite colonoscopy screening raised the question of whether cancers arose rapidly, through a nonadenoma pathway and/or were missed due to poor quality colonoscopy or incomplete polyp resection.

Recent studies have reached divergent conclusions about the role of colonoscopy quality on CRC incidence in Lynch syndrome. In a single-center retrospective study from Finland,[27] the impact of quality metrics (bowel preparation, cecal intubation, and adenoma detection rate) on CRC and advanced neoplasia detection was evaluated. Among 1564 procedures (mean 4.3 per person) in *MLH1, MSH2,* and *MSH6* carriers, 13% had suboptimal bowel preparation, 98.9% intubated the cecum, and adenoma detection rates were 15.8% and 21.9% before and after high-definition scope introduction, respectively. There was no statistical difference in the rate of CRC between high-quality (1.9%) and low-quality (2.6%) examinations, though power might have been inadequate for this endpoint. The conclusion from this study was that examination quality did not explain incident CRC among patients with Finnish.

In contrast, a large, multi-center study in Spain concluded that quality metrics were associated with the incidence of adenomas and postcolonoscopy CRC. In 893 Lynch syndrome carriers, complete colonoscopies to the cecum, adequate preparation, and chromoendoscopy were associated with higher adenoma detection but these metrics were not statistically significant for CRC detection. Intervals of less than 3 years were associated with lower CRC incidence. Notably, there were low rates of complete colonoscopy (89.2%), adequate bowel preparation (50.1%), and use of high definition scopes (12.3%); only 28% of patients had high-quality screening defined by complete colonoscopy, adequate preparation, and 2-year intervals. More data are needed to define appropriate quality metrics in Lynch syndrome screening and to determine the impact of high-quality examinations on adenoma and, importantly, advanced neoplasia incidence based on affected mismatch repair gene, though it makes common sense to strive for high-quality examinations in all patients undergoing colonoscopic CRC screening including those with Lynch syndrome.

Chromoendoscopy involves spraying the colonic mucosa with nonpermanent stains or dyes (eg, methylene blue, indigo carmine) during colonoscopy. As shown in **Table 2**, the outcomes of these procedures are variable in CRC screening for Lynch syndrome likely related to variable study designs and endoscopists. The most recent chromoendoscopy study in Lynch syndrome was an adequately-powered, multi-center randomized controlled noninferiority trial of high-definition white-light endoscopy compared with pan-colonic chromoendoscopy in Lynch syndrome.[28] Overall, there were no statistical differences in adenoma detection rates between the 2 study arms (which were high in both), though chromoendoscopy detected statistically more small serrated lesions, had a nonsignificant higher rate of detection of flat adenomas, and took longer to perform (nearly 8 minutes longer on average). As discussed in the article's accompanying editorial,[29] although the study showed noninferiority, chromoendoscopy could still have a place in Lynch syndrome especially for low adenoma detecting endoscopists and should be considered one potential component of a systematic approach to high-quality screening for Lynch syndrome carriers. The ESGE issued a strong recommendation for the use of high-definition colonoscopes for CRC screening for Lynch syndrome but recommended only consideration for chromoendoscopy based on weak and conflicting evidence to date.[30] **Fig. 4** shows the images of methylene blue dye sprayed on the colonic mucosa during colonoscopy screening in a patient with an *MSH6* pathogenic variant highlighting small hyperplastic polyps in the rectum.

Table 2
Chromoendoscopy studies in Lynch syndrome

Study (Year)	Design	Sample Size	Comparison	Main Outcomes
Lecomte (2005)	Prospective, single-center, tandem, nonrandomized	33	WLE vs CE in proximal colon	CE identified 45 additional polyps; 11 adenomas
Hurlstone (2005)	Prospective, single-center, tandem, nonrandomized	25	WLE vs targeted CE vs pan-colonic CE	CE identified 52 additional polyps; 32 adenomas
Stoffel (2008)	Prospective, multicenter, tandem, randomized	54	WLE vs pan-colonic CE	CE identified more polyps; no difference in adenomas
Hueneburg (2009)	Prospective, multicenter, tandem, nonrandomized	109	WLE vs pan-colonic CE	CE identified 3x more polyps
Rahmi (2015)	Prospective, multicenter, tandem, randomized	78	WLE vs pan-colonic CE	CE identified more adenomas (41% vs 23%)
Haanstra (2019)	Prospective, multicenter, randomized controlled trial (noninferiority)	246	WLE vs CE proximal colon	No difference in neoplasia detection; 30% vs 27% for CE & WLE
Rivero-Sanchez (2020)	Prospective, multicenter, randomized controlled trial (noninferiority)	256	WLE vs pan-colonic CE	No difference in adenoma detection rate; 34.4% vs 28.1% for CE & WLE

Abbreviations: CE, chromoendoscopy; WLE, white-light endoscopy.

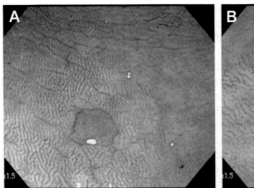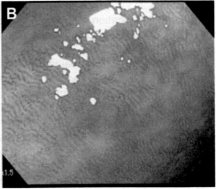

Fig. 4. Chromoendoscopy with methylene blue staining of the colonic mucosa during colonoscopy. Methylene blue dye was sprayed on the colonic mucosa during colonoscopy screening in a patient with an *MSH6* pathogenic variant highlighting small hyperplastic polyps in the rectum (*A, B*).

Computer-aided polyp detection using artificial intelligence has been evaluated in average-risk CRC screening. A randomized controlled trial of 1058 patients found that computer-aided colonoscopy increased adenoma detection rate from 20.3% to 29.1%, though there was no difference in the detection of large polyps.[31] In addition, a larger number of hyperplastic lesions were found with computer-aided technology. An example of a computer-aided finding in a patient with a *PMS2* P/LP variant is shown in **Fig. 5**; it should be noted that the polyp identified by the computer, in this case, was small and nonadenomatous highlighting potential limitations of this technology in the detection of unmeaningful findings. While computer-aided colonoscopy could aid endoscopists with low adenoma detection rates, it is questionable what added benefit this technology will bring to endoscopists who perform high quality

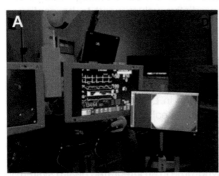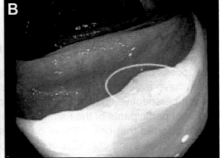

Fig. 5. Computer-assisted colonoscopy in a *PMS2* carrier. A 75-year-old man without a personal history of colorectal cancer was found to carry a familial *PMS2* variant when his nephew was diagnosed with constitutional mismatch repair deficiency syndrome. The patient has had colonoscopy every 2 years since this was identified. He underwent a computer-assisted colonoscopy in the context of a research study. The set-up for this procedure with an additional screen showing computer findings is shown in Figure 5A. The computer identified a polyp in the ascending colon (*yellow circle*) that was also seen on white-light endoscopy. Pathologic condition showed a nonadenomatous polyp (*B*) highlighting potential limitations of this technology.

examinations. In Lynch syndrome specifically, given the possibility of a nonadenoma pathway, the application of technologies to enhance polyp detection during colonoscopy might not prove as beneficial for all patients, but clinical studies in this population are needed.

Several noninvasive screening modalities, both stool- and blood-based, are approved and some are recommended for average-risk screening.[32] Stool-based tests include guaiac, fecal immunochemical test (FIT), and multi-targets stools DNA (panel of fecal gene alterations and FIT). The only blood-based marker approved by the Federal Drug Administration is methylated SEPT9, though this test is not recommended by the USMSTF given poor test characteristics than other modalities.[32] Studies of nonendoscopic screening modalities in Lynch syndrome are currently limited. During restrictions imposed by the COVID-19 pandemic, the United Kingdom launched an initiative to triage patients with Lynch syndrome using a FIT threshold of 10 µg/g of greater to urgent colonoscopy.[33] It is expected that the outcomes of this emergency initiative will be reported in time and could inform the use of FIT as an adjunct in Lynch syndrome CRC screening. A tissue-based study identified highly discriminant DNA methylation markers in Lynch syndrome tumors and showed the highest discrimination with the gene OPLAH, and ALKBH5 was found to be uniquely methylated in Lynch syndrome tumors.[34] These promising results require validation in a larger population and in stool but suggest that Lynch syndrome-specific stool (or blood) biomarkers could be used for early detection and prevention. Finally, mSEPT9 was evaluated in Lynch syndrome-related tumors and blood in a small proof-of-concept study.[35] mSEPT9 was identified in 97.3% and 90.0% of cancers and advanced adenomas, respectively, from patients with Lynch syndrome, suggesting that this could represent a potential biomarker for neoplasia. In a preliminary study of clinical utility, mSEPT9 was found to be 70% sensitive and 100% specific for CRC in Lynch syndrome. Additional validation would be required to determine test characteristics in a larger patient population prospectively undergoing screening. Given the advantages of noninvasive screening modalities in terms of patient adherence and cost, one could envision future hybrid approaches especially among individuals with lower lifetime CRC risk (eg, MSH6 or PMS2 carriers), though test characteristics and positive and negative predictive values need to be confirmed before implementation clinically.

COLORECTAL CANCER SCREENING ADHERENCE IN LYNCH SYNDROME

The success of any screening program depends on uptake and adherence. Several studies have evaluated CRC screening adherence in Lynch syndrome and provide different perspectives based on patient population, health care system, and country. A study of participants of the Family Health Promotion Project who met Amsterdam II criteria reported that only 26% of participants were aware of colonoscopy intervals every 1 to 2 years and only 30% of endoscopists recommended these surveillance intervals.[36] A study of 74 patients with Lynch syndrome in an integrated health system in the US Pacific Northwest found that 96% of patients had colonoscopy recommendations documented in the electronic health record and that adherence to colonoscopy screening was high at 81.5%.[37] A multicenter study of 227 Lynch syndrome carriers in the United Kingdom reported 68% adherence defined as a colonoscopy interval of less than 27 months.[38] Results from the Spanish study of quality metrics and risk of neoplasia in Lynch syndrome noted that 50.7% and 78.5% of patients were adherent to 2- and 3-year intervals, respectively.[39] Effective systematic approaches to CRC screening for Lynch syndrome can facilitate adherence. Implementation of

> **Box 1**
> **Unanswered questions in CRC screening for Lynch syndrome**
>
> 1. Optimal screening approaches tailored to specific mismatch repair genes
> 2. Understanding of gene-specific CRC carcinogenesis pathways
> 3. Definition and impact of colonoscopy quality metrics in Lynch syndrome screening
> 4. Value of adjunct (eg, chromoendoscopy) and nonendoscopic screening modalities
> 5. Implementation strategies for systematic & coordinated care

guideline-based management in family cancer clinics in Australia led to increased adherence to colonoscopy screening among Lynch syndrome carriers.[40] Factors that predict colonoscopy use in Lynch syndrome include individuals' perceived cancer risks and physician recommendation.[41] Systematic implementation of Lynch syndrome management from genetic diagnosis to screening will enable the full realization of the benefits across all patients and populations.

UNANSWERED QUESTIONS AND FUTURE DIRECTIONS IN COLORECTAL CANCER SCREENING FOR LYNCH SYNDROME

Although much progress has been made in our understanding of outcomes of CRC screening for Lynch syndrome, several questions remain unanswered (**Box 1**). First, optimal screening intervals remain to be firmly established. Currently, international guidelines differ regarding gene-specific initiation age and surveillance intervals. Furthermore, appropriate age to stop screening for Lynch syndrome has not been established. Second, a better understanding of carcinogenesis in Lynch syndrome is needed to inform gene-specific screening approaches tailored to specific pathways. Third, a better definition of quality metrics and their impact on CRC screening for Lynch syndrome are needed. Current studies are conflicting about the role of colonoscopy quality on adenoma detection and CRC incidence. Fourth, the role of adjunctive and nonendoscopic screening modalities requires further exploration. Current data do not support an added benefit of chromoendoscopy, though additional studies are needed to confirm these results. Finally, implementation strategies for systematic and coordinated care for patients with Lynch syndrome are needed to ensure that the benefits of CRC screening are realized universally.

CLINICS CARE POINTS

- Initiation age and intervals for colorectal cancer screening in Lynch syndrome depend on affected gene based on recognition of gene-specific differences in lifetime neoplasia risks.
- Colorectal cancer screening decreases incidence and mortality, though recent prospective studies report persistently high lifetime colorectal cancer risk even with regular screening suggesting non-polypoid cancer pathways.
- Adjunctive screening tools such as chromoendoscopy have not been shown to definitively improve high-definition white light examinations in Lynch syndrome.

CONFLICTS OF INTEREST

None.

REFERENCES

1. Pan JY, Haile RW, Templeton A, et al. Worldwide Practice Patterns in Lynch Syndrome Diagnosis and Management, Based on Data From the International Mismatch Repair Consortium. Clin Gastroenterol Hepatol 2018;16:1901.e11.
2. National Comprehensive Cancer Network, Inc. 2021 Genetic/Familial High Risk Assessment: Colorectal v.1.2021. Available at: https://www.nccn.org/guidelines/guidelines-detail?category=2&id=1436. Accessed April 29, 2021.
3. Herzig DO, Buie WD, Weiser MR, et al. Clinical Practice Guidelines for the Surgical Treatment of Patients With Lynch Syndrome. Dis Colon Rectum 2017;60:137–43.
4. Rubenstein JH, Enns R, Heidelbaugh J, et al. American Gastroenterological Association Institute Guideline on the Diagnosis and Management of Lynch Syndrome. Gastroenterology 2015;149:777–82.
5. Syngal S, Brand RE, Church JM, et al. ACG clinical guideline: Genetic testing and management of hereditary gastrointestinal cancer syndromes. Am J Gastroenterol 2015;110:223–63 [quiz: 263].
6. Giardiello FM, Allen JI, Axilbund JE, et al. Guidelines on Genetic Evaluation and Management of Lynch Syndrome: A Consensus Statement by the US Multi-Society Task Force on Colorectal Cancer. Dis Colon Rectum 2014;57(8):1025–48.
7. Stoffel EM, Mangu PB, Gruber SB, et al. Hereditary Colorectal Cancer Syndromes: American Society of Clinical Oncology Clinical Practice Guideline Endorsement of the Familial Risk–Colorectal Cancer: European Society for Medical Oncology Clinical Practice Guidelines. J Clin Oncol 2015;33:209–17.
8. Balmaña J, Balaguer F, Cervantes A, et al. Familial risk-colorectal cancer: ESMO Clinical Practice Guidelines. Ann Oncol 2013;24 Suppl 6:vi73–80.
9. Seppälä TT, Latchford A, Negoi I, et al. European guidelines from the EHTG and ESCP for Lynch syndrome: an updated third edition of the Mallorca guidelines based on gene and gender. Br. J. Surg 2020. https://doi.org/10.1002/bjs.11902.
10. Monahan KJ, Bradshaw N, Dolwani S, et al. Guidelines for the management of hereditary colorectal cancer from the British Society of Gastroenterology (BSG)/Association of Coloproctology of Great Britain and Ireland (ACPGBI)/United Kingdom Cancer Genetics Group (UKCGG). Gut 2020;69:411–44.
11. Leggett, B, Dr Nicola Poplawski, "[Pachter],[NP]", Rosty C., Norton I, Dr Caroline W, Dr Aung Ko Win, Cancer Council Australia Colorectal Cancer Guidelines Working Party. Guidelines:Colorectal cancer/Lynch syndrome . In: Clinical practice guidelines for the prevention, early detection and management of colorectal cancer. Sydney (Australia): Cancer Council Australia. Available at: https://wiki.cancer.org.au/australiawiki/index.php?oldid=175314, Accessed April 29, 2021. https://wiki.cancer.org.au/australia/Guidelines:Colorectal_cancer.
12. Ishida H, Yamaguchi T, Tanakaya K, et al. Japanese Society for Cancer of the Colon and Rectum (JSCCR) Guidelines 2016 for the Clinical Practice of Hereditary Colorectal Cancer (Translated Version). J Anus Rectum Colon 2018;2:S1–51.
13. Järvinen HJ, Aarnio M, Mustonen H, et al. Controlled 15-year trial on screening for colorectal cancer in families with hereditary nonpolyposis colorectal cancer. Gastroenterology 2000;118:829–34.
14. Dove-Edwin I, Sasieni P, Adams J, et al. Prevention of colorectal cancer by colonoscopic surveillance in individuals with a family history of colorectal cancer: 16 year, prospective, follow-up study. BMJ 2005;331:1047.

15. Møller P, Seppälä TT, Bernstein I, et al. Cancer incidence and survival in Lynch syndrome patients receiving colonoscopic and gynaecological surveillance: first report from the prospective Lynch syndrome database. Gut 2017;66:464–72.
16. Dominguez-Valentin M, Sampson JR, Seppälä TT, et al. Cancer risks by gene, age, and gender in 6350 carriers of pathogenic mismatch repair variants: findings from the Prospective Lynch Syndrome Database. Genet Med 2020;22(1): 15–25.
17. Engel C, Vasen HF, Seppälä T, et al. No Difference in Colorectal Cancer Incidence or Stage at Detection by Colonoscopy Among 3 Countries With Different Lynch Syndrome Surveillance Policies. Gastroenterology 2018;155:1400.e2.
18. Ahadova A, Seppälä TT, Engel C, et al. The 'unnatural' history of colorectal cancer in Lynch syndrome: Lessons from colonoscopy surveillance. Int J Cancer 2021; 148(4):800–11.
19. Ahadova A, von Knebel Doeberitz M, Bläker H, et al. CTNNB1-mutant colorectal carcinomas with immediate invasive growth: a model of interval cancers in Lynch syndrome. Fam Cancer 2016;15:579–86.
20. Ahadova A, Gallon R, Gebert J, et al. Three molecular pathways model colorectal carcinogenesis in Lynch syndrome. Int J Cancer 2018;143:139–50.
21. Seppälä TT, Dominguez-Valentin M, Sampson JR, et al. Prospective observational data informs understanding and future management of Lynch syndrome: insights from the Prospective Lynch Syndrome Database (PLSD). Fam Cancer 2021;20(1):35–9.
22. Engel C, Ahadova A, Seppälä TT, et al. Associations of Pathogenic Variants in MLH1, MSH2, and MSH6 With Risk of Colorectal Adenomas and Tumors and With Somatic Mutations in Patients With Lynch Syndrome. Gastroenterology 2020;158:1326–33.
23. Goverde A, Eikenboom EL, Viskil EL, et al. Yield of Lynch Syndrome Surveillance for Patients With Pathogenic Variants in DNA Mismatch Repair Genes. Clin Gastroenterol Hepatol 2020;18:1112.e1.
24. Kastrinos F, Ingram MA, Silver ER, et al. Gene-Specific Variation in Colorectal Cancer Surveillance Strategies for Lynch Syndrome. Gastroenterology 2021. https://doi.org/10.1053/j.gastro.2021.04.010.
25. Kaminski MF, Robertson DJ, Senore C, et al. Optimizing the Quality of Colorectal Cancer Screening Worldwide. Gastroenterology 2020;158:404–17.
26. Rex DK, Schoenfeld PS, Cohen J, et al. Quality indicators for colonoscopy. Gastrointest Endosc 2015;81:31–53.
27. Lappalainen J, Holmström D, Lepistö A, et al. Incident colorectal cancer in Lynch syndrome is usually not preceded by compromised quality of colonoscopy. Scand J Gastroenterol 2019;54:1473–80.
28. Rivero-Sánchez L, Arnau-Collell C, Herrero J, et al. White-Light Endoscopy Is Adequate for Lynch Syndrome Surveillance in a Randomized and Noninferiority Study. Gastroenterology 2020;158:895.e1.
29. Latchford A. How Should Colonoscopy Surveillance in Lynch Syndrome Be Performed? Gastroenterology 2020;158:818–9.
30. van Leerdam ME, Roos VH, van Hooft JE, et al. Endoscopic management of Lynch syndrome and of familial risk of colorectal cancer: European Society of Gastrointestinal Endoscopy (ESGE) Guideline. Endoscopy 2019;51:1082–93.
31. Wang P, Berzin TM, Glissen Brown JR, et al. Real-time automatic detection system increases colonoscopic polyp and adenoma detection rates: a prospective randomised controlled study. Gut 2019;68:1813–9.

32. Rex DK, Boland CR, Dominitz JA, et al. Colorectal Cancer Screening: Recommendations for Physicians and Patients From the U.S. Multi-Society Task Force on Colorectal Cancer. Gastroenterology 2017;153:307–23.
33. Monahan KJ, Lincoln A, East JE, et al. Management strategies for the colonoscopic surveillance of people with Lynch syndrome during the COVID-19 pandemic. Gut 2020;2020:321993.
34. Ballester V, Taylor WR, Slettedahl SW, et al. Novel methylated DNA markers accurately discriminate Lynch syndrome associated colorectal neoplasia. Epigenomics 2020;12(24):2173–87.
35. Hitchins MP, Vogelaar IP, Brennan K, et al. Methylated SEPTIN9 plasma test for colorectal cancer detection may be applicable to Lynch syndrome. BMJ Open Gastroenterol 2019;6:e000299.
36. Patel SG, Ahnen DJ, Kinney AY, et al. Knowledge and Uptake of Genetic Counseling and Colonoscopic Screening Among Individuals at Increased Risk for Lynch Syndrome and their Endoscopists from the Family Health Promotion Project. Am J Gastroenterol 2016;111:285–93.
37. Mittendorf KF, Hunter JE, Schneider JL, et al. Recommended care and care adherence following a diagnosis of Lynch syndrome: a mixed-methods study. Hered Cancer Clin Pract 2019;17:31.
38. Newton K, Green K, Lalloo F, et al. Colonoscopy screening compliance and outcomes in patients with Lynch syndrome. Colorectal Dis 2015;17:38–46.
39. Sánchez A, Roos VH, Navarro M, et al. Quality of Colonoscopy Is Associated With Adenoma Detection and Postcolonoscopy Colorectal Cancer Prevention in Lynch Syndrome. Clin. Gastroenterol. Hepatol. Off. Clin. Pract. J. Am. Gastroenterol. Assoc. 2020. https://doi.org/10.1016/j.cgh.2020.11.002.
40. Meiser B, Kaur R, Kirk J, et al. Evaluation of implementation of risk management guidelines for carriers of pathogenic variants in mismatch repair genes: a nationwide audit of familial cancer clinics. Fam Cancer 2020;19:337–46.
41. Hadley DW, Eliezer D, Addissie Y, et al. Uptake and predictors of colonoscopy use in family members not participating in cascade genetic testing for Lynch syndrome. Sci Rep 2020;10:15959.

Lynch Syndrome-Associated Cancers Beyond Colorectal Cancer

Leah H. Biller, MD[a,b,c], Siobhan A. Creedon, RN, NP[a],
Margaret Klehm, RN, MPH, MSN, FNP[a],
Matthew B. Yurgelun, MD[a,b,c],*

KEYWORDS

• HNPCC • Extra-colonic • Screening

KEY POINTS

- Lynch syndrome (LS) predisposes to a wide array of malignancies beyond colorectal cancer (CRC). Such extracolonic malignancies account for a disproportionate degree of mortality in individuals with LS.
- Specific LS gene, sex, age, and family history of individual LS-associated malignancies can help identify subsets of individuals with LS who may be at particular risk for various extracolonic cancers. Free online tools such as www.PLSD.eu and www.ASK2ME.org can help clinicians understand an individual LS carrier's future risk of specific malignancies, accounting for such personalized risk factors.
- There are limited data on the efficacy of surveillance for most extracolonic cancers in LS. We advocate for clinicians to weigh the potential risks and benefits of such surveillance in each individual LS carrier, including personalized risk factors, when deciding which LS carriers should undergo specific forms of extracolonic cancer surveillance.

INTRODUCTION

Lynch syndrome (LS) is a common, autosomal dominant inherited form of cancer predisposition defined by the presence of pathogenic germline variants (PGVs) in one of the DNA mismatch repair (MMR) genes (*MLH1*, *MSH2*, *MSH6*, or *PMS2*) or *EPCAM*.[1,2] Although LS (formerly known as hereditary nonpolyposis colorectal cancer (CRC), or HNPCC) has been classically linked to its high lifetime risk of CRC, individuals with LS are also at significantly increased risk of a wide variety of other malignancies involving the gastrointestinal, gynecologic, urinary tracts, and other organ systems (**Table 1**).[1,2] This article will review the spectrum of extracolonic manifestations in

[a] Dana-Farber Cancer Institute, 450 Brookline Avenue, Boston, MA 02215, USA; [b] Harvard Medical School, Boston, MA 02215, USA; [c] Brigham & Women's Hospital, Boston, MA 02215, USA
* Corresponding author. Dana-Farber Cancer Institute, 450 Brookline Avenue, Dana 1126, Boston, MA 02215.
E-mail address: matthew_yurgelun@dfci.harvard.edu

Gastrointest Endoscopy Clin N Am 32 (2022) 75–93
https://doi.org/10.1016/j.giec.2021.08.002
1052-5157/22/© 2021 Elsevier Inc. All rights reserved.

Table 1
Gene-specific cumulative risks (to age 75 y) of various Lynch syndrome-associate extracolonic malignancies based on data from the Prospective Lynch Syndrome Database[4,17,69]

Cancer Type	MLH1	MSH2[a]	MSH6	PMS2
Endometrial	37%	49%	41%	13%
Ovarian	11%	17%	11%	3%
Gastric	7%	8%	5%	b
Duodenum	7%	2%	b	b
Pancreatic	6%	<1%	1%	b
Biliary	4%	2%	b	b
Upper Urinary Tract	4%–5%	18%–19%	2%–6%	4%
Bladder	5%–7%	8%–13%	1%–8%	b
Prostate	14%	24%	9%	5%
Brain	1%–2%	3%–8%	1%–2%	b
Osteosarcoma	0.7%	4.2%	b	1.6%

[a] Note that there are minimal data on cancer risks for individuals with *EPCAM*-associated Lynch syndrome, though they are typically assumed to have risks similar to *MSH2*-associated Lynch syndrome.
[b] PLSD data reported 0% cumulative incidence; the authors of this article do not interpret this to mean that there is no risk, but rather that the risk may not be increased than the general population.

individuals with LS, patient-specific factors that may predispose LS carriers to specific malignancies, and evidence-based strategies for surveillance and risk-reduction (**Table 2**). Although there is a rapidly growing body of literature on gene-specific manifestations for individuals with *MLH1*-, *MSH2*-, *MSH6*-, and *PMS2*-associated LS, we acknowledge that there remains a marked lack of data on gene-specific considerations for individuals with *EPCAM*-associated LS, due to the relative rarity of this subset. Because germline deletions involving *EPCAM* induce epigenetic silencing of *MSH2*,[3] it has typically been assumed that the phenotype of *EPCAM*-associated LS mirrors that of *MSH2*-associated LS, though this has not been robustly studied. Until further data are available, we support the practice of individuals with *EPCAM*-associated LS being managed similarly to *MSH2*-associated LS.

LYNCH SYNDROME-ASSOCIATED GYNECOLOGIC CANCERS

Endometrial adenocarcinoma and epithelial ovarian adenocarcinoma, typically with endometrioid-type histologies, are hallmark malignancies associated with LS. Thus, gynecologic cancer risk reduction is an important component of managing female LS carriers. Like other LS-associated malignancies, there are gene-specific differences in the risks of endometrial and ovarian cancers. Based on the data from the multinational Prospective Lynch Syndrome Database (PLSD), female *MLH1*, *MSH2*, and *MSH6* PGV carriers have 37.0%, 48.9%, and 41.1% cumulative risk of endometrial cancer by age 75, respectively, and 11.0%, 17.4%, and 10.8% cumulative risk of ovarian cancer by age 75, respectively.[4] By contrast, female *PMS2* PGV carriers only have a 12.8% risk of endometrial cancer by age 75 and may have no significantly increased risk of ovarian cancer than the general population.[4,5] Beyond gene-specific differences, family history may also help with risk stratification, as one recent study observed that female LS carriers had a roughly 1.4-fold increased likelihood of

Table 2
Authors' recommendations for extracolonic cancer surveillance and risk reduction in individuals with Lynch syndrome

Cancer type	MLH1 PGVs	MSH2 PGVs[a]	MSH6 PGVs	PMS2 PGVs	Comments
Endometrial	• Total hysterectomy reduces cancer incidence; usually not needed before age 40 • Consider annual endometrial biopsy and transvaginal ultrasound starting age 30–35				• Encourage shared decision-making on the optimal timing of surgery
Ovarian	• Salpingo-oopherectomy reduces cancer incidence; usually not needed before age 40 • Consider annual transvaginal ultrasound starting age 30–35 • CA125 not recommended			May not derive benefit from risk-reducing salpingo-oophrectomy	• Encourage shared decision-making on the optimal timing of surgery • Counsel regarding hormone replacement therapy and lifestyle modifications to slow bone loss after oophorectomy and consideration of DXA scan monitoring
Gastric	• EGD every 3–5 y beginning age 30–40, or more frequently based on risk factors; assess for histologic risk factors (eg, H. pylori) at baseline			Baseline EGD between age 30–40 with biopsy for H. pylori and other histologic risk factors	• Risk factors include a family history of gastric cancer, H. pylori, intestinal metaplasia, autoimmune gastritis, Asian ancestry
Small bowel	• Screen duodenum with EGD • VCE not routinely recommended				• Duodenum is the most common site of small bowel cancer • Risk factors include MLH1 PGVs, MSH2

(continued on next page)

Table 2
(continued)

Cancer type	MLH1 PGVs	MSH2 PGVs[a]	MSH6 PGVs	PMS2 PGVs	Comments
					PGVs, and family history
Pancreatic	• Annual MRCP or EUS beginning at age 50, only for those with a family history of pancreatic cancer			Not routinely recommended	
Biliary	• Not routinely recommended				
Urinary tract	Not routinely recommended, unless strong family history (then consider annual urinalysis)	Consider annual urinalysis, especially if there is a family history	Not routinely recommended, unless strong family history (then consider annual urinalysis)	Not routinely recommended	
Prostate	• Consider annual PSA beginning age 40			Benefit is unknown	
Skin	• Annual full-body skin examination				
Breast (female)	• Age-appropriate population-based mammography and clinical breast examination, unless family history warrants more aggressive surveillance				

[a] Note that there are minimal data on cancer risks for individuals with *EPCAM*-associated Lynch syndrome, though they are typically assumed to have risks similar *MSH2*-associated Lynch syndrome; we recommend that *EPCAM*-associated Lynch syndrome be managed the same as *MSH2*-associated Lynch syndrome, pending updated data.

endometrial cancer for each first-and/or second-degree relative with endometrial cancer.[6]

Risk-reducing total hysterectomy (TH) and bilateral salpingo-oophorectomy (BSO) have long been the mainstay of endometrial and ovarian cancer risk-reduction in female LS carriers. The landmark study[7] demonstrating the efficacy of risk-reducing gynecologic surgery in LS examined 315 female LS carriers and observed 0 endometrial cancers in those who had undergone risk-reducing TH versus 0.045 cases/woman-year (69 cases among 210 participants over an average 7.4 years follow-up) in those who had not. Similarly, there were no ovarian cancers diagnosed among the 47 female LS carriers who had undergone risk-reducing BSO versus 0.005 cases per woman-year among those who had (12 cases among 223 participants over an average 10.6 years follow-up).

Risk-reducing gynecologic surgery is not without risk or consequence, however. For premenopausal female LS carriers who undergo BSO, the abrupt withdrawal of hormones can lead to adverse effects including vasomotor symptoms, sexual dysfunction, heart disease, bone loss, and cognitive changes over both the short- and long-term. Much of the data about symptoms and medical consequences from risk-reducing BSO come from the literature on female *BRCA1* and *BRCA2* PGV carriers undergoing such surgery, though these lessons likely apply to LS carriers as well. Multiple such studies have demonstrated significant declines in bone mineral density in the first 2 years after risk-reducing BSO in premenopausal women with inherited ovarian cancer risk.[8,9] Data have also shown that estrogen-based hormone replacement therapy can significantly mitigate bone loss in this setting,[8,9] use of which is supported by various clinical practice guidelines until the age of expected natural menopause,[10,11] though uptake seems to be variable.[12]

For many female LS carriers, the question of the optimal timing of risk-reducing TH/BSO is particularly difficult, given these hormonal considerations as well as the implications for childbearing. Data from the *PLSD*[13] demonstrated only a 2% cumulative endometrial cancer risk from age 25 to 40 for female *MLH1*, *MSH2*, and *MSH6* PGV carriers, but an 11% to 16% risk for these carriers from ages 40 to 50. Risks of ovarian cancer are likewise higher in the 40 to 50 year age range for *MLH1* and *MSH2* PGV carriers than the 25 to 40 year age range.[13] However, even for individuals with LS who are diagnosed with gynecologic cancer, the prognosis is often favorable, with 89% 5- and 10-year survival for LS-associated endometrial cancer and 84% 5- and 10-year survival for LS-associated ovarian cancer.[4] PLSD data[13] have suggested that risk-reducing TH at age 40 will prevent endometrial cancer in 13%, 16%, and 11% of female *MLH1*, *MSH2*, and *MSH6* PGV carriers, respectively, but with only 1%, 2%, and 1% reduction in mortality, respectively. Risk-reducing BSO at age 40 in this study[13] would have prevented death in 1% of *MLH1* and *MSH2* female PGV carriers, but with no appreciable preventive impact for *MSH6* PGV carriers. Given the exceedingly low incidence of premenopausal endometrial and ovarian cancer, these data[13] demonstrated no preventative benefit to risk-reducing TH/BSO at age 40 for female *PMS2* PGV carriers, because nearly all of the endometrial cancer diagnoses in these carriers occurred after age 50.

Our approach to gynecologic cancer risk-reduction includes emphasis on the importance of shared decision-making with female LS carriers regarding TH/BSO, particularly with regards to the timing of surgery. Risk-reducing TH/BSO is typically not needed before age 40 for female LS carriers, though could be considered in individual circumstances based on patient preference or particular risks for early-onset gynecologic malignancy (eg, family history of young-onset gynecologic cancer). At and after age 40, TH/BSO is an effective means of gynecologic cancer prevention for female *MLH1*, *MSH2*, and *MSH6* PGV carriers, though the precise age at which to pursue risk-reducing surgery should factor in patient preference regarding risk tolerance, lifestyle/childbearing plans, and symptomatic hormonal considerations. To facilitate such shared decision-making, we encourage clinicians to use free online tools that demonstrate age-, gene-, and sex-specific short- and long-term risks of specific cancers for LS carriers, including www.plsd.eu and www.ASK2ME.org. There are no data to suggest that female *PMS2* PGV carriers derive significant preventative benefit from risk-reducing BSO.

For female LS carriers who pursue risk-reducing BSO, especially before menopause, we recommend the consideration of obtaining a dual-energy x-ray absorptiometry (DXA) scan 1 to 2 years after BSO. Female LS carriers should be advised that hormone replacement therapy can help mitigate bone loss and other menopausal symptoms, and that there are no LS-related contraindications to such treatment. We also recommend counseling regarding lifestyle modifications to slow further bone loss, including weight-bearing exercise and supplementation with vitamin D3 and calcium.

Although there are no robust data demonstrating the efficacy of gynecologic cancer screening in female LS carriers, we agree with current recommendations from the National Comprehensive Cancer Network (NCCN) NCCN and others to consider annual transvaginal ultrasound and endometrial biopsy on an annual basis at age 30 to 35 until the time of risk-reducing surgery. We do not routinely perform CA-125 screening in female LS carriers.

LYNCH SYNDROME-ASSOCIATED GASTROINTESTINAL CANCERS
Gastric Cancer

In the original reports of Family G, widely recognized as being the first major published the description of what is now known as LS, gastric cancer was recognized as one of the most common malignancies in the family.[14–16] Interestingly, however, more recent analyses of Family G[15] have shown gastric cancer to have become notably less common in recent generations, paralleling recent epidemiologic trends in the general population.[14] In spite of this apparent decrease in incidence, however, gastric cancer remains a significant threat to individuals with LS, with 72% 5-year survival (lower than that seen with LS-associated colon, rectal, endometrial, ovarian, urinary tract, and small bowel cancers) in recent data from the PLSD.[4] Data from the PLSD have also demonstrated a cumulative incidence of gastric cancer to age 75 of 7.1%, 7.7%, and 5.3% for LS carriers with *MLH1*, *MSH2*, and *MSH6* PGVs, respectively.[17] By contrast, data from the PLSD and others have demonstrated that LS carriers with *PMS2* PGVs may have no significantly increased risk gastric cancer than the general population.[5,17]

Recent data from a large laboratory-based cohort of more than 3800 individuals with LS demonstrated that male sex (odds ratio [OR] >2.8 than females)[6,18] is a significant risk factor for LS-associated gastric cancer and also confirmed the finding that individuals with *MLH1* (OR: 6.5) and *MSH2* (OR: 5.2) PGVs are significantly more likely to develop gastric cancer than those with *MSH6* or *PMS2* PGVs. Controlling for age-, gene-, and sex-specific considerations, these data also demonstrated that familial burden (the number of affected first- and second-degree relatives) of gastric cancer is independently associated with an LS carrier's own likelihood of developing gastric cancer, with a near doubling of one's likelihood of gastric cancer for each affected relative.[6]

Histologic findings at the time of esophagogastroduodenoscopy (EGD) can also identify LS carriers with particularly increased risks of gastric cancer. One single-site study of 255 individuals with LS identified 7 cases of gastric cancer, 6 (86%) of whom had intestinal metaplasia of the gastric mucosa and 5 (71%) of whom had autoimmune gastritis on histology.[19] Interestingly, none of the 7 cases had evidence of *Helicobacter pylori* infection.[19] By contrast, a recent study of Japanese patients with LS found *H. pylori* in 6 of 10 cases of resected gastric cancer and also calculated a cumulative 5.5% incidence of gastric cancer by age 50 (vs 0%–0.8% cumulative incidence by age 50 in the PLSD[17]), supporting the theory that Asian individuals with LS may have higher risks of gastric cancer than non–Asian individuals.[20] Another multicenter study[21] of 172 LS carriers with at least one prior EGD observed that LS carriers with *H. pylori* infection were significantly more likely to have gastric cancer or premalignant gastric findings on EGD than those who were *H. pylori* negative.

In spite of this growing knowledge on patient-specific risk factors for LS-associated gastric cancer, there has remained a striking paucity of data on the efficacy of gastric cancer surveillance in LS up until recently. One recent report from the German Consortium for Familial Intestinal Cancer suggested an important downstaging effect to regular EGD surveillance.[22] In this study, 47 LS carriers were diagnosed with gastric cancer from among 1128 such individuals undergoing EGD, and 78% of gastric cancers diagnosed within 30 months of a prior EGD were stage I malignancies, versus only 23% of those diagnosed greater than 30 months from their most recent EGD.[22] A separate single-institution study[23] likewise reported 6 gastric cancers from among 217 LS carriers undergoing EGD, 3 of which were detected in the setting of asymptomatic surveillance.

For surveillance and risk reduction of LS-related gastric cancer, we recommend at least a one-time baseline EGD for individuals with LS, including biopsy of the gastric mucosa for *H. pylori* (with appropriate therapy and follow-up to confirm eradication in those found to test positive) and intestinal metaplasia. The optimal age at which to begin EGD-based surveillance is not well-defined, but we recommend that baseline EGD takes place between ages 30 and 40. For LS carriers with *MLH1*, *MSH2*, or *MSH6* PGVs, we recommend the continuation of surveillance EGDs every 3 to 5 years, with more frequent EGDs for individuals with additional risk factors (eg, family history of gastric cancer, prior *H. pylori* infection, intestinal metaplasia, autoimmune gastritis, and/or Asian ancestry).

Small Bowel Cancer

Small bowel carcinomas (SBCs), including those of the duodenum, jejunum, and ileum, are rare malignancies of the gastrointestinal tract, with an estimated 11,300 new cases in the United States in 2021.[24] Among LS carriers, however, rates of SBC are markedly increased, with an estimated 100-fold increased risk and a cumulative lifetime of roughly 4%.[25,26] In LS carriers who develop SBCs, it is also frequently the first cancer to develop.[27] Understanding which individuals with LS are at highest risk for developing SBCs is therefore important, especially because this is an uncommon cancer among the general population with limited effective screening modalities and with inferior survival than more common LS-associated malignancies (eg, colon, endometrial, and ovarian cancers).[4]

A study of 2118 LS carriers from the Dutch and German national LS registries identified male sex to be significantly associated with SBC risk in LS carriers (hazard ratio 2.52).[26] This and other studies have also observed that LS carriers with *MLH1* and *MSH2* PGVs are at higher risk of SBCs (6.5% and 2.0% cumulative incidence of duodenal cancer to age 75, respectively, in the PLSD[17]) versus those with *MSH6*[17,26,28] and *PMS2* PGVs.[17] In addition to these gene- and sex-specific differences in SBC risk, a recent analysis of 3828 LS carriers additionally identified familial burden of SBCs as being independently and incrementally associated with LS carriers' likelihood of SBCs, with more than a 3-fold increased likelihood of SBCs for each affected first- and/or second-degree relative.[6]

As the most common site of SBCs among LS carriers is the duodenum,[27,29,30] which can be visualized during routine EGD, multiple professional society guidelines[10,31,32] include recommendations for EGD to at least be considered for both gastric and duodenal cancer surveillance in LS carriers, though data regarding the efficacy of such SBC screening are limited. In a single-site retrospective analysis[23] of 217 LS carriers undergoing EGD, 4 duodenal adenocarcinomas were identified, 2 of which were within 2 years from the last EGD, and 4 duodenal adenomas were identified. In this analysis,[23] the presence of a duodenal adenoma was significantly associated with the development of an upper GI malignancy on univariable analysis. An abstract[33] describing 125 SBCs from 112 LS carriers within the German Consortium for Intestinal Cancer database found that LS carriers with duodenal cancer were significantly more likely to be diagnosed with stage I–II disease if they were undergoing EGD surveillance versus those diagnosed based on symptoms, whereas EGD surveillance was not associated with earlier stages at diagnosis for those with jejunal/ileal cancers.

There are likewise relatively scant data about whether the visualization of the more distal small bowel is useful for LS-associated SBC surveillance. A prospective study of 200 asymptomatic LS carriers undergoing video capsule endoscopy (VCE) detected 2 small bowel neoplasms (duodenal adenocarcinoma and a duodenal adenoma), but also presumably missed a duodenal adenocarcinoma detected 7 months after negative VCE.[34] After 2 years, 155 of the original 200 participants underwent a second VCE and, despite 17 (11%) individuals having suspicious VCE findings, no small bowel neoplasms were identified on follow-up evaluation by EGD or balloon-assisted enteroscopy.[35] Another study of 135 LS carriers undergoing VCE identified 3 small bowel adenomas and 3 SBCs (4.6% of participants) at baseline VCE, with another 2 small bowel adenomas and 2 SBCs identified among 87 participants (4.6%) who underwent repeat VCE at 2 years' follow-up (all of whom had had normal findings at baseline).[36] As these studies were conducted among asymptomatic LS carriers without stratification for higher risk clinical features (males, those with *MLH1* or *MSH2* PGVs, and/or those with family histories of SBCs), it is possible that the targeted screening of LS individuals with some of these specific SBC risk factors would improve the efficacy of such surveillance.

For SBC surveillance, we recommend thorough evaluation of the duodenum at the time of surveillance EGD for individuals with LS. Given the low incidence of distal SBCs and a paucity of data on VCE efficacy, we do not recommend routine VCE surveillance for most individuals with LS, though it can be considered on an individual basis for those with specific features that may indicate a particularly elevated risk of SBCs (eg, family history of SBCs and *MLH1* or *MSH2* PGVs).

Pancreatic and Biliary Cancers

Studies have found that 0.2%–3.6% of individuals diagnosed with pancreatic cancer[37–40] have LS, and data from the PLSD[17] have calculated a cumulative pancreatic cancer incidence by age 75 of 6.2%, 0.5%, and 1.4% for those with *MLH1*, *MSH2*, and *MSH6* PGVs, respectively (note that LS carriers with *PMS2* PGVs may not have a significantly increased risk of pancreatic cancer than the general population). Thus, pancreatic cancer is an uncommon manifestation of LS, but nonetheless an important one due to its particularly poor prognosis. Data from the PLSD[4] have demonstrated a 29% 5-year survival for LS carriers with pancreatic cancer, making it one of the deadliest LS-associated malignancies.

Cancer of the biliary tree (including intra- and extrahepatic cholangiocarcinomas, gallbladder cancers, and ampullary cancers) are likewise uncommon manifestations of LS. Data from the PLSD have shown a cumulative 3.7% and 1.7% incidence of bile duct and gallbladder cancers for those with *MLH1* and *MSH2* PGVs, respectively, with no apparent increased risk of biliary tract cancers in those with *MSH6* and *PMS2* PGVs, and with a 5-year survival of 42%.[4,17]

In spite of their potential lethality, there are limited data on how to risk-stratify individuals with LS to better understand which may be at particular risk for pancreatic and biliary cancers, beyond the aforementioned gene-specific considerations. One recent analysis demonstrated that increasing age and family history are independently associated with the likelihood of pancreaticobiliary cancers in LS carriers, with more than a 2-fold increased likelihood of pancreaticobiliary cancer per affected first- and/or second-degree relative.[6]

There has been a rapidly growing amount of data on surveillance for pancreatic cancer using upper endoscopic ultrasound (EUS) and magnetic resonance cholangiopancreatography (MRCP) in individuals with increased pancreatic cancer risk due to various genetic syndromes, including LS. Prospective data from the Cancer of the Pancreas Screening (CAPS) studies[41] calculated a 1.6% per year rate of neoplastic progression among 354 high-risk individuals undergoing MRCP and/or EUS-guided surveillance, including 14 pancreatic cancers and 10 individuals with high-grade precursor lesions (intraductal papillary mucinous neoplasms with high-grade dysplasia or pancreatic intraepithelial neoplasia-3). Encouragingly, 9 of the 10 screen-detected pancreatic cancers were resectable at diagnosis (the other 4 cancers were diagnosed in individuals who had been lost to follow-up). Three-year overall survival was 85% for individuals with screen-detected pancreatic cancer and 100% for those with high-grade precursor lesions, suggesting clinical benefit for high-risk individuals undergoing pancreatic cancer surveillance. None of the individuals in this study who were diagnosed with pancreatic cancer or high-grade precursor lesions, however, had a diagnosis of LS, so the efficacy of surveillance in this population remains undefined.

Based on such encouraging data, clinical practice guidelines from the NCCN[42] and the International CAPS consortium[43] endorse annual pancreatic cancer screening for high-risk individuals, including those with *MLH1*, *MSH2*, or *MSH6* PGVs who have a close family history of pancreatic cancer, beginning at age 50 to 55 or 10 years younger than the youngest affected relative.

Our approach to pancreatic cancer surveillance in LS is to offer annual surveillance (with EUS, MRCP, or alternating between the 2 modalities) for high-risk subsets of individuals with LS, beginning at age 50 or 10 years younger than the youngest diagnosis in the family. We define high-risk LS carriers as being those with *MLH1*, *MSH2*, or *MSH6* PGVs who have one or more first- and/or second-degree relatives from the same side of the family that has LS. For individuals with *PMS2*-associated LS, however, there may not be a statistically increased risk of pancreatic cancer and the benefits of surveillance are unclear, even if there is a family history of pancreatic cancer. As part of the counseling about the risks and uncertainties about pancreatic cancer surveillance in LS, we also strongly encourage providers to discuss with patients with LS the high rate (>38%) of detecting cystic lesions in the pancreas, the vast majority of which are low risk for malignancy and do not require intervention.[44] There are no data supporting any form of routine biliary tract cancer surveillance in LS, though attention to the ampulla should be given at the time of routine EGD, especially for those with family histories of pancreaticobiliary cancer.

LYNCH SYNDROME-ASSOCIATED GENITOURINARY CANCERS
Urothelial Cancer

Individuals with LS are at increased risk of transitional cell carcinoma of the urothelial tract, including the ureter/renal pelvis, bladder, and urethra. One recent analysis demonstrated that such urinary tract cancers (UTCs) are the second- and fourth-most common type of malignancies in male and female LS carriers, respectively, after colorectal, endometrial, and ovarian cancers.[45] Data from the PLSD have shown that individuals with LS-associated UTCs have 81% to 86% and 67% to 68% 5- and 10-year survival rates, respectively.[4]

Data have consistently shown that individuals with *MSH2* PGVs are at a particularly increased risk of UTCs than other LS carriers (OR: ~4.0) for reasons that are unclear.[4,6,25,45–48] Analyses from the PLSD[4] have calculated a cumulative 18.7% and 17.6% incidence of ureter and "kidney" cancer (see discussion on "kidney" cancer below) by age 75 for female and male *MSH2* PGV carriers, respectively, than 1.7% to 5.5% for other LS PGV carriers. Likewise, they found a cumulative 7.9% and 12.8% incidence of bladder cancer by age 75 for female and male *MSH2* PGV carriers.[4]

Beyond gene-specific factors, other analyses have shown increasing age (OR: 2.4 per decade), male sex (OR: 1.9), and familial burden of UTCs (OR: 2.7 per affected first-/second-degree relative) to be significantly and independently associated with UTC in LS carriers.[6,45] Individuals with LS-associated UTC may be particularly likely to develop metachronous UTC, as demonstrated by a Danish national registry study which found that 12.4% of individuals with LS-associated UTC developed an additional subsequent urothelial carcinoma.[48] Although smoking is a clear risk factor for UTC in the general population, it is unclear whether smoking or other behavioral factors are associated with risks of LS-associated UTC.

Although UTCs are relatively common manifestations of LS, particularly for individuals with *MSH2* PGVs, evidence-based approaches to surveillance risk-reduction are lacking. One large study[49] from the National Danish Hereditary Nonpolyposis Colorectal Cancer Register evaluating more than 1800 urine cytology specimens from nearly 1000 individuals with LS found that only 0.11% of specimens diagnosed asymptomatic UTC, with 11-times more false positives than true positives. This study[49] also described multiple cases of LS carriers diagnosed with UTC within 3 years of normal urine cytology. Overall, these data strongly suggest that urine cytology surveillance in asymptomatic LS carriers has particularly poor sensitivity and specificity.

Based on these data, we do not recommend routine UTC surveillance in all asymptomatic individuals with LS. We do recommend that LS carriers be counseled about the risk of UTCs and the need for prompt evaluation if hematuria develops. For LS carriers with particularly high risks of UTC (eg, those with *MSH2* PGVs and/or a significant family history of UTC), we discuss the paucity of data and the uncertainties about asymptomatic surveillance, including risks of "false positives," and will offer annual urinalysis to screen for microscopic hematuria for individuals who agree to such surveillance in spite of these uncertainties. Given the particular risk of metachronous UTCs in LS, we recommend the consideration of annual cystoscopic evaluation for LS carriers with a prior personal history of UTC.

Although registry data have classically included "kidney cancer" among the spectrum of LS-associated malignancies, there is suspicion that most such cancers actually represent urothelial malignancies of the renal pelvis rather than renal cell carcinomas.[45,50] One recent study of paired germline and molecular testing across a wide spectrum of malignancies found that only 2.4% of renal cell carcinoma specimens had microsatellite instability (MSI), none of whom had LS on germline testing.[51] As such, we do not recommend routine imaging (eg, ultrasound, CT, or MRI) of the kidneys for LS-related surveillance, given the absence of data on such screening as well as the dubious link between LS and renal cell carcinoma risk.

Prostate Cancer

Multiple studies have demonstrated that male carriers of *MLH1*, *MSH2*, and *MSH6* PGVs have modestly increased risks of prostate cancer, than the general population, with a median age at diagnosis in the mid-60s.[52–56] The PLSD[4] has reported a cumulative prostate cancer incidence of 13.8%, 23.8%, and 8.9% for *MLH1*, *MSH2*, and *MSH6* PGV carriers, respectively, though the confidence intervals for these risks overlap with the estimated 11.6% cumulative lifetime risk for the general population.[10] It is unknown whether or not LS-associated prostate cancer has a differential prognosis versus sporadic prostate cancer, as is seen with *BRCA1/2*-associated prostate cancer, whereby outcomes are significantly worse in the setting of PGVs.[54] To help understand the optimal approach to prostate cancer surveillance in asymptomatic men with LS, the Identification of Men with a genetic predisposition to the ProstAte Cancer (IMPACT) study[57] has been expanded to include annual PSA screening in male ages 40 to 69 with *MLH1*, *MSH2*, or *MSH6* PGVs, in addition to *BRCA1* and *BRCA2* PGVs.

Pending results from this study, we recommend that men with *MLH1*-, *MSH2*-, and *MSH6*-associated LS consider annual PSA-based prostate cancer surveillance beginning at age 40.

OTHER LYNCH SYNDROME-ASSOCIATED MALIGNANCIES
Cutaneous Neoplasms

In the 1960s, E.G. Muir and Douglas Torre individually reported cutaneous sebaceous neoplasia associated with gastrointestinal malignancy which later came to be known as Muir–Torre syndrome (MTS).[58,59] MTS is now recognized as a subset of LS, with cutaneous neoplasms including sebaceous adenomas, sebaceous carcinomas, keratoacanthomas, and sebaceous epitheliomas occurring in roughly 9% of individuals with LS.[60] Data have shown that LS carriers with *MSH2* PGVs are particularly at risk for these cutaneous neoplasms, and they seem to cluster in specific LS families.[6] A recent study demonstrated that LS carriers have more than a 7-fold increased likelihood of cutaneous sebaceous neoplasms for each first- and second-degree relative with a sebaceous neoplasm.[6] Another recent analysis[61] concluded that cutaneous squamous cell carcinomas, which are not typically part of the MTS spectrum of skin neoplasms, may also be LS-associated malignancies, particularly in individuals with histories of other cutaneous neoplasia.

Although there are no data on the risks and benefits of routine dermatologic surveillance in LS, we recommend full-body skin examinations for all individuals with LS, particularly those with a family history of LS-associated cutaneous neoplasia. We also recommend routine counseling on skin cancer prevention, including use of sunblock and avoidance of tanning bed usage and other forms of UV radiation.

Brain Malignancies

In 1959, surgeon Jacques Turcot described a link between CRC and brain malignancy, which later became known as Turcot syndrome.[62] It was, eventually, recognized that some cases of Turcot syndrome were attributable to germline *APC* PGVs and are thus actually a subset of familial adenomatous polyposis, whereas other cases were subsets of what is now known as LS.[63] Thus, to avoid confusion, we recommend against the use of the term "Turcot syndrome."

In spite of this longstanding recognition, however, there remains a paucity of data on the clinical phenotype of LS carriers with brain malignancies. One study examining data from the National Danish Hereditary Nonpolyposis Colorectal Cancer Register identified 47 primary brain neoplasms in 42 (14%) of 288 families examined.[64] Thirty-four of the brain neoplasms were diagnosed in individuals known to be mono-allelic carriers of LS PGVs (or first-degree relatives of known carriers), including 26 from families with *MSH2* PGVs, including 9 with the c.942+3A>T *MSH2* variant. Glioblastomas were the most common histology of primary brain neoplasm diagnosed (56% of all cases) in LS carriers in this study, though astrocytomas and oligodendrogliomas were also observed. The authors calculated a cumulative risk of developing a primary brain neoplasm by age 70 years of 0.5%, 2.5%, and 0.8% for LS carriers with *MLH1*, *MSH2*, and *MSH6* PGVs, respectively.

Data from a study[65] estimating the nationwide prevalence of LS in the country of Iceland identified the c.1754T>C (p.Leu585Pro) *MSH6* PGV as a common Icelandic founder variant (estimated Icelandic population prevalence 0.08%) associated with a roughly 12% cumulative 10.7% and 13.4% lifetime incidence of gliomas for female and male carriers, respectively (OR: 8.9 vs the general population).

The PLSD investigators[4] have calculated the cumulative incidence of brain malignancies to age 75 as being the highest for *MSH2* PGV carriers (2.9% for females and 7.7% for males), with less than 2% cumulative incidence for *MLH1* and *MSH6* PGV carriers. LS carriers with *PMS2* PGVs seem to have no increased risk of brain malignancies,[4,5] though brain malignancies are a significant manifestation of constitutional mismatch repair deficiency (CMMR-D), which occurs when an individual inherits biallelic PGVs in the same MMR gene (most commonly biallelic *PMS2* PGVs).[66]

Given the relative rarity of brain malignancies in LS as well as the absence of effective strategies for early detection, we do not recommend routine surveillance in asymptomatic LS carriers.

Sarcomas

Sarcomas are a rare and diverse collection of malignancies that, until recently, had not been linked to LS. Multi-institutional data from 7 different cancer genetics programs presented as an abstract in 2015, however, began to suggest that sarcomas may be rare LS-associated malignancies.[67] This abstract reported on data from 958 families with known LS, 55 (5.7%) of which included ≥1 "possible" or "likely" sarcoma diagnosis in 58 different individuals. The mean age of sarcoma diagnosis in this study was 47.1 years (range 4–87 years) with 62% of sarcomas being diagnosed in families with *MSH2/EPCAM* PGVs and 21% diagnosed in LS families with *MLH1* PGVs.

Data from a single-institution analysis that systematically assessed MSI status and germline LS status across more than 15,000 patients with cancer (including >50 types of malignancies) found high-level MSI (MSI-H) in 45 (5.7%) of 785 soft tissue sarcomas, 2 (0.3%) of which were in individuals found to have LS (both with *MSH2* PGVs).[51] Another single-institution analysis[68] identified MSI-H/MMR-deficiency in 7/304 (2.3%) sarcomas, including 4 pleomorphic and/or otherwise unclassified sarcomas, 1 epithelioid leiomyosarcoma, 1 malignant PEComa, and 1 pleomorphic rhabdomyosarcoma. Only the individual with the pleomorphic rhabdomyosarcoma was known to have LS with an *MSH2* PGV, and the remaining 6 cases were confirmed or suspected to have somatic origins to their MSI-H/MMR-D.

Perhaps the most compelling data to date linking sarcoma to LS comes from data from the multinational PLSD, in which 14 sarcoma diagnoses (including 10 osteosarcomas) have been observed among 1808 prospectively identified malignancies in the database.[69] 57% of the sarcomas were in LS carriers with *MSH2* PGVs and another 21% were in *MLH1* PGV carriers. Investigators calculated a cumulative osteosarcoma incidence to age 75 years of 4.24% (95% confidence interval (CI): 0.54–7.93) for LS carriers with *MSH2* PGVs, which is more than 42-fold higher than the general population.

Although these data provide compelling evidence that sarcomas are, indeed, LS-associated malignancies, we do not currently recommend any formal surveillance for sarcomas, due to the low absolute incidence and the absence of proven surveillance strategies.

Other Rare Lynch Syndrome-Associated Malignancies

A study evaluating paired germline LS testing and somatic MSI testing of more than 15,000 individuals with more than 50 different types of primary cancer shed important light on the concept that the full spectrum of LS-associated malignancies may still not yet be fully defined.[51] In addition to the classic LS-associated gastrointestinal, gynecologic, and genitourinary cancers described above, investigators reported isolated cases of cancers with high-level MSI and germline LS PGVs that were not classically LS-associated malignancies, including melanoma, mesothelioma, and adrenocortical carcinoma. Another single institution study[70] identified LS in 3 (3.2%) of 94 patients with adrenocortical carcinoma who prospectively underwent clinical germline genetic testing while also retrospectively identifying 2 (1.5%) of 135 LS carriers in the institutional registry as having had a diagnosis of adrenocortical carcinoma. Of the 5 patients with adrenocortical carcinoma in this study with LS, 3 had *MSH2* PGVs and MMR-D was identified in 3 of 4 available tumor specimens. There have also been isolated case reports[71,72] of MSI-H thymic carcinoma in individuals with *MLH1* PGVs, hinting that these may also be rare manifestations of LS.

Given the apparent rarity of such cancers and their as yet unclear link to LS, we do not recommend surveillance for these malignancies in asymptomatic LS carriers.

BREAST CANCER AND LYNCH SYNDROME – A CONTROVERSIAL LINK

The question of whether or not there exists a link between LS and female breast cancer has been a matter of debate for decades.[73] This debate has recently been resurrected with the emergence and widespread use of multigene panel testing for inherited cancer risk assessment. A diagnosis of female breast cancer is one of the most common indications for multigene panel testing, and some data[74] have suggested that *MSH6* and *PMS2* PGVs are found more commonly in female breast patients with cancer than would otherwise be expected by chance. Complicating such analyses, however, is the fact that *MSH6* and *PMS2* PGVs are far and away from the most common forms of LS in the overall population,[75] and it is not entirely clear if a woman's *MSH6* or *PMS2* PGV is truly the etiologic factor when she is diagnosed with breast cancer, or if this simply represents independent co-occurrence of 2 common phenomena (breast cancer and *MSH6* or *PMS2* PGVs). In the previously described study[51] of greater than 15,000 individuals with paired germline LS testing and MSI analyses, none of the 150 breast cancer diagnoses identified in female LS carriers harbored MSI-H biology, suggesting that most such diagnoses are unrelated to the individual's underlying LS.

One recent analysis[76] of greater than 440,000 females undergoing multigene panel testing for inherited cancer risk at a large commercial laboratory found that female LS carriers were actually less likely to have breast cancer than those in the general population (standardized incidence ratio [SIR] 0.88, 95% CI: 0.81 to 0.96). When stratified by individual LS gene, there was likewise no significantly increased incidence of breast cancer in female LS carriers though, interestingly, MSH6 and PMS2 PGVs were more commonly identified in females undergoing germline testing for suspected hereditary breast/ovarian cancer rather than suspected LS, again suggesting that the previously reported link between these genes and breast cancer risk may simply reflect ascertainment bias.[76] Two other recent large case–control studies[77,78] likewise demonstrated no increased risk of breast cancer among females with MLH1 or MSH2 PGVs, though one[78] of these 2 studies did detect a modestly increased risk of breast cancer in female MSH6 PGV carriers (OR: 1.96; 95% CI: 1.15–3.33).

Data from the PLSD have demonstrated cumulative risks of breast cancer to age 75 of 12.3%, 14.6%, 13.7%, and 15.2% for female MLH1, MSH2, MSH6, and PMS2 PGV carriers, respectively.[4] Note that the 95% confidence intervals for each of these estimates cross the estimated 12.8% cumulative lifetime breast cancer incidence reported for the general population.[10]

Based on the current state of the data, we counsel female LS carriers that the link between LS and breast cancer remains uncertain but that, if such a link does exist, it seems to be a mild predisposition at worst. We recommend that female LS carriers undergo breast cancer surveillance beginning at age 40 with annual mammography and clinical breast examination, consistent with population-based guidelines, unless they have a family history of breast cancer that would warrant earlier or otherwise more aggressive surveillance. To date, there has been no known purported association between LS and risks of male breast cancer.

SUMMARY

LS is a common form of inherited cancer risk that predisposes to a wide array of malignancies beyond CRC. In spite of the long and ever-growing list of associated cancer risks, there is a growing body of literature on specific clinical factors (eg, sex, gene, familial burden, and other features) that can help clinicians identify which LS carriers need specialized surveillance for particular LS malignancies. We advocate for clinicians to consider such personalized risk factors as well as the efficacy (or lack thereof) of organ-specific cancer surveillance techniques in determining who and how to screen for such extracolonic cancer risks in LS, rather than a "one size fits all" approach in which all LS carriers are screened for every possible associated malignancy.

CLINICS CARE POINTS

- LS carriers are at increased risk for an increasing number of noncolorectal malignancies. For most of these extracolonic malignancies, there is a paucity of data on how to best screen for these cancers.

- It is important to obtain a complete family history of cancer for first- and second-degree relatives of LS carriers, as familial burden of certain cancers has been associated with an increased personal risk of those cancers in LS.

- Personalized risk stratification (based on LS gene, age, sex, and family history) can help identify LS carriers at increased risk for specific types of extracolonic cancer. Free online resources (such as this) can be used to help with this risk stratification.

- Shared decision making remains critical in discussing cancer risk reduction strategies for LS carriers, particularly in situations where there is a lack of high-quality data on optimal surveillance and prevention approaches. Patients should be encouraged to participate in clinical trials for surveillance when possible.

DISCLOSURE

Dr M.B. Yurgelun reports consulting/scientific advisory board fees and research funding from Janssen Pharmaceuticals as well as payments for peer review services from UpToDate. The authors have nothing to disclose.

REFERENCES

1. Boland PM, Yurgelun MB, Boland CR. Recent progress in Lynch syndrome and other familial colorectal cancer syndromes. CA Cancer J Clin 2018;68(3):217–31.
2. Biller LH, Syngal S, Yurgelun MB. Recent advances in Lynch syndrome. Fam Cancer 2019;18(2):211–9.
3. Ligtenberg MJ, Kuiper RP, Chan TL, et al. Heritable somatic methylation and inactivation of MSH2 in families with Lynch syndrome due to deletion of the 3' exons of TACSTD1. Nat Genet 2009;41(1):112–7.
4. Dominguez-Valentin M, Sampson JR, Seppala TT, et al. Cancer risks by gene, age, and gender in 6350 carriers of pathogenic mismatch repair variants: findings from the Prospective Lynch Syndrome Database. Genet Med 2020;22(1): 15–25.
5. ten Broeke SW, van der Klift HM, Tops CMJ, et al. Cancer risks for PMS2-associated lynch syndrome. J Clin Oncol 2018;36(29):2961–8.
6. Biller LH, Horiguchi M, Uno H, et al. Familial burden and other clinical factors associated with various types of cancer in individuals with lynch syndrome. Gastroenterology 2021;161(1):143–50.e4.
7. Schmeler KM, Lynch HT, Chen LM, et al. Prophylactic surgery to reduce the risk of gynecologic cancers in the Lynch syndrome. N Engl J Med 2006;354(3):261–9.
8. Jiang H, Robinson DL, Lee PVS, et al. Loss of bone density and bone strength following premenopausal risk-reducing bilateral salpingo-oophorectomy: a prospective controlled study (WHAM Study). Osteoporos Int 2021;32(1):101–12.
9. Kotsopoulos J, Hall E, Finch A, et al. Changes in bone mineral density after prophylactic bilateral salpingo-oophorectomy in carriers of a BRCA mutation. JAMA Netw Open 2019;2(8):e198420.
10. National comprehensive cancer network clinical practice guidelines - genetic/familial high-risk assessment: colorectal (Version 1.2021). Available at: https://www.nccn.org/professionals/physician_gls/pdf/genetics_colon.pdf. Accessed June 23, 2021.
11. Crosbie EJ, Ryan NAJ, Arends MJ, et al. The Manchester International Consensus Group recommendations for the management of gynecological cancers in Lynch syndrome. Genet Med 2019;21(10):2390–400.
12. Dominguez-Valentin M, Seppala TT, Engel C, et al. Risk-reducing gynecological surgery in lynch syndrome: results of an international survey from the prospective lynch syndrome database. J Clin Med 2020;9(7):2290.
13. Dominguez-Valentin M, Crosbie EJ, Engel C, et al. Risk-reducing hysterectomy and bilateral salpingo-oophorectomy in female heterozygotes of pathogenic mismatch repair variants: a Prospective Lynch Syndrome Database report. Genet Med 2021;23(4):705–12.

14. Boland CR, Yurgelun MB. Historical perspective on familial gastric cancer. Cell Mol Gastroenterol Hepatol 2017;3(2):192–200.
15. Douglas JA, Gruber SB, Meister KA, et al. History and molecular genetics of Lynch syndrome in family G: a century later. JAMA 2005;294(17):2195–202.
16. Warthin AS. Heredity with reference to carcinoma as shown by the study of teh cases examined in the Pathological Laboratory of the University of Michigan, 1895-1912. Arch Int Med 1913;12:546–55.
17. Møller P, Seppälä TT, Bernstein I, et al. Cancer risk and survival in path_MMR carriers by gene and gender up to 75 years of age: a report from the Prospective Lynch Syndrome Database. Gut 2018;67(7):1306–16.
18. Kim J, Braun D, Ukaegbu C, et al. Clinical factors associated with gastric cancer in individuals with lynch syndrome. Clin Gastroenterol Hepatol 2020;18(4):830–7.e1.
19. Adar T, Friedman M, Rodgers LH, et al. Gastric cancer in Lynch syndrome is associated with underlying immune gastritis. J Med Genet 2019;56(12):844–5.
20. Saita C, Yamaguchi T, Horiguchi SI, et al. Tumor development in Japanese patients with Lynch syndrome. PLoS One 2018;13(4):e0195572.
21. Chautard R, Malka D, Samaha E, et al. Upper gastrointestinal lesions during endoscopy surveillance in patients with Lynch syndrome: a multicentre cohort study. Cancers (Basel) 2021;13(7):1657.
22. Ladigan-Badura S, Vangala DB, Engel C, et al. Value of upper gastrointestinal endoscopy for gastric cancer surveillance in patients with Lynch syndrome. Int J Cancer 2021;148(1):106–14.
23. Kumar S, Dudzik CM, Reed M, et al. Upper endoscopic surveillance in lynch syndrome detects gastric and duodenal adenocarcinomas. Cancer Prev Res (Phila) 2020;13(12):1047–54.
24. Siegel RL, Miller KD, Fuchs HE, et al. Cancer statistics, 2021. CA Cancer J Clin 2021;71(1):7–33.
25. Engel C, Loeffler M, Steinke V, et al. Risks of less common cancers in proven mutation carriers with lynch syndrome. J Clin Oncol 2012;30(35):4409–15.
26. ten Kate GL, Kleibeuker JH, Nagengast FM, et al. Is surveillance of the small bowel indicated for Lynch syndrome families? Gut 2007;56(9):1198–201.
27. Koornstra JJ, Kleibeuker JH, Vasen HF. Small-bowel cancer in Lynch syndrome: is it time for surveillance? Lancet Oncol 2008;9(9):901–5.
28. Karimi M, von Salome J, Aravidis C, et al. A retrospective study of extracolonic, non-endometrial cancer in Swedish Lynch syndrome families. Hered Cancer Clin Pract 2018;16:16.
29. Latham A, Shia J, Patel Z, et al. Characterization and clinical outcomes of DNA mismatch repair-deficient small bowel adenocarcinoma. Clin Cancer Res 2021;27(5):1429–37.
30. Aparicio T, Henriques J, Manfredi S, et al. Small bowel adenocarcinoma: results from a nationwide prospective ARCAD-NADEGE cohort study of 347 patients. Int J Cancer 2020;147(4):967–77.
31. Syngal S, Brand RE, Church JM, et al. ACG clinical guideline: Genetic testing and management of hereditary gastrointestinal cancer syndromes. Am J Gastroenterol 2015;110(2):223–62 [quiz 263].
32. Giardiello FM, Allen JI, Axilbund JE, et al. Guidelines on genetic evaluation and management of Lynch syndrome: a consensus statement by the US Multi-Society Task Force on colorectal cancer. Gastroenterology 2014;147(2):502–26.

33. Vangala DB, Pox C, Ladigan S, et al. Clinical characteristics and EGD surveillance in lynch syndrome patients with small bowel/duodenal carcinomas. J Clin Oncol 2018;36(15_suppl):1555.
34. Haanstra JF, Al-Toma A, Dekker E, et al. Prevalence of small-bowel neoplasia in Lynch syndrome assessed by video capsule endoscopy. Gut 2015;64(10):1578–83.
35. Haanstra JF, Al-Toma A, Dekker E, et al. Incidence of small bowel neoplasia in Lynch syndrome assessed by video capsule endoscopy. Endosc Int Open 2017;5(7):E622–6.
36. Perrod G, Samaha E, Perez-Cuadrado-Robles E, et al. Effectiveness of a dedicated small bowel neoplasia screening program by capsule endoscopy in Lynch syndrome: 5 years results from a tertiary care center. Therap Adv Gastroenterol 2020;13. 1756284820934314.
37. Hu C, Hart SN, Polley EC, et al. Association between inherited germline mutations in cancer predisposition genes and risk of pancreatic cancer. JAMA 2018;319(23):2401–9.
38. Yurgelun MB, Chittenden AB, Morales-Oyarvide V, et al. Germline cancer susceptibility gene variants, somatic second hits, and survival outcomes in patients with resected pancreatic cancer. Genet Med 2019;21(1):213–23.
39. Brand R, Borazanci E, Speare V, et al. Prospective study of germline genetic testing in incident cases of pancreatic adenocarcinoma. Cancer 2018;124(17):3520–7.
40. Shindo K, Yu J, Suenaga M, et al. Deleterious germline mutations in patients with apparently sporadic pancreatic adenocarcinoma. J Clin Oncol 2017;35(30):3382–90.
41. Canto MI, Almario JA, Schulick RD, et al. Risk of neoplastic progression in individuals at high risk for pancreatic cancer undergoing long-term surveillance. Gastroenterology 2018;155(3):740–51.e2.
42. National comprehensive cancer network clinical practice guidelines - genetic/familial high-risk assessment: Breast, Ovarian, and Pancreatic (Version 2.2021). Available at: http://www.nccn.org/professionals/physician_gls/pdf/genetics_bop.pdf. Accessed June 23, 2021.
43. Goggins M, Overbeek KA, Brand R, et al. Management of patients with increased risk for familial pancreatic cancer: updated recommendations from the International Cancer of the Pancreas Screening (CAPS) Consortium. Gut 2020;69(1):7–17.
44. Canto MI, Hruban RH, Fishman EK, et al. Frequent detection of pancreatic lesions in asymptomatic high-risk individuals. Gastroenterology 2012;142(4):796–804 [quiz e714–95].
45. Wischhusen JW, Ukaegbu C, Dhingra TG, et al. Clinical factors associated with urinary tract cancer in individuals with Lynch syndrome. Cancer Epidemiol Biomarkers Prev 2020;29(1):193–9.
46. van der Post RS, Kiemeney LA, Ligtenberg MJ, et al. Risk of urothelial bladder cancer in Lynch syndrome is increased, in particular among MSH2 mutation carriers. J Med Genet 2010;47(7):464–70.
47. Aarnio M, Saily M, Juhola M, et al. Uroepithelial and kidney carcinoma in Lynch syndrome. Fam Cancer 2012;11(3):395–401.
48. Joost P, Therkildsen C, Dominguez-Valentin M, et al. Urinary tract cancer in lynch syndrome; increased risk in carriers of MSH2 mutations. Urology 2015;86(6):1212–7.

49. Myrhøj T, Andersen MB, Bernstein I. Screening for urinary tract cancer with urine cytology in Lynch syndrome and familial colorectal cancer. Fam Cancer 2008; 7(4):303–7.

50. Matin SF, Coleman JA. Misclassification of upper tract urothelial carcinoma in patients with lynch syndrome. JAMA Oncol 2018;4(7):1010.

51. Latham A, Srinivasan P, Kemel Y, et al. Microsatellite instability is associated with the presence of lynch syndrome pan-cancer. J Clin Oncol 2019;37(4):286–95.

52. Raymond VM, Mukherjee B, Wang F, et al. Elevated risk of prostate cancer among men with Lynch syndrome. J Clin Oncol 2013;31(14):1713–8.

53. Dominguez-Valentin M, Joost P, Therkildsen C, et al. Frequent mismatch-repair defects link prostate cancer to Lynch syndrome. BMC Urol 2016;16:15.

54. Giri VN, Knudsen KE, Kelly WK, et al. Role of genetic testing for inherited prostate cancer risk: philadelphia prostate cancer consensus conference 2017. J Clin Oncol 2018;36(4):414–24.

55. Haraldsdottir S, Hampel H, Wei L, et al. Prostate cancer incidence in males with Lynch syndrome. Genet Med 2014;16(7):553–7.

56. Grindedal EM, Moller P, Eeles R, et al. Germ-line mutations in mismatch repair genes associated with prostate cancer. Cancer Epidemiol Biomarkers Prev 2009;18(9):2460–7.

57. Page EC, Bancroft EK, Brook MN, et al. Interim results from the IMPACT study: evidence for prostate-specific antigen screening in BRCA2 mutation carriers. Eur Urol 2019;76(6):831–42.

58. Muir EG, Bell AJ, Barlow KA. Multiple primary carcinomata of the colon, duodenum, and larynx associated with kerato-acanthomata of the face. Br J Surg 1967;54(3):191–5.

59. Torre D. Multiple sebaceous tumors. Arch Dermatol 1968;98(5):549–51.

60. South CD, Hampel H, Comeras I, et al. The frequency of Muir-Torre syndrome among Lynch syndrome families. J Natl Cancer Inst 2008;100(4):277–81.

61. Ykema BLM, Adan F, Crijns MB, et al. Cutaneous squamous cell carcinoma is associated with Lynch syndrome: widening the spectrum of Lynch syndrome-associated tumours. Br J Dermatol 2021;185(2):462–3.

62. Turcot J, Despres JP, St Pierre F. Malignant tumors of the central nervous system associated with familial polyposis of the colon: report of two cases. Dis Colon Rectum 1959;2:465–8.

63. Hamilton SR, Liu B, Parsons RE, et al. The molecular basis of Turcot's syndrome. N Engl J Med 1995;332(13):839–47.

64. Therkildsen C, Ladelund S, Rambech E, et al. Glioblastomas, astrocytomas and oligodendrogliomas linked to Lynch syndrome. Eur J Neurol 2015;22(4):717–24.

65. Haraldsdottir S, Rafnar T, Frankel WL, et al. Comprehensive population-wide analysis of Lynch syndrome in Iceland reveals founder mutations in MSH6 and PMS2. Nat Commun 2017;8:14755.

66. Durno C, Boland CR, Cohen S, et al. Recommendations on surveillance and management of biallelic mismatch repair deficiency (BMMRD) syndrome: a consensus statement by the US multi-society task force on colorectal cancer. Gastroenterology 2017;152(6):1605–14.

67. Kaczmar JM, Everett J, Ruth K, et al. Sarcoma: A Lynch Syndrome (LS)-associated malignancy? J Clin Oncol 2015;33(15_suppl):1516.

68. Doyle LA, Nowak JA, Nathenson MJ, et al. Characteristics of mismatch repair deficiency in sarcomas. Mod Pathol 2019;32(7):977–87.

69. Dominguez-Valentin M, Sampson JR, Moller P, et al. Analysis in the prospective lynch syndrome database identifies sarcoma as part of the Lynch syndrome tumor spectrum. Int J Cancer 2021;148(2):512–3.
70. Raymond VM, Everett JN, Furtado LV, et al. Adrenocortical carcinoma is a lynch syndrome-associated cancer. J Clin Oncol 2013;31(24):3012–8.
71. Repetto M, Conforti F, Pirola S, et al. Thymic carcinoma with Lynch syndrome or microsatellite instability, a rare entity responsive to immunotherapy. Eur J Cancer 2021;153:162–7.
72. Pandey D, Shepro DS. Thymic cancer in lynch syndrome: an unusual association. BMJ Case Rep 2020;13(4):e230241.
73. Watson P, Lynch HT. Extracolonic cancer in hereditary nonpolyposis colorectal cancer. Cancer 1993;71(3):677–85.
74. Roberts ME, Jackson SA, Susswein LR, et al. MSH6 and PMS2 germ-line pathogenic variants implicated in Lynch syndrome are associated with breast cancer. Genet Med 2018;20(10):1167–74.
75. Win AK, Jenkins MA, Dowty JG, et al. Prevalence and penetrance of major genes and polygenes for colorectal cancer. Cancer Epidemiol Biomarkers Prev 2017;26(3):404–12.
76. Stoll J, Rosenthal E, Cummings S, et al. No evidence of increased risk of breast cancer in women with lynch syndrome identified by multigene panel testing. JCO Precis Oncol 2020;4:51–60.
77. Hu C, Hart SN, Gnanaolivu R, et al. A population-based study of genes previously implicated in breast cancer. N Engl J Med 2021;384(5):440–51.
78. Breast Cancer Association C, Dorling L, Carvalho S, et al. Breast cancer risk genes - association analysis in more than 113,000 women. N Engl J Med 2021;384(5):428–39.

Evaluation of Classic, Attenuated, and Oligopolyposis of the Colon

Jessica M. Long, MS, CGC[a,1], Jacquelyn M. Powers, MS, CGC[a,1], Bryson W. Katona, MD, PhD[b,*]

KEYWORDS

- Colon polyps • Adenomatous polyposis • Genetic testing
- Hereditary colorectal cancer syndrome

KEY POINTS

- Genetic evaluation and testing are warranted for colonic polyposis, including for any individual with 10 or more cumulative adenomatous polyps.
- Given overlapping and emerging phenotypes, multi-gene panel testing is an efficient and advantageous strategy for the genetic testing of colonic polyposis.
- Accurate diagnosis of colonic polyposis syndromes is the key to the development of a comprehensive cancer screening and risk-reduction plan for affected individuals, as well as to guide the risk assessment and management of at-risk relatives.

INTRODUCTION

Colorectal cancer (CRC) is one of the most common forms of cancer worldwide,[1] and it is estimated that 2% to 8% of CRC cases are attributed to well-defined, inherited monogenic cancer predisposition syndromes, including Lynch syndrome (LS), familial adenomatous polyposis (FAP), MUTYH-associated polyposis (MAP), and other less frequent CRC predisposing syndromes, including those characterized by the presence of hamartomatous polyps.[2] Colonic polyposis is frequently classified by the histologic subtype of the predominant polyps and the number of polyps that develop in the colon. For adenomatous polyposis, which is the most common type of colonic polyposis, classic polyposis often refers to the development of 100 or more colonic

[a] Division of Hematology/Oncology, Department of Medicine, University of Pennsylvania, Philadelphia, PA, USA; [b] Division of Gastroenterology and Hepatology, Department of Medicine, University of Pennsylvania Perelman School of Medicine, Philadelphia, PA, USA
[1] Authors contributed equally.
* Corresponding author. Perelman Center for Advanced Medicine, 3400 Civic Center Boulevard, 751 South Pavilion, Philadelphia, PA 19104.
E-mail address: bryson.katona@pennmedicine.upenn.edu

Gastrointest Endoscopy Clin N Am 32 (2022) 95–112
https://doi.org/10.1016/j.giec.2021.08.003
1052-5157/22/© 2021 Elsevier Inc. All rights reserved.

giendo.theclinics.com

adenomas, whereas attenuated polyposis or oligopolyposis refers to having between 10–20 and 99 colonic adenomas.

Despite advances in the field, much of the genetic predisposition to CRC and polyposis remains unexplained. In recent years, significant advancements have been made to identify rare causal genes associated with CRC and polyposis, which have been vital in the risk stratification and clinical management of affected individuals and their families.[2] Herein, we focus on the evaluation of adenomatous polyposis of the colon, including well-established syndromes as well as those newly characterized. Up-to-date referral criteria for genetic evaluation and guidance for testing are also highlighted and organized based on adenoma and nonadenoma indications. Lastly, the ordering and outcomes of genetic testing in adenomatous colonic polyposis cohorts, as well as a brief synopsis on management and critical elements of follow-up care will be covered.

DIFFERENTIAL DIAGNOSIS OF COLONIC ADENOMATOUS POLYPOSIS

Multiple hereditary gastrointestinal cancer syndromes are associated with the propensity to develop colonic and extra-colonic polyps, and these are discretely characterized based on polyp pathology and burden, as well as specific disease-causing genetic variants (**Fig. 1**). Understanding the nuances of these syndromes is important to help narrow the differential diagnosis in affected patients.

Familial Adenomatous Polyposis

Familial adenomatous polyposis (FAP) is the most common and well-understood adenomatous polyposis syndrome, accounting for ~1% of CRC cases. FAP results

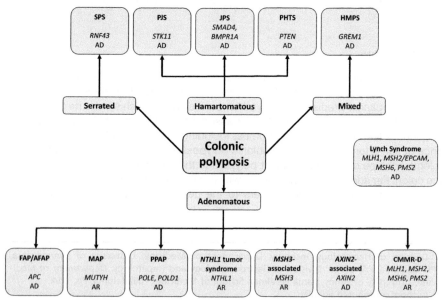

Fig. 1. Overview of polyposis syndromes. AD, Autosomal dominant; AFAP, Attenuated familial adenomatous polyposis; AR, Autosomal recessive; CMMRD, Constitutional mismatch repair-deficiency; FAP, Familial adenomatous polyposis; HMPS, Hereditary mixed polyposis syndrome; JPS, Juvenile polyposis syndrome; MAP, *MUTYH*-associated polyposis; PHTS, *PTEN* hamartoma tumor syndrome; PJS, Peutz–Jeghers syndrome; PPAP, Polymerase proofreading-associated polyposis; SPS, Serrated polyposis syndrome.

from heterozygous germline pathogenic/likely pathogenic (P/LP) variants in the *APC* gene demonstrating an autosomal dominant inheritance pattern.[3,4] Classic FAP leads to the development of 100s to 1000s of colonic adenomas, typically presenting in early adolescence, with a nearly 100% chance of developing CRC if left untreated.[5] The less severe form of this disease, known as attenuated FAP (AFAP), is associated with smaller adenoma burden (often <100), delayed onset, and lower overall risk for CRC (~70%).[3,4,6] In FAP and AFAP there is also increased risk of duodenal/ampullary, gastric, and thyroid cancers.[7,8] Genotype–phenotype relationships may influence polyp severity and location, as well as the presence or absence of extra-intestinal manifestations including congenital hypertrophy of the retinal pigmented epithelium (CHRPE), osteomas, supernumerary teeth, and desmoid tumors.[9] Though FAP/AFAP is typically familial, approximately 30% of P/LP variants in *APC* are *de novo*, and therefore, FAP/AFAP can be observed in the absence of a family history of polyposis.[10]

MUTYH-Associated Polyposis

MAP is another well-characterized adenomatous polyposis syndrome. Unlike FAP/AFAP, MAP is autosomal recessive, caused by biallelic *MUTYH* P/LP variants; thus, it is typically observed in one generation of a family, but not successive generations.[11] The MAP phenotype overlaps most closely with AFAP as most individuals have less than 100 adenomas, with some exceptions spanning the entire spectrum (ie, CRC in the absence of polyps and in cases with 100+ adenomas).[12,13] Biallelic *MUTYH* P/LP variants rarely are associated with thousands of polyps as seen in classic FAP.[12] Of note, serrated polyps have also been observed along with adenomas among individuals with MAP.[14] The overall lifetime risk to develop CRC without intervention approaches 70%, and there is increased risk for duodenal cancer as well as the reports of sebaceous adenomas and other extracolonic features reported at low frequency.[13,15] Though *MUTYH* P/LP variants are pan-ethnic, 2 founder pathogenic variants (p.Tyr179Cys and p.Gly396Asp) account for approximately 73% of P/LP *MUTYH* variants detected among those with European ancestry.[16] Importantly, monoallelic *MUTYH* P/LP variants do not cause MAP. In those with monoallelic *MUTYH* germline P/LP variants, the risk of cancer continues to be debated.[13]

Lynch Syndrome and Constitutional Mismatch Repair-Deficiency Syndrome

Lynch syndrome (LS) is among the most common hereditary cancer predisposition syndromes, affecting 1 in 279 people and accounting for 2% to 3% of all CRC and 2% of all endometrial cancer (EC) cases.[17,18] Affected individuals carry heterozygous germline P/LP variants in a DNA mismatch repair (MMR) gene (*MLH1, MSH2, MSH6, PMS2*) or *EPCAM* (causing epigenetic inactivation of *MSH2*).[19,20] Although CRC is the most common LS tumor, risks for neoplasms of the endometrium and ovaries, extracolonic gastrointestinal tract (stomach and small intestine, pancreas, biliary tract), urinary tract, brain (glioblastoma), and skin (keratoacanthoma and sebaceous adenoma/carcinoma) are also increased.[21] Historically, personal and family history-based risk assessments, specifically Amsterdam I/II clinical diagnostic criteria, have consistently underperformed in identifying LS.[22–24] Because MMR deficiency (dMMR) causes microsatellite instability (MSI) in cancers, multiple organizations now recommend universal dMMR testing of all patients with newly diagnosed CRC or EC via immunohistochemistry or MSI analysis to better aid in LS diagnosis.[25–29] Though previously known as hereditary nonpolyposis colorectal cancer, or HNPCC, LS can cause multiple adenomas in a single individual; therefore, while 10 or more adenomas generate suspicion for polyposis, LS should also be considered with this clinical presentation.[30] LS shares overlap with MAP in terms of potential for solitary CRCs, lower adenoma count, and extracolonic features such as sebaceous neoplasm.[15] A more severe cancer phenotype known as constitutional mismatch repair deficiency (CMMR-D) syndrome results from biallelic P/LP variants within the same MMR gene.[31,32] Individuals with CMMR-D have increased risk for CRC, hematologic, and brain malignancies and may present with other clinical features, such as café-au-lait hyperpigmented lesions, agenesis of the corpus callosum, and immunoglobulin deficiency.[33,34] Although LS causes adult-onset cancer susceptibility, CMMR-D leads to significant anticipation of symptoms and early onset of polyposis.[33] A large proportion of patients with CMMR-D develop multiple synchronous adenomas ranging from a few to greater than 100 polyps, mimicking attenuated FAP.[2]

Polymerase Proofreading-Associated Polyposis

Polymerase proofreading-associated polyposis (PPAP) was first characterized in 2013 as being associated with a dominantly inherited syndrome that confers increased risk of CRC as well as adenomatous polyposis due to germline P/LP variants in the exonuclease (proofreading) domain of DNA polymerases Pol δ (*POLD1* gene) and Pol ε (*POLE* gene).[35] The PPAP phenotype typically consists of an attenuated or oligopolyposis (10 to <100 adenomas), as well as increased incidence of duodenal adenomas and potential proclivity toward EC and glioblastoma.[36–38] One case report described a germline *POLE* pathogenic variant in a 14-year-old boy with early-onset CRC, adenomas, and café-au-lait macules, whose MMR germline testing was negative, lending some preliminary data that PPAP could present with a CMMR-D-like phenotype.[38] Overall, *POLE* and *POLD1* germline P/LP variants have been heavily investigated in cohorts of polyposis or Amsterdam I/II positive families with negative germline *APC, MUTYH,* and MMR genetic testing; therefore, there is some concern for ascertainment bias.[36] *POLE* p.Leu424Val and *POLD1* p.Ser478Asn are 2 well-established recurrent PVs, though others have been detected.[35,36] Regarding age-stratified CRC risk, Buchanan and colleagues have reported a 28% and 90% chance by age 70 for *POLE* and *POLD1* P/LP variant carriers, respectively.[38] Lastly, most PPAP-associated tumors are mismatch repair (MMR) proficient, microsatellite stable (MSS), and confer ultrahigh Somatic tumor mutational burden (TMB) with base substitutions (or polymerase replicative mutations) greater than 100 mutations per megabase (>100 Mut/Mb).[39–41]

Hereditary Mixed Polyposis Syndrome

Hereditary mixed polyposis syndrome (HMPS) was described originally as an autosomal dominant syndrome associated with multiple polyps of differing histologies (tubular/villous/tubulovillous adenomas, serrated lesions, as well as hyperplastic and hamartomatous polyps), as well as enrichment for CRC.[42–45] A genetic etiology for HMPS was first described in 2012, when a 40kb duplication in the 5' regulatory region of the *GREM1* gene was identified as the causal PV in Ashkenazi Jewish families with shared haplotypes, suggesting a potential founder effect.[46] Subsequently, other duplications have been characterized.[43,47,48] The data gathered to date indicate that *GREM1* duplications may occur in individuals with or without polyposis. The onset of polyposis usually occurs in adulthood (late 20s or older), although there are reports of polyps earlier in life. The phenotype may overlap with FAP or LS, and extracolonic tumors have been reported.[42,43,49]

NTHL1 Tumor Syndrome

Through whole-exome sequencing of select adenomatous polyposis cases, Weren and colleagues described the second autosomal recessive form of attenuated adenomatous polyposis, caused by biallelic P/LP variants in the DNA base excision repair gene, NTHL1.[50] Previously called NTHL1-associated polyposis, "NTHL1 tumor syndrome" has been proposed based on the observed increased risk to develop variable extracolonic benign and malignant tumor types, including but not limited to breast, endometrial, and urothelial cancers, as well as duodenal polyps and meningiomas.[51] The attenuated polyposis phenotype (<100 polyps) and increased CRC risk are the most robustly described features, whereas the extracolonic risks remain less well-defined. In total, only 31 individuals from 23 families have been characterized with inevitable ascertainment bias.[50–58] More than 90% of the reported NTHL1 biallelic families carry the c.268 C>T (p.Gln90*) stop-gain variant, first appreciated in the Netherlands and Germany, but since found across other ethnicities.[53] Overall, the allele frequency of this PV in European populations is 0.24%, whereas, in other populations (ie, Asian, African, or Hispanic), the frequency decreases below 0.05%.[59]

MSH3-Associated Polyposis

Similar to the NTHL1 gene discovery, Adam and colleagues identified a rare cause of autosomal recessive adenomatous polyposis via whole-exome sequencing in a cohort of individuals with unexplained disease (N = 102, majority <100 adenomas).[60] These efforts led to the discovery of biallelic pathogenic variants in the MMR gene, MSH3, in 2 unrelated individuals. Consistent with MMR deficiency, tumor tissue in biallelic carriers revealed high MSI and complete loss of MSH3 protein staining in both tumor and normal tissues.[60] The polyposis phenotype is most consistent with attenuated disease, although the full spectrum of risks remains ill-defined. Early documented cases report duodenal adenomas in addition to colonic polyps, as well as singular reporting of astrocytoma, uterine leiomyomas, cutaneous fibrolipoma, and ovarian dermoid cyst.[60]

AXIN2-Associated Polyposis

The AXIN2 gene plays a crucial role in the morphogenesis of the craniofacial area and is essential for tooth development. Monoallelic germline P/LP variants in the AXIN2 gene are most well-known for their implication in oligodontia and ectodermal dysplasia, both in isolation and co-occurrence, and with variable severity.[61] However, AXIN2 has also been implicated in risk for cancer, predominantly CRC, as well as adenomatous polyps, with or without the aforementioned features.[61,62] The association with colorectal neoplasia was first described in a 4 generation Finnish family whereby multiple carriers of AXIN2 c.1966C>T (p.Arg656*) displayed severe oligodontia, polyposis, and/or CRC.[63] The polyposis observed in this family as well as in subsequent studies has ranged from 10s to greater than 100 polyps and the observed polyp subtypes include both adenomatous and serrated polyps.[63–65] There has also been documentation of duodenal and gastric polyps, as well as breast, lung, prostate, and hepatocellular carcinoma.[61] There are very few AXIN2 families reported in the literature and there is ongoing work to better characterize the spectrum of AXIN2-associated risks.[66]

Colonic Polyposis of Unknown Etiology/Oligopolyposis of Unknown Etiology

For some individuals clinically presenting with classic, attenuated, or oligopolyposis, current genetic testing methods may prove uninformative with no detectable P/LP variant in a known polyposis gene. It has been estimated that 30% to 50% of individuals evaluated for FAP, MAP, and PPAP may lack a molecular diagnosis, and somatic mosaicism has been suggested as one possible underlying cause for a minority of these unexplained cases.[67] Nevertheless, individuals with colonic polyposis of unknown etiology (CPUE) or oligopolyposis of unknown etiology (OPUE) and their relatives must be followed closely, and a recent review has summarized the available literature regarding medical management, including colonic and extracolonic surveillance, in this scenario.[68]

REFERRAL INDICATIONS FOR GENETIC EVALUATION AND TESTING FOR ADENOMATOUS POLYPOSIS

Proper referral of patients with colonic polyposis for genetic evaluation is critical to allow for the identification of a potential hereditary polyposis syndrome, which has implications for both the patient and relatives. Current practice guidelines from the National Society of Genetic Counselors (NSGC), the American College of Medical Genetics (ACMG), the American College of Gastroenterology (ACG), the European Society for Medical Oncology (ESMO), and American Society of Clinical Oncology (ASCO) have established positions to offer germline genetic testing for FAP and MAP when an individual has 10 or more cumulative colonic adenomas.[69–72] However, these guidelines, which were published within the last 5 to 6 years, do not integrate more newly appreciated adenomatous polyposis genes. More recently, the National Comprehensive Cancer Network (NCCN) suggests the consideration of multigene panel testing (MGPT) for a personal history of 10 to 19 colonic adenomas, and recommends MGPT when more than 20 cumulative adenomas are identified.[25] Similarly, the Collaborative Group of the Americas on Inherited Gastrointestinal Cancer (CGA-IGC) Position Statement on MGPT now recommends the consideration of MGPT for any individual with 10 or more cumulative colonic adenomas.[73] Considerations for differential diagnoses and gene inclusion are listed in **Table 1**. Although polyposis remains the central feature of phenotype for referral and genetic evaluation, extra-colonic indications also may merit referral and genetic testing (see **Table 1**). These features may be present in isolation or in combination with others. The extracolonic features, as previously described, are best characterized in FAP, LS/CMMRD, and *AXIN2*-associated polyposis (see **Table 1**). Lastly, regardless of the patient's known medical history, genetic evaluation and testing are warranted when there is a family history of a known P/LP variant in an adenomatous polyposis gene in a relative, as well as when there is a family history of suspected polyposis syndrome without the ability to test the affected relative.[25]

GENETIC TESTING CONSIDERATIONS FOR ADENOMATOUS POLYPOSIS

Once a patient has been referred for genetic evaluation with concern for a polyposis syndrome, there are numerous considerations that should be addressed before ordering genetic testing, including what type of genetic testing should be offered, when to order genetic testing, and family planning considerations related to genetic testing.

Genetic Testing Options

Historically, genetic evaluation has occurred via single gene analysis for a specific hereditary polyposis syndrome based on the risk assessment of the personal and family history, including the polyp pathology type. For families with a P/LP variant in a single gene, single-site analysis for the familial P/LP variant is a highly informative predictive test to directly determine whether an individual inherited the known hereditary syndrome in the family.[25] Additionally in the past, when the personal/family history was suspicious, but a defined hereditary condition had not yet been molecularly confirmed, polyposis syndromes in the differential diagnosis were sequentially assessed in order of prior probability. Furthermore, the apparent inheritance pattern could influence the testing strategy, such as the decision to evaluate first for MAP in situations whereby the phenotype seemed autosomal recessive (eg, clinical polyposis only in siblings).[25] Once technology advancements enabled multi-gene panel testing (MGPT) through next-generation sequencing, the time- and cost-burden of genetic testing decreased dramatically, enabling multiple hereditary polyposis syndromes to be evaluated

Table 1
Referral indications for genetic evaluation for adenomatous polyposis syndromes

Referral Based on the Personal History of Adenomatous Polyps	Genetic Testing to Consider
≥10 cumulative colonic adenomas, age-independent	MGPT for CRC/polyposis predisposition, minimally including FAP (*APC*),
Personal history of colonic adenoma(s) and duodenal/ampullary adenoma(s), age-independent	MAP (*MUTYH*), LS (*MLH1, MSH2, MSH6, PMS2, EPCAM*), PPAP (*POLE, POLD1*),
Young-onset colonic adenomas (<10 cumulative)[a]	HMPS (*GREM1*), NTLH1, MSH3, AXIN2[b]
Meets clinical criteria for serrated polyposis syndrome and also has some colonic adenomas	

Referral Based on Family History	Genetic Testing to Consider
Family history of polyposis syndrome with a known pathogenic/likely pathogenic (P/LP) gene variant	Single gene testing (or MGPT if other concerning family history)
Family history of polyposis syndrome without a known P/LP gene variant	MGPT, if affected relative unavailable for testing

Syndrome-Specific and Extracolonic Referral Considerations	Syndrome(s) to consider[c]
Congenital hypertrophy of the retinal epithelium (CHRPE) (unilateral or bilateral)	FAP (*APC*)
Desmoid tumor(s)	
Cribriform-morular variant of papillary thyroid cancer	
Hepatoblastoma (<5 y of age)	
Epidermal cysts	
Osteomas	
Endometrial cancer or CRC cancer < 50, or Synchronous or metachronous CRC or endometrial cancer any age, or Personal/family history satisfying Amsterdam I/II or Revised Bethesda criteria	LS (*MLH1, MSH2, MSH6, PMS2, EPCAM*), PPAP (*POLE, POLD1*), NTHL1, MSH3[d]
Tumor (any type) suggesting mismatch repair deficiency (via IHC, MSI, or somatic testing)	LS (*MLH1, MSH2, MSH6, PMS2, EPCAM*)
Hyper- to ultramutated CRC suggesting polymerase proofreading deficiency	PPAP (*POLE, POLD1*)

(continued on next page)

Table 1
(continued)

Syndrome-Specific and Extracolonic Referral Considerations	Syndrome(s) to consider[c]
≥ 10 polyps of more than 1 histologic type (adenomas, hyperplastic, and juvenile)	HMPS (*GREM1*)
Personal history of brain tumor < 18, and Café-au-lait macules, or Adenoma(s) (typically ≥ 10), or Family history of Lynch-associated cancer or childhood cancer, or Consanguineous parents	CMMR-D *(biallelic P/LP variants in MLH1, MSH2, MSH6, PMS2 or EPCAM)*
Personal history of oligodontia, and/or Ectodermal dysplasia	*AXIN2*

Abbreviations: CMMR-D, Constitutional mismatch repair-deficiency syndrome; CRC, colorectal cancer; FAP, familial adenomatous polyposis; HMPS, hereditary mixed polyposis syndrome; IHC, immunohistochemistry; LS, Lynch syndrome; MAP, *MUTYH*-associated polyposis; MGPT, Multi-gene panel testing; MSI, microsatellite instability; NGS, tumor next-generation sequencing; PPAP, Polymerase proofreading-associated polyposis (PPAP); SSP, sessile serrated polyposis.

[a] Serial follow-up to assess the presence or absence of additional adenoma development (+/− changes to other personal/family history) may also be considered as a sufficient alternative to up-front MGPT. Should the clinical scenario evolve and suspicions heighten for a polyposis syndrome, genetic testing could then be considered and facilitated.

[b] Non-adenomatosis polyposis syndrome genes (*STK11, BMPR1A, SMAD4, PTEN, RNF43*), non-polyposis CRC genes (eg, *CHEK2, TP53*), and emerging evidence genes (*RPS20, GALNT12, MLH3*) may also be included.

[c] Other polyposis genes (as per the previous footnote) and syndromes may be considered as part of MGPT.

[d] Current data on PPAP, *NTHL1* tumor syndrome, and *MSH3*-associated polyposis support seminal feature as adenomatous polyps in most cases.

simultaneously through a single test.[74] Given the phenotypic overlap between various hereditary colorectal/polyposis syndromes, the improved efficiency of MGPT has led to increased use in the clinic, although the advantages and disadvantages of this approach and test options must be carefully weighed.[75] Current best practices and considerations for multi-gene panel testing in hereditary colorectal cancer and/or polyposis risk assessment have been described in the recent position statement published by the CGA-IGC.[73] Moreover, multiple professional societies and guidelines, including the NCCN, the American Society of Colon and Rectal Surgeons (ASCRS), ASCO, the NSGC and the ACMG encourage pre- and post-test genetic counseling by individuals with relevant genetic expertise.[25,69,71,73,76,77]

At present, decisions regarding genetic testing in terms of single syndrome evaluation or MGPT, as well as which genes to include, rely on clinical judgment, commercial laboratory test options, and patient preferences, including insurance criteria and cost. As MGPT became increasingly available and affordable before evidence-based standards, careful consideration must be given to advantages, disadvantages, and limitations of various test options, as described in detail elsewhere,[78] and ideally should occur in the context of genetic counseling with a provider having related expertise, to promote informed decision-making by the patient.[25,75,79,80] For the patient presenting with multiple adenomatous colon polyps, the differential diagnosis is broad, and thus multi-gene panel testing may be a more efficient and cost-effective method to pursue the genetic evaluation.[25,73]

In terms of gene selection for MGPT, the CGA-IGC recommends a minimum set for the evaluation of colorectal cancer and/or polyposis, which includes the following genes associated with well-described, high penetrance hereditary syndromes: *APC, BMPR1A, EPCAM, MLH1, MSH2, MSH6, MUTYH, PMS2, PTEN, SMAD4, STK11.*[73] The CGA Position Statement also delineates that in specific circumstances, consideration may be given to genes with low to moderately increased CRC risk (*ATM, CHEK2, TP53*) or those with preliminary but limited data (*GREM1, POLD1, POLE, AXIN2, NTHL1, MSH3, GALNT12, RPS20*). Current NCCN guidelines recommend strong consideration of all known polyposis and CRC predisposition genes as outlined in the Stanich and colleagues 2019 study (described in detail in the genetic testing outcomes section of this review), particularly before managing an individual as having CPUE.[25]

When to Order Genetic Testing

The approach to genetic evaluation also must consider the appropriateness of timing, that is, when the results will impact medical management and/or reproductive decision-making for the patient. According to the American Academy of Pediatrics and American Society of Human Genetics, predictive genetic testing is not recommended in children below age 18 if results would not impact immediate risk assessment or medial management.[81,82] Similarly, NSGC's Position Statement specifically indicates predictive genetic testing for adult-onset conditions "should optimally be deferred until the individual has the capacity to weigh the associated risks, benefits, and limitations of this information, taking his/her circumstances, preferences, and beliefs into account to preserve his/her autonomy and right to an open future."[83] Of the hereditary adenomatous polyposis syndromes, however, there are several for which diagnosis in childhood does confer important medical interventions, including FAP and CMMR-D.[25] Because the initiation of endoscopy surveillance is recommended in childhood for classic FAP, for example, it is advisable to offer predictive genetic testing for a familial *APC* P/LP variant by age 10 to 12, to determine whether surveillance is necessary; furthermore, if hepatoblastoma screening is to be considered, testing for a familial *APC* P/LP variant may even be considered in infancy.[25] Children who test "true negative" for a known familial P/LP variant, in the absence of other concerning signs/symptoms, will not need to undergo enhanced surveillance or other unnecessary procedures, hence predictive genetic testing is an important tool in childhood for families with FAP and CMMR-D. For adolescents and young adults suspected of having hereditary polyposis, genetic counseling is strongly recommended in conjunction with genetic testing, as outlined by a recent report with recommendations issued by the American College of Gastroenterology.[84]

Family Planning Considerations

Another important time point for genetic evaluation relates to family planning decisions. Preimplantation genetic testing-monogenic (PGT-M) may be used to test for a specific hereditary condition when a known familial P/LP variant has previously been identified in a single gene.[85] Thus, using PGT-M can allow selective implantation of embryos that lack the familial P/LP variant, therefore, preventing this hereditary condition from being passed on. Among individuals with FAP or other hereditary cancer syndromes, surveyed respondents have indicated a willingness to consider PGT-M to prevent the transmission of a known hereditary syndrome in the family, and a majority felt PGT-M should be available, even if they themselves would be unlikely to pursue.[86,87] Given that some individuals acquire a clinical diagnosis of polyposis based on the number and pathology of polyps, genetic testing in these individuals remains important to identify the specific familial P/LP variant, to provide the option of informed family planning, as well as for the purposes of highly informative, cascade testing in at-risk relatives.

GENETIC TESTING OUTCOMES IN ADENOMATOUS POLYPOSIS

Understanding the outcomes of genetic testing in individuals with colonic adenoma-tous polyposis is also important to inform expectations for both patients and pro-viders. Before the availability of MGPT, Grover and colleagues evaluated single gene APC and MUTYH analysis conducted at a single commercial genetics laboratory for 7225 individuals with colonic adenomas; these individuals were specifically referred for genetic evaluation for polyposis based on personal/family history.[12] The prevalence of pathogenic variants in APC or MUTYH varied by cumulative adenoma burden. Among 119 individuals with classic polyposis with more than 1000 cumulative adenomas, 80% had an APC pathogenic variant and 2% had biallelic MUTYH patho-genic variants. For 1338 individuals with a cumulative adenoma burden of 100 to 999, 56% and 7%, respectively, had an APC pathogenic variant or biallelic MUTYH path-ogenic variants. Among the oligopolyposis cohort with 20 to 99 adenomas, 10% of 3253 individuals had an APC pathogenic variant, and 7% had biallelic MUTYH path-ogenic variants. Even among those with 10 to 19 cumulative adenomas, 9% had a molecularly confirmed diagnosis of AFAP or MAP (5% with an APC pathogenic variant and 4% with biallelic MUTYH pathogenic variants). Although there is certainly ascer-tainment bias in this cohort, these results provided initial support for the recommen-dation to offer genetic evaluation to individuals with at least 20 cumulative adenomas and to consider genetic testing for those with 10 to 19 cumulative ade-nomas, dependent on additional factors such as the age of onset and family history.[25]

More recently using MGPT, Stanich and colleagues summarized 3789 individuals with at least 10 colon polyps (adenomas and/or hamartomas), who were tested at a commercial genetics laboratory from 2012 to 2016 via evaluation of at least 14 genes associated with polyposis and/or colorectal cancer (APC, BMPR1A, CDH1, CHEK2, EPCAM, MLH1, MSH2, MSH6, MUTYH, PMS2, PTEN, SMAD4, STK11, TP53), including a subset also having testing of GREM1, POLD1 and POLE.[88] These results similarly supported genetic testing for individuals with at least 10 cumulative ade-nomas, because regardless of the age of onset or total polyp burden the prevalence of pathogenic variants in these genes exceeded 5%.

Challenges arising from greater availability of MGPT include increased identification of lower penetrance alleles as well as individuals identified as "carriers" (having het-erozygous pathogenic variants) for autosomal recessive polyposis. Although P/LP var-iants in APC are associated with FAP/AFAP and very significantly elevated risk for CRC and polyposis, the APC p.I1307K variant, detected in 6% to 11% of individuals with Ashkenazi Jewish heritage, definitively does not lead to FAP/AFAP, but is asso-ciated with modestly increased risk for CRC.[89] In a meta-analysis in 2013, the pooled odds ratio for the association between the APC p.I1307K variant and CRC was 2.17, suggesting that individuals of Ashkenazi Jewish ancestry who have the APC p.I1307K variant are at significantly increased CRC risk.[90] Evidence regarding the level of risk for those with the APC p.I1307K variant without Ashkenazi heritage remains limited. Based on the available data to date, it has been recommended that individuals with the APC p.I1307K variant initiate colonoscopy surveillance at age 40 and repeat every 5 years, given that this estimation of risk is similar to those with a first-degree relative with CRC.[25,91] Similarly, some studies have demonstrated a modest increase in CRC risk among individuals with heterozygous MUTYH P/LP variants (carriers, but not themselves affected with MAP); however, results from other studies have not supported this association.[92–96] This is important as heterozygous *MUTYH* P/LP mutations are identified in 1% to 2% of the general population, thus making it one of the most commonly identified variants on hereditary cancer multi-gene panels.[18,97] For the more recently identified autosomal recessive syndromes, *NTHL1* tumor syndrome and *MSH3*-associated polyposis, data regarding colorectal cancer risk for heterozygous carriers are scant, and specific recommendations are not available at present.[98] Given the challenges related to integrating these results in clinical decision-making, careful counseling regarding the potential for these types of findings is recommended when including these genes on MGPT.[99]

MANAGEMENT OF ADENOMATOUS POLYPOSIS

For individuals with a molecular (P/LP variant) or clinical (negative genetic testing) diagnosis of an adenomatous polyposis syndrome, medical management recommendations should follow current existing guidelines for the specific condition, which also typically include guidance for at-risk relatives, the details of which are beyond the scope of this review.[25,34,69–72,76,100,101] The multi-system nature of adenomatous polyposis syndromes requires the generation of a comprehensive management plan, ideally developed by a provider with expertise in the condition; this may require referral to a specialty center, given the rarity of these syndromes. Genetic testing to identify a familial P/LP variant and subsequent cascade testing in relatives remain paramount tools to effectively determine which relatives need enhanced surveillance and risk-reduction and which do not; although limited studies at present have focused on cascade testing specific to adenomatous polyposis, cascade testing is standard practice in clinical genetics, and there has been substantial focus on this for families with LS.[102]

SUMMARY

For individuals presenting with adenomatous colonic polyposis, recognition and accurate identification of an underlying genetic susceptibility are necessary to help define a comprehensive, multi-system management plan relevant to the risks associated with the defined polyposis syndrome. As well, accurate and thorough genetic counseling is needed to determine which relatives in the family may also be at risk and would benefit from highly informative, predictive genetic testing. Advances in germline genetic testing via multi-gene panels and newly recognized syndromes have bolstered the ability to properly identify hereditary polyposis risk, while also presenting challenges. Individuals and families suspected of having an inherited adenomatous polyposis syndrome would benefit from a genetic evaluation with a multi-disciplinary team, including genetic counselors and physicians specializing in hereditary polyposis syndromes, to effectively diagnose and manage for enhanced cancer surveillance and risk-reduction.

CLINICS CARE POINTS

- For individuals with adenomatous polyposis, accurate identification of an underlying hereditary syndrome is necessary to guide appropriate colonic and extracolonic surveillance and cancer risk management.
- Multiple cancer risk syndromes caused by hereditary pathogenic variants in different genes can be associated with adenomatous polyposis.

- Studies on outcomes of genetic testing for adenomatous polyposis support offering genetic testing to individuals presenting with 10 or more cumulative adenomas, regardless of age.
- Multi-gene panel testing may be the most comprehensive and efficient strategy to simultaneously evaluate for multiple adenomatous polyposis syndromes; the implications and limitations of multi-gene panel testing should be addressed before testing to ensure informed consent.
- Identification of a pathogenic variant in a gene related to adenomatous polyposis enables accurate risk assessment and highly informative predictive genetic testing in at-risk relatives.

ACKNOWLEDGMENTS

NIH/NIDDK grant R03DK120946 (B.W. Katona) and the Jason and Julie Borrelli Lynch Syndrome Research Fund (B.W. Katona).

DISCLOSURE

J.M. Long – None; J.M. Powers - Consulting (Carevive Systems, Inc.), Honoraria (Myriad Genetics and Ambry Genetics); B.W. Katona - Consulting (Exact Sciences), Travel (Janssen).

REFERENCES

1. Siegel RL, Miller KD, Fuchs HE, et al. Cancer Statistics, 2021. CA Cancer J Clin 2021;71(1):7–33.
2. Valle L, de Voer RM, Goldberg Y, et al. Update on genetic predisposition to colorectal cancer and polyposis. Mol Aspects Med 2019;69:10–26.
3. Basso G, Bianchi P, Malesci A, et al. Hereditary or sporadic polyposis syndromes. Best Pract Res Clin Gastroenterol 2017;31(4):409–17.
4. Byrne RM, Tsikitis VL. Colorectal polyposis and inherited colorectal cancer syndromes. Ann Gastroenterol 2018;31(1):24–34.
5. Jasperson KW, Tuohy TM, Neklason DW, et al. Hereditary and familial colon cancer. Gastroenterology 2010;138(6):2044–58.
6. Burt RW, Leppert MF, Slattery ML, et al. Genetic testing and phenotype in a large kindred with attenuated familial adenomatous polyposis. Gastroenterology 2004;127(2):444–51.
7. Feng X, Milas M, O'Malley M, et al. Characteristics of benign and malignant thyroid disease in familial adenomatous polyposis patients and recommendations for disease surveillance. Thyroid 2015;25(3):325–32.
8. Knudsen AL, Bulow S, Tomlinson I, et al. Attenuated familial adenomatous polyposis: results from an international collaborative study. Colorectal Dis 2010; 12(10 Online):e243–9.
9. Jasperson KW. Genetic testing by cancer site: colon (polyposis syndromes). Cancer J 2012;18(4):328–33.
10. Aretz S, Uhlhaas S, Caspari R, et al. Frequency and parental origin of de novo APC mutations in familial adenomatous polyposis. Eur J Hum Genet 2004; 12(1):52–8.
11. Sieber OM, Lipton L, Crabtree M, et al. Multiple colorectal adenomas, classic adenomatous polyposis, and germ-line mutations in MYH. N Engl J Med 2003;348(9):791–9.

12. Grover S, Kastrinos F, Steyerberg EW, et al. Prevalence and phenotypes of APC and MUTYH mutations in patients with multiple colorectal adenomas. JAMA 2012;308(5):485–92.
13. Samadder NJ, Baffy N, Giridhar KV, et al. Hereditary Cancer Syndromes-A Primer on Diagnosis and Management, Part 2: Gastrointestinal Cancer Syndromes. Mayo Clin Proc 2019;94(6):1099–116.
14. Guarinos C, Juarez M, Egoavil C, et al. Prevalence and characteristics of MUTYH-associated polyposis in patients with multiple adenomatous and serrated polyps. Clin Cancer Res 2014;20(5):1158–68.
15. Vogt S, Jones N, Christian D, et al. Expanded extracolonic tumor spectrum in MUTYH-associated polyposis. Gastroenterology 2009;137(6):1976–85.e1-10.
16. Cheadle JP, Sampson JR. MUTYH-associated polyposis–from defect in base excision repair to clinical genetic testing. DNA Repair (Amst) 2007;6(3):274–9.
17. Carethers JM, Stoffel EM. Lynch syndrome and Lynch syndrome mimics: The growing complex landscape of hereditary colon cancer. World J Gastroenterol 2015;21(31):9253–61.
18. Win AK, Jenkins MA, Dowty JG, et al. Prevalence and Penetrance of Major Genes and Polygenes for Colorectal Cancer. Cancer Epidemiol Biomarkers Prev 2017;26(3):404–12.
19. Ligtenberg MJ, Kuiper RP, Chan TL, et al. Heritable somatic methylation and inactivation of MSH2 in families with Lynch syndrome due to deletion of the 3' exons of TACSTD1. Nat Genet 2009;41(1):112–7.
20. Lynch HT, Snyder CL, Shaw TG, et al. Milestones of Lynch syndrome: 1895-2015. Nat Rev Cancer 2015;15(3):181–94.
21. Stoffel EM, Kastrinos F. Familial colorectal cancer, beyond Lynch syndrome. Clin Gastroenterol Hepatol 2014;12(7):1059–68.
22. Sinicrope FA. Lynch Syndrome-Associated Colorectal Cancer. N Engl J Med 2018;379(8):764–73.
23. Vasen HF, Mecklin JP, Khan PM, et al. The International Collaborative Group on Hereditary Non-Polyposis Colorectal Cancer (ICG-HNPCC). Dis Colon Rectum 1991;34(5):424–5.
24. Vasen HF, Watson P, Mecklin JP, et al. New clinical criteria for hereditary nonpolyposis colorectal cancer (HNPCC, Lynch syndrome) proposed by the International Collaborative group on HNPCC. Gastroenterology 1999;116(6):1453–6.
25. NCCN. National Comprehensive Cancer Network Guidelines, Version 1.2021. Genetic/Familial High Risk Assessment: Colorectal. 2021. Available at: https://www.nccn.org/professionals/physician_gls/pdf/genetics_colon.pdf. Accessed May 24, 2021.
26. Evaluation of Genomic Applications in P, Prevention Working G. Recommendations from the EGAPP Working Group: genetic testing strategies in newly diagnosed individuals with colorectal cancer aimed at reducing morbidity and mortality from Lynch syndrome in relatives. Genet Med 2009;11(1):35–41.
27. Lancaster JM, Powell CB, Chen L-m, et al. Society of Gynecologic Oncology statement on risk assessment for inherited gynecologic cancer predispositions. Gynecol Oncol 2015;136(1):3–7.
28. Thibodeau SN, Bren G, Schaid D. Microsatellite instability in cancer of the proximal colon. Science 1993;260(5109):816–9.
29. ACOG Practice Bulletin No. 147: Lynch syndrome. Obstet Gynecol 2014;124(5):1042–54.
30. Kalady MF, Kravochuck SE, Heald B, et al. Defining the adenoma burden in lynch syndrome. Dis Colon Rectum 2015;58(4):388–92.

31. Ricciardone MD, Ozcelik T, Cevher B, et al. Human MLH1 deficiency predisposes to hematological malignancy and neurofibromatosis type 1. Cancer Res 1999;59(2):290–3.

32. Wang Q, Lasset C, Desseigne F, et al. Neurofibromatosis and early onset of cancers in hMLH1-deficient children. Cancer Res 1999;59(2):294–7.

33. MacFarland SP, Zelley K, Katona BW, et al. Gastrointestinal Polyposis in Pediatric Patients. J Pediatr Gastroenterol Nutr 2019;69(3):273–80.

34. Tabori U, Hansford JR, Achatz MI, et al. Clinical Management and Tumor Surveillance Recommendations of Inherited Mismatch Repair Deficiency in Childhood. Clin Cancer Res 2017;23(11):e32–7.

35. Palles C, Cazier JB, Howarth KM, et al. Germline mutations affecting the proofreading domains of POLE and POLD1 predispose to colorectal adenomas and carcinomas. Nat Genet 2013;45(2):136–44.

36. Bellido F, Pineda M, Aiza G, et al. POLE and POLD1 mutations in 529 kindred with familial colorectal cancer and/or polyposis: review of reported cases and recommendations for genetic testing and surveillance. Genet Med 2016;18(4): 325–32.

37. Vande Perre P, Siegfried A, Corsini C, et al. Germline mutation p.N363K in POLE is associated with an increased risk of colorectal cancer and giant cell glioblastoma. Fam Cancer 2019;18(2):173–8.

38. Buchanan DD, Stewart JR, Clendenning M, et al. Risk of colorectal cancer for carriers of a germ-line mutation in POLE or POLD1. Genet Med 2018;20(8): 890–5.

39. Campbell BB, Light N, Fabrizio D, et al. Comprehensive Analysis of Hypermutation in Human Cancer. Cell 2017;171(5):1042–56.e10.

40. Cancer Genome Atlas N. Comprehensive molecular characterization of human colon and rectal cancer. Nature 2012;487(7407):330–7.

41. Cancer Genome Atlas Research N, Kandoth C, Schultz N, et al. Integrated genomic characterization of endometrial carcinoma. Nature 2013;497(7447): 67–73.

42. Daca Alvarez M, Quintana I, Terradas M, et al. The inherited and familial component of early-onset colorectal cancer. Cells 2021;10(3):710.

43. McKenna DB, Van Den Akker J, Zhou AY, et al. Identification of a novel GREM1 duplication in a patient with multiple colon polyps. Fam Cancer 2019;18(1):63–6.

44. Whitelaw SC, Murday VA, Tomlinson IP, et al. Clinical and molecular features of the hereditary mixed polyposis syndrome. Gastroenterology 1997;112(2): 327–34.

45. Thomas HJ, Whitelaw SC, Cottrell SE, et al. Genetic mapping of hereditary mixed polyposis syndrome to chromosome 6q. Am J Hum Genet 1996;58(4): 770–6.

46. Jaeger E, Leedham S, Lewis A, et al. Hereditary mixed polyposis syndrome is caused by a 40-kb upstream duplication that leads to increased and ectopic expression of the BMP antagonist GREM1. Nat Genet 2012;44(6):699–703.

47. Rohlin A, Eiengard F, Lundstam U, et al. GREM1 and POLE variants in hereditary colorectal cancer syndromes. Genes Chromosomes Cancer 2016;55(1): 95–106.

48. Venkatachalam R, Verwiel ET, Kamping EJ, et al. Identification of candidate predisposing copy number variants in familial and early-onset colorectal cancer patients. Int J Cancer 2011;129(7):1635–42.

49. Lieberman S, Walsh T, Schechter M, et al. Features of Patients With Hereditary Mixed Polyposis Syndrome Caused by Duplication of GREM1 and Implications for Screening and Surveillance. Gastroenterology 2017;152(8):1876–80.e1.
50. Weren RD, Ligtenberg MJ, Kets CM, et al. A germline homozygous mutation in the base-excision repair gene NTHL1 causes adenomatous polyposis and colorectal cancer. Nat Genet 2015;47(6):668–71.
51. Grolleman JE, de Voer RM, Elsayed FA, et al. Mutational Signature Analysis Reveals NTHL1 Deficiency to Cause a Multi-tumor Phenotype. Cancer Cell 2019; 35(2):256–66.e5.
52. Altaraihi M, Gerdes AM, Wadt K. A new family with a homozygous nonsense variant in NTHL1 further delineated the clinical phenotype of NTHL1-associated polyposis. Hum Genome Var 2019;6:46.
53. Belhadj S, Mur P, Navarro M, et al. Delineating the Phenotypic Spectrum of the NTHL1-Associated Polyposis. Clin Gastroenterol Hepatol 2017;15(3):461–2.
54. Belhadj S, Quintana I, Mur P, et al. NTHL1 biallelic mutations seldom cause colorectal cancer, serrated polyposis or a multi-tumor phenotype, in absence of colorectal adenomas. Sci Rep 2019;9(1):9020.
55. Broderick P, Dobbins SE, Chubb D, et al. Validation of Recently Proposed Colorectal Cancer Susceptibility Gene Variants in an Analysis of Families and Patients-a Systematic Review. Gastroenterology 2017;152(1):75–7.e74.
56. Fostira F, Kontopodis E, Apostolou P, et al. Extending the clinical phenotype associated with biallelic NTHL1 germline mutations. Clin Genet 2018;94(6): 588–9.
57. Groves A, Gleeson M, Spigelman AD. NTHL1-associate polyposis: first Australian case report. Fam Cancer 2019;18(2):179–82.
58. Rivera B, Castellsague E, Bah I, et al. Biallelic NTHL1 Mutations in a Woman with Multiple Primary Tumors. N Engl J Med 2015;373(20):1985–6.
59. Karczewski KJ, Weisburd B, Thomas B, et al. The ExAC browser: displaying reference data information from over 60 000 exomes. Nucleic Acids Res 2017;45(D1):D840–5.
60. Adam R, Spier I, Zhao B, et al. Exome Sequencing Identifies Biallelic MSH3 Germline Mutations as a Recessive Subtype of Colorectal Adenomatous Polyposis. Am J Hum Genet 2016;99(2):337–51.
61. Hlouskova A, Bielik P, Bonczek O, et al. Mutations in AXIN2 gene as a risk factor for tooth agenesis and cancer: A review. Neuro Endocrinol Lett 2017;38(3): 131–7.
62. Marvin ML, Mazzoni SM, Herron CM, et al. AXIN2-associated autosomal dominant ectodermal dysplasia and neoplastic syndrome. Am J Med Genet A 2011; 155A(4):898–902.
63. Lammi L, Arte S, Somer M, et al. Mutations in AXIN2 cause familial tooth agenesis and predispose to colorectal cancer. Am J Hum Genet 2004;74(5): 1043–50.
64. Beard C, Purvis R, Winship IM, et al. Phenotypic confirmation of oligodontia, colorectal polyposis and cancer in a family carrying an exon 7 nonsense variant in the AXIN2 gene. Fam Cancer 2019;18(3):311–5.
65. Rivera B, Perea J, Sanchez E, et al. A novel AXIN2 germline variant associated with attenuated FAP without signs of oligondontia or ectodermal dysplasia. Eur J Hum Genet 2014;22(3):423–6.
66. Macklin-Mantia SK, Hines SL, Chaichana KL, et al. Case report expanding the germline AXIN2- related phenotype to include olfactory neuroblastoma and gastric adenoma. BMC Med Genet 2020;21(1):161.

67. Spier I, Drichel D, Kerick M, et al. Low-level APC mutational mosaicism is the underlying cause in a substantial fraction of unexplained colorectal adenomatous polyposis cases. J Med Genet 2016;53(3):172–9.
68. Long JM, Powers JM, Stanich PP, et al. Clinical management of oligopolyposis of unknown etiology. Current Treat Options Gastroenterol 2021;183–97.
69. Hampel H, Bennett RL, Buchanan A, et al. A practice guideline from the American College of Medical Genetics and Genomics and the National Society of Genetic Counselors: referral indications for cancer predisposition assessment. Genet Med 2015;17(1):70–87.
70. Balmana J, Balaguer F, Cervantes A, et al. Familial risk-colorectal cancer: ESMO Clinical Practice Guidelines. Ann Oncol 2013;24(Suppl 6):vi73–80.
71. Stoffel EM, Mangu PB, Gruber SB, et al. Hereditary colorectal cancer syndromes: American Society of Clinical Oncology Clinical Practice Guideline endorsement of the familial risk-colorectal cancer: European Society for Medical Oncology Clinical Practice Guidelines. J Clin Oncol 2015;33(2):209–17.
72. Syngal S, Brand RE, Church JM, et al. ACG clinical guideline: Genetic testing and management of hereditary gastrointestinal cancer syndromes. Am J Gastroenterol 2015;110(2):223–62 [quiz: 263].
73. Heald B, Hampel H, Church J, et al. Collaborative Group of the Americas on Inherited Gastrointestinal Cancer Position statement on multigene panel testing for patients with colorectal cancer and/or polyposis. Fam Cancer 2020;19(3):223–39.
74. Pritchard CC, Smith C, Salipante SJ, et al. ColoSeq provides comprehensive lynch and polyposis syndrome mutational analysis using massively parallel sequencing. J Mol Diagn 2012;14(4):357–66.
75. Fecteau H, Vogel KJ, Hanson K, et al. The evolution of cancer risk assessment in the era of next generation sequencing. J Genet Couns 2014;23(4):633–9.
76. Herzig D, Hardiman K, Weiser M, et al. The American Society of Colon and Rectal Surgeons Clinical Practice Guidelines for the Management of Inherited Polyposis Syndromes. Dis Colon Rectum 2017;60(9):881–94.
77. Robson ME, Bradbury AR, Arun B, et al. American Society of Clinical Oncology Policy Statement Update: Genetic and Genomic Testing for Cancer Susceptibility. J Clin Oncol 2015;33(31):3660–7.
78. Powers JM, Ebrahimzadeh JE, Katona BW. Genetic testing for hereditary gastrointestinal cancer syndromes: Interpreting results in today's practice. Curr Treat Options Gastroenterol 2019;17(4):636–49.
79. Kurian AW, Ford JM. Multigene Panel Testing in Oncology Practice: How Should We Respond? JAMA Oncol 2015;1(3):277–8.
80. Lorans M, Dow E, Macrae FA, et al. Update on Hereditary Colorectal Cancer: Improving the Clinical Utility of Multigene Panel Testing. Clin Colorectal Cancer 2018;17(2):e293–305.
81. Committee On B. Committee On Genetics AND, American College Of Medical Genetics AND, Genomics S, Ethical, Legal Issues C. Ethical and policy issues in genetic testing and screening of children. Pediatrics 2013;131(3):620–2.
82. Botkin JR, Belmont JW, Berg JS, et al. Points to Consider: Ethical, Legal, and Psychosocial Implications of Genetic Testing in Children and Adolescents. Am J Hum Genet 2015;97(1):6–21.
83. Statement NSoGCP. 2021. Available at: https://www.nsgc.org/Policy-Research-and-Publications/Position-Statements/Position-Statements/Post/genetic-testing-of-minors-for-adult-onset-conditions. Accessed May 24, 2021.

84. Attard TM, Burke CA, Hyer W, et al. ACG Clinical Report and Recommendations on Transition of Care in Children and Adolescents With Hereditary Polyposis Syndromes. Am J Gastroenterol 2021;116(4):638–46.

85. Preimplantation Genetic Testing: ACOG Committee Opinion, Number 799. Obstet Gynecol 2020;135(3):e133–7.

86. Kastrinos F, Stoffel EM, Balmana J, et al. Attitudes toward prenatal genetic testing in patients with familial adenomatous polyposis. Am J Gastroenterol 2007;102(6):1284–90.

87. Rich TA, Liu M, Etzel CJ, et al. Comparison of attitudes regarding preimplantation genetic diagnosis among patients with hereditary cancer syndromes. Fam Cancer 2014;13(2):291–9.

88. Stanich PP, Pearlman R, Hinton A, et al. Prevalence of Germline Mutations in Polyposis and Colorectal Cancer-Associated Genes in Patients With Multiple Colorectal Polyps. Clin Gastroenterol Hepatol 2019;17(10):2008–15.e3.

89. Rennert G, Almog R, Tomsho LP, et al. Colorectal polyps in carriers of the APC I1307K polymorphism. Dis Colon Rectum 2005;48(12):2317–21.

90. Liang J, Lin C, Hu F, et al. APC polymorphisms and the risk of colorectal neoplasia: a HuGE review and meta-analysis. Am J Epidemiol 2013;177(11):1169–79.

91. Boursi B, Sella T, Liberman E, et al. The APC p.I1307K polymorphism is a significant risk factor for CRC in average risk Ashkenazi Jews. Eur J Cancer 2013;49(17):3680–5.

92. Theodoratou E, Campbell H, Tenesa A, et al. A large-scale meta-analysis to refine colorectal cancer risk estimates associated with MUTYH variants. Br J Cancer 2010;103(12):1875–84.

93. Win AK, Dowty JG, Cleary SP, et al. Risk of colorectal cancer for carriers of mutations in MUTYH, with and without a family history of cancer. Gastroenterology 2014;146(5):1208–11.e1-5.

94. Win AK, Hopper JL, Jenkins MA. Association between monoallelic MUTYH mutation and colorectal cancer risk: a meta-regression analysis. Fam Cancer 2011;10(1):1–9.

95. Ma X, Zhang B, Zheng W. Genetic variants associated with colorectal cancer risk: comprehensive research synopsis, meta-analysis, and epidemiological evidence. Gut 2014;63(2):326–36.

96. Lubbe SJ, Di Bernardo MC, Chandler IP, et al. Clinical implications of the colorectal cancer risk associated with MUTYH mutation. J Clin Oncol 2009;27(24):3975–80.

97. Samadder NJ, Riegert-Johnson D, Boardman L, et al. Comparison of Universal Genetic Testing vs Guideline-Directed Targeted Testing for Patients With Hereditary Cancer Syndrome. JAMA Oncol 2021;7(2):230–7.

98. Elsayed FA, Grolleman JE, Ragunathan A, et al. Monoallelic NTHL1 Loss-of-Function Variants and Risk of Polyposis and Colorectal Cancer. Gastroenterology 2020;159(6):2241–3.e6.

99. Katona BW, Yurgelun MB, Garber JE, et al. A counseling framework for moderate-penetrance colorectal cancer susceptibility genes. Genet Med 2018;20(11):1324–7.

100. Monahan KJ, Bradshaw N, Dolwani S, et al. Guidelines for the management of hereditary colorectal cancer from the British Society of Gastroenterology (BSG)/Association of Coloproctology of Great Britain and Ireland (ACPGBI)/United Kingdom Cancer Genetics Group (UKCGG). Gut 2020;69(3):411–44.

101. Yang J, Gurudu SR, Koptiuch C, et al. American Society for Gastrointestinal Endoscopy guideline on the role of endoscopy in familial adenomatous polyposis syndromes. Gastrointest Endosc 2020;91(5):963–82.e2.
102. Roberts MC, Dotson WD, DeVore CS, et al. Delivery Of Cascade Screening For Hereditary Conditions: A Scoping Review Of The Literature. Health Aff (Millwood) 2018;37(5):801–8.

Endoscopic Management and Surgical Considerations for Familial Adenomatous Polyposis

Peter P. Stanich, MD[a],*, Brian Sullivan, MD, MHS[b], Alex C. Kim, MD[c], Matthew F. Kalady, MD[d]

KEYWORDS

- Adenomatous polyposis coli • Colonic neoplasms • Disease management
- Duodenal neoplasms • Genetic predisposition to disease

KEY POINTS

- In classic familial adenomatous polyposis, colorectal cancer screening is generally recommended to start at age 10 to 12 years with colonoscopy every 1 to 2 years.
- Absolute indications for colectomy are the presence of cancer or significant colorectal symptoms and relative indications include increasing number of polyps over serial examinations or the presence of large, advanced polyps.
- Colorectal cancer surveillance should continue at least every 1 to 2 years after colectomy.
- Duodenal, ampullary, and gastric screening is generally recommended to start with upper endoscopy with ampullary visualization at age 20 to 25 years with surveillance interval determined by findings.
- Malignancy, Spigelman stage IV duodenal polyposis, and advanced duodenal polyps that are not endoscopically resectable are indications for surgical resection with either pancreas-sparing duodenectomy or pancreatoduodenectomy.

[a] Division of Gastroenterology, Hepatology & Nutrition, The Ohio State University Wexner Medical Center, 395 West 12th Avenue, Suite 200, Columbus, OH 43210, USA; [b] Division of Gastroenterology, Duke University Medical Center, 2301 Erwin Road, Durham, NC 27710, USA; [c] Division of Surgical Oncology, The Ohio State University Wexner Medical Center, N924 Doan Hall, 410 West 10th Avenue, Columbus, OH 43210, USA; [d] Division of Colorectal Surgery, The Ohio State University Wexner Medical Center, 737 Doan Hall, 410 West 10th Avenue, Columbus, OH 43210, USA
* Corresponding author.
E-mail address: Peter.Stanich@osumc.edu
Twitter: @DocStanich (P.P.S.); @gi_sullivan (B.S.); @CRS_HIPEC (A.C.K.); @MattKaladyMD (M.F.K.)

Gastrointest Endoscopy Clin N Am 32 (2022) 113–130
https://doi.org/10.1016/j.giec.2021.08.007
1052-5157/22/© 2021 Elsevier Inc. All rights reserved.

INTRODUCTION

Familial adenomatous polyposis (FAP) is primarily characterized by the development of a multitude of adenomatous polyps in the colon and rectum and the resultant extremely high risk for colorectal cancer (CRC), but duodenal and gastric neoplasia is also very common and becomes increasingly impactful as patients age. FAP is commonly reported to have an incidence of about 1 in 10,000.[1] It is caused by germline pathogenic variants in the adenomatous polyposis coli (*APC*) gene, with disease phenotype correlating with the location of the mutation, and is inherited in an autosomal dominant fashion.[1]

This article focuses on current endoscopic and surgical management recommendations in FAP. Multiple national guidelines are discussed, with recently updated recommendations published by the American Society for Gastrointestinal Endoscopy (ASGE), European Society of Gastrointestinal Endoscopy (ESGE), National Comprehensive Cancer Network (NCCN), and British Society of Gastroenterology/Association of Coloproctology of Great Britain and Ireland/United Kingdom Cancer Genetics Group (UK).[2–5] Note that a referral to a specialized center with expertise in hereditary CRC syndrome management is recommended once a diagnosis of FAP is made. Among the benefits of these programs is the ability to offer multidisciplinary care including personalized endoscopic and surgical treatment protocols, as well as providing genetic counseling and predictive testing for at-risk family members.

DISCUSSION
Endoscopic Management

Colon and rectum
Clinical characteristics. Classic FAP is highly penetrant, with diffuse colon adenomatous polyposis and CRC occurring in nearly 100% of untreated individuals. The median age at CRC diagnosis is approximately 35 to 45 years.[6,7] Attenuated FAP (AFAP) has a lower penetrance than classic FAP and is typically characterized by a later onset (around age 30 years) of fewer colonic adenomas (<100, although >100 may occur by later ages), which often have a predilection for the right colon.[8,9] The risk of developing CRC is also lower, estimated to be around 70% by age 80 years, with the average age of CRC diagnosis at approximately 50 to 60 years.[8,10–12]

Observational studies of patients with FAP from centralized registries suggest a significant reduction in CRC incidence and mortality from endoscopic surveillance and prophylactic colectomy programs. Results from the Danish Polyposis Registry showed that CRC risk in individuals with FAP under surveillance was approximately 2%, compared with about 62% in those not undergoing close follow-up. Furthermore, all cases of CRC in patients under surveillance were identified at the time of FAP diagnosis, with none occurring during the follow-up program.[13] In the same registry, the 10-year cumulative survival was 94% in patients with FAP undergoing follow-up, compared with 41% in those without programmatic surveillance.[14] In a systematic review, all 33 included studies showed a significant reduction in CRC incidence and mortality with FAP programmatic surveillance.[15] It should be noted that these observational studies evaluated patients enrolled in programs that provided regular call-up reminders and access to a variety of treatment options (including endoscopy, surgery, and chemoprevention).

Endoscopic screening and surveillance
Classic In patients with classic FAP, guidelines generally recommend to begin a CRC screening program at around puberty, or between ages 10 and 15 years

Table 1
Recommendations for presurgical colorectal cancer screening and surveillance

	Starting Age (y)	Modality	Frequency (y)
ASGE[4]	10–12	Colonoscopy or sigmoidoscopy[b]	1–2
ESGE[3]	12–14	Colonoscopy	1–2
NCCN 2021[a,2]	10–15	Colonoscopy (preferred) or sigmoidoscopy[b]	Annual
UK[5]	12–14	Colonoscopy	1–3

[a] If surgery is delayed.
[b] Colonoscopy if polyps are found on sigmoidoscopy.

(**Table 1**).[2–5] This recommendation is based on data from various FAP registries, in which the median age of polyp occurrence was early adolescence.[16,17] CRC is rare before this starting age range, with a combined European registry data reporting no CRC before age 10 years, 0.2% before age 15 years, and 1.3% before age 20 years.[17]

At screening initiation, colonoscopy is generally the recommended modality.[3,5] Sigmoidoscopy may be an acceptable alternative given that the rectum is usually involved if polyposis is present, but a full colonic evaluation is warranted once an adenoma is identified.[2,4] There can be significant heterogeneity in polyposis phenotype and CRC risk related to specific *APC* gene mutations.[8,18] In high-risk individuals, polyps of various sizes may carpet the entire colon, making individual polypectomy difficult, but others can present with more polyps amenable to resection. An increasing understanding of the wide spectrum of risk, as well as improvements in endoscopic techniques, has provided justification for the development of presurgical endoscopic surveillance strategies. Patients with mild polyposis, or those unwilling to undergo surgery, may be candidates for these intensive endoscopic surveillance programs.

After an initial screening examination, follow-up intervals are typically every 1 to 2 years, depending on polyp burden, although some guidelines support every 3 years based on phenotypic and genotypic risk (see **Table 1**). At a minimum, all polyps larger than 5 mm should be removed at each endoscopy. In patients with a manageable polyp burden, surveillance colonoscopy is safe, and limited data suggest invasive CRC can be prevented through at least 5 years of adherent follow-up.[19] A relative indication for surgery is the presence of polyps that are no longer manageable endoscopically. Guidelines define small/manageable adenoma burden somewhat arbitrarily as fewer than 20 small (<6–10 mm) adenomas without advanced histology.[2–5] Furthermore, these guidelines do not apply to symptomatic patients, because immediate endoscopy and surgical referral is recommended in patients presenting with new rectal bleeding, anemia, or change in bowel habits.

Chromoendoscopy is performed by spraying a dye, commonly methylene blue or indigo carmine, onto the mucosa with the aim of increasing polyp detection and delineation of polyp borders. Although this significantly increases the detection of diminutive adenomas in patients with FAP, this technique is not routinely recommended because it is unlikely to dramatically change outcomes in an intensive FAP surveillance program.[20]

Attenuated Although the ESGE guidelines recommend similar management strategies for AFAP as for classic FAP, the ASGE and NCCN recommend starting screening in the later teenage years given that CRC seems to occur 1 to 2 decades later in AFAP.[2–4] Given the proximal nature of polyps in AFAP, colonoscopy is recommended,

Table 2 Recommendations for postsurgical colorectal cancer surveillance intervals			
	IRA	**IPAA**	**Ileostomy**
ASGE[4]	6–12 mo	1–2 y[a]	1–2 y
ESGE[3]	1–2 y	1–2 y	1–2 y
NCCN 2021[2]	6–12 mo	Annual[a]	Annual
UK[5]	Annual	Annual	Annual

[a] Shortened to every 6 months if large, flat polyps with villous histology and/or high-grade dysplasia.

at an interval of every 1 to 2 years. Prior studies suggest that endoscopic surveillance and polypectomy may delay or even prevent the need for surgery in individuals with AFAP and a manageable polyp burden.[8,12,21] However, the same surgical indications for FAP apply to the AFAP phenotype as well.

Postsurgery After colectomy, endoscopic surveillance is still required throughout the individual's lifetime. Adenomas can develop in the retained rectal cuff after ileorectal anastomosis (IRA), the anal transition zone, or ileal pouch after ileal pouch-anal anastomosis (IPAA), or in the stoma and neoterminal ileum after end ileostomy. Although the cumulative risk of rectal cancer in the retained rectal cuff after IRA may have been as high as 24% in the prepouch area, with careful patient selection the cancer risk after IRA is much lower and may be close to zero with ongoing surveillance.[22,23] In patients undergoing IPAA, subsequent cancer risk in the pouch is about 1%, with most (75%) cancers developing in the anal transition zone.[24] The cumulative risk for adenoma development in the pouch may be as high as 45% (including 12% with advanced histology), and ongoing endoscopic surveillance with polypectomy is recommended.[25]

Guidelines recommend endoscopic surveillance in accordance with the type of colectomy (**Table 2**).[2–5] More frequent surveillance is recommended after IRA, typically every 12 months, although intervals should be shortened to 6 months if large and/or advanced polyps are identified. Less frequent surveillance is recommended after IPAA or end ileostomy, although, again, intervals are shortened based on the presence of advanced endoscopic findings. At each examination, endoscopic evaluation should include a close examination of the anal transition zone, including the use of retroflexion. Management should include the removal of all polyps larger than 5 mm. Although robust data supporting endoscopic surveillance remain limited, available long-term observational studies suggest that the risk of advanced endoscopic findings, including cancer and need for subsequent surgery or treatment, remains low in patients adherent to surveillance.[22,26,27] Experts have reported that even dense rectal and pouch polyposis in postsurgical patients with FAP can be successfully managed with endoscopic polypectomy, with significantly reduced polyp burden and no cancer identified at follow-up.[28]

Duodenum and ampulla
Clinical characteristics. Premalignant lesions in the duodenum are extremely common in FAP. Studies indicate that duodenal polyposis occurs in 88% to 98% of patients, whereas duodenal cancer risk is estimated to be 18% by age 75 years.[29,30] Ampullary adenomas are less prevalent but are still found in 66% of patients with FAP, with the risk of periampullary cancer estimated to be 10% by age 60 years.[29,31] Therefore,

endoscopic screening and surveillance of the upper gastrointestinal (GI) tract is widely recommended by relevant clinical guidelines. This approach has been associated with improved outcomes, including a reduced need for surgical interventions.[30,32]

Endoscopic screening and surveillance

Duodenum. Current guidelines have small variations in their recommendations for age to initiate duodenal and ampullary endoscopic screening. The ASGE and NCCN recommend starting screening at age 20 to 25 years (with caveats to consider starting earlier if colectomy is planned per the ASGE, or if there is a family history of aggressive duodenal polyp burden or cancer per the NCCN).[2,4] The ESGE and UK guidelines suggest screening initiation at age 25 years.[3,5] Note that the colon phenotype does not affect these recommendations.

The Spigelman scoring system remains the backbone of all guidelines focused on endoscopic assessment and surveillance of the duodenal manifestations of FAP.[33] It uses duodenal polyp number, size, histology, and dysplasia grade to categorize patients into stages 0 to IV (**Table 3**). Some guidelines now use a slightly modified version that removes the pathology requirement and allows optical diagnosis of histology.[2–4] Although Spigelman staging has generally been found to perform well, malignancy may still occur without preceding advanced findings, and future optimization may be needed.[34,35]

In general, guidelines for surveillance based on Spigelman staging are largely consistent. The ASGE, ESGE, and UK guidelines all recommend a 5-year interval for stage 0 and I polyposis, a 3-year interval for stage II, at least annual endoscopy for stage III, and at least every 6 months with consideration of surgical therapy for stage IV (**Table 4**).[3–5] The NCCN recommendations have more aggressive recommendations, with an interval of 3 to 5 years for stage 0, 2 to 3 years for stage I, 1 to 2 years for stage II, 6 to 12 months for stage III, and every 3 to 6 months for stage IV.[2]

Ampulla Ampullary sampling was included in the original Spigelman and colleagues[33] surveillance protocol. However, most guidelines now recommend evaluation of ampullary findings separately when determining an appropriate surveillance

Table 3
Duodenal staging and surveillance intervals

	Spigelman Staging		
Points	1	2	2
Number of Duodenal Polyps	1–4	5–20	>20
Duodenal Polyp Size	1–4 mm	5–10 mm	>10 mm
Histology	Tubular	Tubulovillous	Villous
Degree of Dysplasia	Mild (low grade)	Moderate	Severe (high grade)

Stage	Total Points	Surveillance Interval
Stage 0	0	5 y
Stage I	1–4	5 y
Stage II	5–6	3 y
Stage III	7–8	6–12 mo
Stage IV	9–12	3–6 mo and surgical evaluation

Data from Refs.[4,33]

Table 4
Ampullary staging and surveillance intervals

Stage	Ampullary Assessment:	Surveillance Interval
Normal	Normal	5 y
Minor	Size<1 cm, tubular adenoma, and low-grade dysplasia	3 y
Major	Size>1 cm, any villous histology, or high-grade dysplasia	1 y and consideration of ampullectomy in an expert center

Data from Refs.[3,33]

interval or management strategy.[3,5] The grading system for ampullary adenomas proposed by Kashiwagi and colleagues[36] is commonly used and has 3 categories based on size and histology. The authors favor this approach, because there are endoscopic techniques for ampullectomy that are independent of duodenal disease burden.

Distinct recommendations for ampullary surveillance are included in the ESGE and UK guidelines. A surveillance interval of 5 years is recommended with a normal ampulla (in line with their recommendations for stage 0–I duodenal polyposis), 3 years for minor ampullary adenomas, and 1 year for major ampullary adenomas with large size or advanced histology (**Table 5**).[3,5]

Postsurgery Surveillance after surgery for duodenal polyposis is not standardized. Polyposis in residual duodenum after duodenectomy or in biliopancreatic and jejunal limbs after pancreatodoudenectomy is common.[37] The NCCN recommends annual surveillance after surgery for advanced duodenal polyposis or malignancy.[2] Although it is unclear whether this short interval is necessary on an ongoing basis, it is clear that continued monitoring through use of enteroscopy should be performed and intervals shorter than standard should be considered.

Similarly, surveillance after ampullectomy is not standardized. Recurrence of adenoma after endoscopic ampullectomy can be expected, especially if the lesion was larger than 1 cm.[38] A commonly used approach is a short, 3-month interval to ensure complete resection and then at least annual monitoring thereafter.

Endoscopic management

Duodenum Although all guidelines agree on endoscopic monitoring of the duodenum for the detection and staging of polyps, there is some disagreement on the optimal next step. The ASGE supports the resection of adenomatous polyps with the goal of downstaging disease in line with the standard clinical practice in the United States.[4] The ESGE are more conservative and only favor removal of adenomas larger than 1 cm because of concern for fibrosis with the frequent removal of smaller lesions, which may limit future endoscopic resection attempts of more clinically significant lesions.[3] Standard polypectomy techniques, including cold snaring and endoscopic mucosal resection, should be used, but care needs to be taken given the complexities of duodenal polyp resection. Alternatives to polypectomy, such as argon plasma coagulation and band ligation, have been suggested but are not widely used.

Chromoendoscopy has been shown to increase identification of duodenal adenomas and lead to higher Spigelman scores in a prospective tandem endoscopy study.[39] This technique is not yet widely endorsed or performed. Virtual chromoendoscopy, which is less cumbersome to use, also has shown potential and could be considered.[40] However, it remains unclear whether these techniques improve outcomes.

Table 5
Gastric polyp characteristics and recommended surveillance intervals

Histology	Size	Dysplasia	Surveillance Interval
Fundic gland polyps	<1 cm	None or low grade	3 y
	≥1 cm	None or low grade	6–12 mo
	Any size	High grade	3–6 mo and surgical evaluation
Tubular adenomas	<1 cm	Low grade	1 y
	≥1 cm	Low grade	6–12 mo
	Any size	High grade	3–6 mo and surgical evaluation
Pyloric gland adenomas	<1 cm	Low grade	1 y
	≥1 cm	Low grade	6–12 mo
	Any size	High grade	3–6 mo and surgical evaluation

Adapted from Mankaney G, Leone P, Cruise M, LaGuardia L, O'Malley M, Bhatt A, et al. Gastric cancer in FAP: a concerning rise in incidence. Fam Cancer. 2017;16(3):371-6.

Ampulla It is critical to adequately visualize the ampulla during upper endoscopy in FAP because this has been shown to dramatically increase the detection of neoplasia.[33] The traditional method is through use of a side-viewing duodenoscope. However, many endoscopists only rarely use this device. Recently, the use of a clear distal attachment cap on a standard forward-viewing gastroscope has been shown to allow complete visualization of the ampulla in almost all patients with FAP and was noninferior to the use of a duodenoscope in a randomized controlled trial (**Fig. 1**).[41] This option is attractive because it allows the use of a single gastroscope to assess the duodenum and ampulla and avoids the risk of passing a second, less familiar device. Evaluation of the ampulla can include biopsy, which has been shown to be safe, with a risk of pancreatitis less than 1%.[42] Current guidelines do not endorse routine biopsy, but there should be a low threshold to sample any endoscopically abnormal ampulla.[3,4]

Endoscopic ampullectomy should only be considered for adenomas larger than 1 cm or with advanced histology. Small ampullary adenomas in FAP generally follow a benign course and do not need resection.[43] Further, endoscopic ampullectomy carries a high rate of adverse events, with expert centers reporting complications in up to 41% of cases, and therefore should only be performed by experienced endoscopists.[32]

Endoscopic ultrasonography (EUS) has not consistently been found to be of benefit in the routine assessment of duodenal or ampullary adenomas.[44,45] However, if there is a concern for malignancy, then EUS can help determine depth of invasion and inform decisions regarding optimal surgical approach. Also of note, surgical resection is more favored than endoscopic resection if there is a concern for malignancy.

Stomach
Clinical characteristics. Gastric polyps are common in FAP. Fundic gland polyps (FGPs) are most common (reported in up to 88% of patients with FAP) and can be innumerable in the proximal stomach with antral sparing (**Fig. 2**).[46] FGPs are often found to harbor low-grade dysplasia, although this has not been shown to be a sign of progression.[47] High-grade dysplasia is found in less than 5% of patients with FGPs, whereas the development of adenocarcinoma from FGPs is exceedingly rare.[46,48]

Neoplastic polyps, such as tubular adenomas and pyloric gland adenomas, are less common than FGPs. They can be found in any segment of the stomach but are more

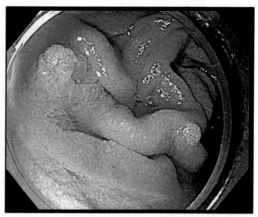

Fig. 1. A clear distal attachment cap is used to gain clear visualization of a small ampullary adenoma. Also noted is a diminutive duodenal adenoma.

common in the antrum.[4] One series from a large FAP registry reported 23% of patients with FAP with gastric tubular adenomas and 6% with pyloric gland adenomas. Proximal occurrences of these polyps mixed in with the many FGPs are thought to be related to an increasing incidence of gastric cancer.[49] A recent analysis of a large registry noted an increased gastric cancer incidence of 1.3% in patients with FAP, with a resultant standardized incidence ratio of 140 compared with the general population in the Surveillance, Epidemiology, and End Results (SEER) database.[50]

Despite this increasing incidence, there are no data showing a benefit to gastric screening and surveillance. Two recent series from large registries have noted that most gastric cancers were advanced at the time of diagnosis and had developed in the midst of active surveillance.[50,51] Thus, the prevention of gastric cancer in patients with FAP is an area of active research.

Endoscopic screening and surveillance. Most current guidelines do not have well-developed gastric cancer screening or surveillance recommendations. They favor incorporating gastric monitoring into the previously discussed duodenal protocols. Mankaney and colleagues[50] in 2017 proposed surveillance guidelines for patients with FAP with gastric polyps that have been adopted into clinical practice. They take into account the polyp number, size, histology, level of dysplasia, and presence of other high-risk features to determine surveillance intervals (see **Table 5**).[50]

Postsurgery If a partial gastrectomy is performed because of antral neoplasia or as part of another surgical procedure, then standard gastric surveillance recommendations should be continued for the residual stomach.

Endoscopic management. Typically, the great number of polyps in the fundus and body precludes complete endoscopic resection. The generally recommended strategy is to resect polyps 1 cm or larger as well as any polyps that appear concerning for advanced histology. Random sampling of the smaller, bland-appearing polyps by multiple biopsies or cold snare resections should also be performed.[4,46,50]

Criteria have been proposed by Mankaney and colleagues[52] to aid identification of high-risk polyps in the proximal stomach. A polyp can be classified as high risk if it includes 1 or more of the following features: lighter or darker shade than surrounding mucosa, open pit pattern, irregular surface, or a similar appearance on examination

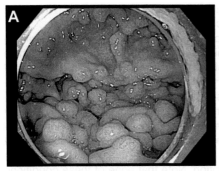 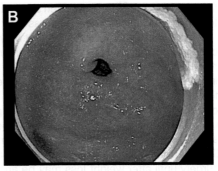

Fig. 2. Multiple FGPs visualized in the gastric body (*A*) of a patient with FAP with antral sparing (*B*).

with white light and virtual chromoendoscopy.[52] Resection or at least directed sampling should be performed on polyps with high-risk features, with plans for complete resection if high-risk pathologic findings are confirmed.

Additional features associated with the development of gastric cancer include mounding or carpeting of polyps in the proximal stomach.[49,51] These characteristics should be recognized as a marker of increased risk independent of histologic findings on biopsy. Mounding in particular may limit the accuracy of endoscopic surveillance. Further investigation with EUS and cross-sectional imaging has been recommended if this feature is noted, with consideration of gastrectomy if other high-risk characteristics are also present.[50]

Because adenomas predominate in the antrum, snare resection or endoscopic mucosal resection of all polyps in this location is recommended.[4] Although it is less investigated than in the duodenum, chromoendoscopy and virtual endoscopy may also hold promise for increased gastric adenoma detection.[39,40]

Distal small bowel

Jejunal and ileal adenomas may occur in FAP, but the occurrence of adenocarcinoma in the distal small bowel is exceedingly rare.[53] The benefit of small bowel screening distal to the proximal duodenum is unclear and it is not widely recommended. ASGE recommends capsule endoscopy or MRI enterography every 2 to 4 years in patients with Spigelman stage III or IV duodenal disease and before duodenectomy.[4] Other guidelines do not endorse small bowel screening because of the low rate of malignancy and the lack of evidence showing benefit to surveillance.

Surgical Management

Colon and rectum

Indications for surgery. Without intervention, the development of CRC in FAP is 100%, and thus surgical resection remains the cornerstone of treatment. Although surgery is inevitable, the timing of surgery should be determined after an individualized discussion. The primary goal of colorectal surgery in FAP is to mitigate cancer risk or less optimally treat cancer. Accordingly, the presence of cancer or significant colorectal symptoms such as bleeding are absolute indications for colectomy. Relative indications include increase in the number of polyps from one examination to the next, multiple polyps larger than 1 cm, and polyps with high-grade dysplasia. Cancer before age 20 years is extremely rare, and deferring surgery until the late teens, when patients are more physically, emotionally, and socially mature, is reasonable in the absence of these indications.[54] Patients often select a natural break or transition time in their lives to undergo elective surgery, such as after completing high school or college.

There are other circumstances that may be considered when discussing the timing of surgery. If a patient has a personal or family history of desmoid disease or is at high risk for developing desmoids, then a delay of surgery should be considered. Almost all intra-abdominal desmoids form after surgery, and thus the longer surgery can be deferred in these patients the lower this risk is. Pelvic surgery decreases female fecundity, and thus female patients who require proctocolectomy may wish to delay surgery until after their families are complete.[55] Obesity in patients with FAP is another circumstance worth mentioning. Particularly in men with a narrow pelvis, proctectomy and ileoanal pouch formation may be technically challenging and infeasible. Thus, delaying surgery until after weight loss may be an option. Note that none of these conditions present an absolute need for deferral, and the priority still remains mitigating CRC risk. Delaying surgery should only be done in asymptomatic patients that are motivated and complaint with surveillance protocols.

Surgical techniques In addition to the primary goal of cancer prevention, preserving and maximizing quality of life is important. The extent of resection relies on a balance of reducing future cancer risk while preserving bowel function and quality of life. Surgical options include total proctocolectomy (TPC) with restoration of GI tract via an IPAA or with end ileostomy; or total abdominal colectomy (TAC) with IRA, thus preserving the rectum. Note that any of these procedures can be done with minimally invasive approaches such as laparoscopy or robotic surgery. The first decision point between TPC and TAC is usually the polyp burden, with the main attention on the rectum.

Many surgeons have used the rule that the rectum can be maintained and surveyed if there are 20 adenomas or fewer in the rectum.[56] The need for future proctectomy in this situation was zero at median follow-up of 12 years in 1 study.[57] This finding is not absolute, and even rectums with higher numbers of polyps may be preserved with appropriate surveillance and polypectomy. A TAC-IRA may be considered in patients who might benefit from avoiding IPAA, including the conditions mentioned earlier. For example, recent data show that the risk of desmoid formation is less after TAC-IRA than TPC and IPAA.[58]

Total proctocolectomy is warranted in patients with profuse polyposis of the colon with more than 20 adenomas in the rectum. Obviously, the presence of rectal cancer also warrants a TPC. Some surgeons consider genotype in making decisions for a TPC, with *APC* mutations at codon 1309 and 1328 noted as independent risk factors for secondary proctectomy following TAC-IRA.[59] An IPAA may also be created after a TAC-IRA if the rectum develops unmanageable adenoma burden or rectal cancer. In this case, the IRA is disconnected, the rectum is removed, and an IPAA is created from the terminal ileum.

There is debate regarding the anal transition zone during TPC and IPAA with regard to performing a mucosectomy and handsewn anastomosis versus a stapled anastomosis, leaving a small anorectal cuff. A mucosectomy conceivably removes all at-risk mucosa, but 14% of patients still developed adenomas in the anal transition zone compared with 28% in the doubled-stapled group.[60] Mucosectomy has functional consequences, with higher incontinence and seepage rates compared with the stapled approach.[61] Thus, the authors favor a double-stapled approach as long as there is an area of anal transition zone that is free of polyposis.

Surgical considerations There are relative advantages and disadvantages of TAC-IRA and TPC. A TAC-IRA is less extensive and does not enter deep into the pelvis and thus takes less time, is associated with less complications, and does not affect fecundity or sexual or urinary function. It is usually done as a single operation and does not require a diverting stoma. The functional expectation is about 4 bowel movements per day and has an overall improved quality of life compared with an IPAA. The main disadvantage of a TAC-IRA is that the remaining rectum still requires annual surveillance and is at risk for developing subsequent neoplasia and cancer.

An IPAA is a more complex surgery and has a high rate of urinary and sexual dysfunction, causes decreased fecundity, and may result in some anal seepage or incontinence.[62,63] Patients have about 6 bowel movements daily. Even though the cancer risk is greatly reduced, neoplasia and cancer can still develop in the anal transition zone and within the ileal pouch, and annual surveillance is required. One other disadvantage of an IPAA is that the anastomosis is often covered with a temporary diverting ileostomy and thus the patient requires a second surgery to close it after 3 months.

A TPC and end ileostomy is rarely used but may be indicated for patients with rectal cancer involving the sphincter complex, patients with poor sphincter control, or patients that prefer an ileostomy to a pelvic pouch.

Duodenum and ampulla
Indications for surgery Duodenal and ampullary cancer and advanced neoplasia are commonly encountered in FAP. Patients with Spigelman stage III polyposis with severe dysplasia or stage IV classifications are recommended to undergo prophylactic surgical resection with either pancreas-sparing duodenectomy (PSD) or pancreato-duodenectomy (PD).[34,64,65] For patients diagnosed with invasive cancer, the choice of surgical approach remains unclear. However, radical resection with PD remains the standard approach.[66,67]

Surgical techniques There are multiple operative approaches with varying rates of organ preservation and associated morbidities for patients with duodenal manifestations of FAP. Complex resection requiring segmental duodenectomy (SD), PSD, or PD should be performed at high-volume centers with expertise in management of hereditary GI cancer syndromes.[68] In patients with single or low numbers of polyps in favorable intestinal distributions, duodenectomy with polypectomy or SD was previously performed.[69,70] Augustin and colleagues[69] reported SD even in patients with a distal duodenal/jejunal cancer diagnosis with negative margins and adequate lymph node assessment. However, this approach often results in high rates of recurrence, especially in patients with severe duodenal polyposis.[69,70] As such, SD is not recommended for proximal duodenal lesions but can be considered for distal duodenal or proximal jejunal lesions.

In patients with extensive periampullary involvement, a more extensive operation including PD or PSD is required.[65,69,71,72] Standard PD involves resection of the distal stomach, duodenum, head of the pancreas, gallbladder, and bile duct, with subsequent reconstruction entailing pancreatojejunostomy, choledochojejunostomy, and gastrojejunostomy. In contrast, PSD was first described by Chung and colleagues[74] with subsequent optimization by multiple groups.[65,69,71,73–75] The operation begins with the division of the distal jejunum beyond the ligament of Treitz (LOT). The mesentery of the bowel is then divided close to the mesenteric border working proximally to the duodenum. Cholecystectomy is performed and the cystic duct is then cannulated with a Fogarty catheter to appropriately localize the ampulla. Next, the proximal duodenum is transected just distal to the pylorus. The dissection of the ampullary complex is then performed. The complex is completely resected en bloc with any polypoid tissue extending to the bile duct or pancreatic duct. The ductal reconstruction is performed in a single-layer anastomosis between the common channel and the jejunum. In addition, end-to-side anastomosis with the very short segment of proximal duodenum and the jejunum, just distal to the pancreaticobiliary anastomosis, is performed to establish intestinal continuity.[65,71,74] Walsh and colleagues[65] revealed comparable results between PD and PSD for extensive polyposis. As such, PSD was established as a reasonable option for prophylactic resection for patients with high-risk features. However, the role of PD versus PSD in patients with preoperative diagnosis of invasive cancer remains unclear, particularly regarding adequate regional lymph node sampling. As such, PD remains the optimal choice for patients with invasive cancer diagnosis.

Surgical considerations SD, PSD, and PD are complex operations with associated significant morbidity. In the United States, the mortality following PD is less than 3%, with lower risk in high-volume centers. SD represents a less morbid approach, especially for patients with distal duodenal or jejunal involvement. Multiple studies examining PSD and PD revealed similar risks of postoperative complications, including pancreatic fistula, early pancreatitis, delayed gastric emptying, and surgical site infections.[65,70] Interestingly, examination of the long-term outcomes of PSD or PD revealed association of late acute pancreatitis with PSD (16% PSD vs 0% PD, $P = .012$) and of exocrine pancreatic insufficiency (11% PSD vs 30% PD, $P = .034$).[65]

Stomach
Indications for surgery Gastric cancer is an uncommon extracolonic manifestation of FAP, particularly outside Asia.[76] Prophylactic gastrectomy should be considered if there are polyps with high-grade dysplasia.[46,50,77] Gastrectomy is clearly indicated for intramucosal or invasive cancer.[50]

Surgical techniques The surgical approach for patients with FAP with high-risk gastric lesions or invasive cancer is a total gastrectomy with regional lymphadenectomy and intestinal reconstruction by either open or minimally invasive platform (laparoscopic vs robot assisted). The gastrectomy specimen should be intraoperatively confirmed for proximal margin with esophageal mucosa and distal margin with duodenal mucosa. The risk of regional lymph node metastasis in high-risk lesions in patients with FAP undergoing prophylactic gastrectomy is unclear. Roux-en-Y esophagojejunostomy is the most widely accepted reconstruction option following total gastrectomy.

Duodenal and ampullary surveillance remains critical in FAP, and Roux-en-Y reconstruction involves endoscopic access challenges. Recently, 2 reconstruction methods were described to better accommodate future endoscopic duodenal and ampullary surveillance. Zuin and colleagues[78] described an isoperistaltic jejunal loop interposition reconstruction. First, end-to-side esophagojejunostomy between the esophagus and the jejunal loop is established. The distal end of the jejunal loop was then anastomosed to the duodenum in an end-to-end fashion. The intestinal continuity below the LOT was restored with end-to-end jejunojejunostomy. The 2 patients who underwent this operation did not experience any early or late complications and experienced good short-term and long-term outcomes.[78] Otsuka and colleagues[79] described another intestinal restoration called double-tract reconstruction. The distal jejunal limb was directly brought up to the esophagus to establish end-to-side esophagojejunostomy. Next, a side-to-side jejunoduodenostomy was performed using a delta-shaped anastomosis (a technique developed for B1 reconstruction following distal gastrectomy), approximately 15 cm distal to the esophagojejunostomy. Last, a side-to-side jejunostomy was created 30 cm distal to the jejunoduodenostomy. All patients recovered well after some initial complications and underwent routine duodenal endoscopies without any difficulties.[79]

Surgical considerations Total gastrectomy is a major surgical intervention associated with significant morbidity and impact on health-related quality of life. In the United States, total gastrectomy is associated with 30-day mortality of approximately 5%, with lower rates observed in high-volume centers.[68,80,81] Postoperative complications, including anastomotic leak or dumping syndrome, can contribute to nutritional deficiencies requiring parenteral nutrition, prolonged hospital stay, and readmissions.[81] Ongoing duodenal and ampullary surveillance may become difficult because of the intestinal reconstruction from total gastrectomy, and these patients are at high risk of reoperation in the future, especially if the duodenum and ampulla are left intact at the time of gastrectomy.

SUMMARY

FAP is a commonly encountered hereditary cancer syndrome with extremely high risk of colon cancer as well as an increased risk of duodenal and ampullary cancer and an increasing risk for gastric cancer. Endoscopic and surgical management is complicated and is best performed in a specialized center with an experienced multidisciplinary team.

Endoscopic surveillance of the colon with timely colectomy significantly improves outcomes. CRC screening is generally recommended to start at age 10 to 12 years with colonoscopy every 1 to 2 years. Colectomy is indicated in the presence of cancer or significant colorectal symptoms, and relative indications include increasing number of polyps over serial examinations or the presence of large advanced polyps. After colectomy, endoscopic surveillance is still critical and should continue at least every 1 to 2 years (with some variation depending on what surgery was performed).

Duodenal, ampullary, and gastric screening is generally recommended with upper endoscopy with ampullary visualization starting at age 20 to 25 years. Ampullary visualization can be accomplished with a side-viewing duodenoscope or with the use of a clear-cap distal attachment. Surveillance intervals are generally determined by staging of duodenal polyposis, but guidelines are increasingly factoring in ampullary and gastric manifestations. Although advanced duodenal adenomas should be removed endoscopically when possible, the management of smaller polyps is debated. Endoscopic ampullectomy should only be considered when larger than 1 cm or with advanced histology. Close inspection and sampling of gastric polyps is needed with resection or biopsy of any polyps with suspicious features. Surgical management of advanced duodenal, ampullary, and gastric manifestations may also be needed, and there are multiple surgical options.

CLINICS CARE POINTS

- Ampullary visualization is crucial during upper endoscopies and can be accomplished with use of a clear-cap distal attachment or a side-viewing duodenoscope
- Endoscopic ampullectomy should only be considered for adenomas larger than 1 cm or with advanced histology
- Gastric cancer risk is increasing, and close inspection and sampling of gastric polyps is needed with resection or biopsy of any polyps with suspicious features
- Mounding or carpeting of polyps in the proximal stomach is a marker of increased risk for gastric cancer and should lead to more sampling of these areas

DISCLOSURES

P.P.S. receives research support from Emtora Biosciences, Freenome Holdings Inc, Janssen Pharmaceuticals Inc., Pfizer Inc., and the PTEN Research foundation. B.S. reports support from Exact Sciences, which is outside the submitted work. A.C.K. has no disclosures. M.F.K. has no disclosures.

REFERENCES

1. Nieuwenhuis MH, Vasen HF. Correlations between mutation site in APC and phenotype of familial adenomatous polyposis (FAP): a review of the literature. Crit Rev Oncol Hematol 2007;61(2):153–61.
2. National Comprehensive Cancer Network. Genetic/familial high-risk assessment: colorectal version 1.2021. Available at: https://www.nccn.org/professionals/physician_gls/pdf/genetics_colon.pdf. Accessed May 22, 2021.
3. van Leerdam ME, Roos VH, van Hooft JE, et al. Endoscopic management of polyposis syndromes: European Society of Gastrointestinal Endoscopy (ESGE) Guideline. Endoscopy 2019;51(9):877–95.
4. Yang J, Gurudu SR, Koptiuch C, et al. American Society for Gastrointestinal Endoscopy guideline on the role of endoscopy in familial adenomatous polyposis syndromes. Gastrointest Endosc 2020;91(5):963–82.e2.
5. Monahan KJ, Bradshaw N, Dolwani S, et al. Guidelines for the management of hereditary colorectal cancer from the British Society of Gastroenterology (BSG)/ Association of Coloproctology of Great Britain and Ireland (ACPGBI)/United Kingdom Cancer Genetics Group (UKCGG). Gut 2020;69(3):411–44.
6. Jasperson KW, Patel SG, Ahnen DJ. APC-associated polyposis conditions. In: Adam MP, Ardinger HH, Pagon RA, et al, editors. GeneReviews(®). Seattle (WA): University of Washington, Seattle; 1993.
7. Bussey HJR. Familial polyposis coli: family studies, histopathology, differential diagnosis, and results of treatment. Baltimore: Johns Hopkins University Press; 1975.
8. Burt RW, Leppert MF, Slattery ML, et al. Genetic testing and phenotype in a large kindred with attenuated familial adenomatous polyposis. Gastroenterology 2004; 127(2):444–51.
9. Galiatsatos P, Foulkes WD. Familial adenomatous polyposis. Am J Gastroenterol 2006;101(2):385–98.
10. Neklason DW, Stevens J, Boucher KM, et al. American founder mutation for attenuated familial adenomatous polyposis. Clin Gastroenterol Hepatol 2008;6(1): 46–52.
11. Giardiello FM, Brensinger JD, Petersen GM, et al. The use and interpretation of commercial APC gene testing for familial adenomatous polyposis. N Engl J Med 1997;336(12):823–7.
12. Knudsen AL, Bülow S, Tomlinson I, et al. Attenuated familial adenomatous polyposis: results from an international collaborative study. Colorectal Dis 2010;12(10 Online):e243–9.
13. Karstensen JG, Burisch J, Pommergaard HC, et al. Colorectal Cancer in Individuals With Familial Adenomatous Polyposis, Based on Analysis of the Danish Polyposis Registry. Clin Gastroenterol Hepatol 2019;17(11):2294–300.e1.
14. Bülow S, Bülow C, Nielsen TF, et al. Centralized registration, prophylactic examination, and treatment results in improved prognosis in familial adenomatous polyposis. Results from the Danish Polyposis Register. Scand J Gastroenterol 1995; 30(10):989–93.

15. Barrow P, Khan M, Lalloo F, et al. Systematic review of the impact of registration and screening on colorectal cancer incidence and mortality in familial adenomatous polyposis and Lynch syndrome. Br J Surg 2013;100(13):1719–31.
16. Kennedy RD, Potter DD, Moir CR, et al. The natural history of familial adenomatous polyposis syndrome: a 24 year review of a single center experience in screening, diagnosis, and outcomes. J Pediatr Surg 2014;49(1):82–6.
17. Vasen HFA, Möslein G, Alonso A, et al. Guidelines for the clinical management of familial adenomatous polyposis (FAP). Gut 2008;57(5):704–13.
18. Giardiello FM, Krush AJ, Petersen GM, et al. Phenotypic variability of familial adenomatous polyposis in 11 unrelated families with identical APC gene mutation. Gastroenterology 1994;106(6):1542–7.
19. Ishikawa H, Mutoh M, Iwama T, et al. Endoscopic management of familial adenomatous polyposis in patients refusing colectomy. Endoscopy 2016;48(1):51–5.
20. Matsumoto T, Esaki M, Fujisawa R, et al. Chromoendoscopy, narrow-band imaging colonoscopy, and autofluorescence colonoscopy for detection of diminutive colorectal neoplasia in familial adenomatous polyposis. Dis Colon Rectum 2009;52(6).
21. Kinney AY, Hicken B, Simonsen SE, et al. Colorectal cancer surveillance behaviors among members of typical and attenuated FAP families. Am J Gastroenterol 2007;102(1):153–62.
22. Church J, Burke C, McGannon E, et al. Risk of rectal cancer in patients after colectomy and ileorectal anastomosis for familial adenomatous polyposis. Dis Colon Rectum 2003;46(9):1175–81.
23. Koskenvuo L, Renkonen-Sinisalo L, Järvinen HJ, et al. Risk of cancer and secondary proctectomy after colectomy and ileorectal anastomosis in familial adenomatous polyposis. Int J Colorectal Dis 2014;29(2):225–30.
24. Smith JC, Schäffer MW, Ballard BR, et al. Adenocarcinomas after prophylactic surgery for familial adenomatous polyposis. J Cancer Ther 2013;4(1):260–70.
25. Friederich P, de Jong AE, Mathus–Vliegen LM, et al. Risk of developing adenomas and carcinomas in the ileal pouch in patients with familial adenomatous polyposis. Clin Gastroenterol Hepatol 2008;6(11):1237–42.
26. Gleeson FC, Papachristou GI, Riegert-Johnson DL, et al. Progression to advanced neoplasia is infrequent in post colectomy familial adenomatous polyposis patients under endoscopic surveillance. Fam Cancer 2009;8(1):33–8.
27. Saurin JC, Napoleon B, Gay G, et al. Endoscopic management of patients with familial adenomatous polyposis (FAP) following a colectomy. Endoscopy 2005;37(5):499–501.
28. Patel NJ, Ponugoti PL, Rex DK. Cold snare polypectomy effectively reduces polyp burden in familial adenomatous polyposis. Endosc Int Open 2016;4(4):E472–4.
29. Bjork J, Akerbrant H, Iselius L, et al. Periampullary adenomas and adenocarcinomas in familial adenomatous polyposis: cumulative risks and APC gene mutations. Gastroenterology 2001;121(5):1127–35.
30. Bulow S, Christensen IJ, Hojen H, et al. Duodenal surveillance improves the prognosis after duodenal cancer in familial adenomatous polyposis. Colorectal Dis 2012;14(8):947–52.
31. Burke CA, Beck GJ, Church JM, et al. The natural history of untreated duodenal and ampullary adenomas in patients with familial adenomatous polyposis followed in an endoscopic surveillance program. Gastrointest Endosc 1999;49(3 Pt 1):358–64.

32. Roos VH, Bastiaansen BA, Kallenberg FGJ, et al. Endoscopic management of duodenal adenomas in patients with familial adenomatous polyposis. Gastrointest Endosc 2021;93(2):457–66.
33. Spigelman AD, Williams CB, Talbot IC, et al. Upper gastrointestinal cancer in patients with familial adenomatous polyposis. Lancet 1989;2(8666):783–5.
34. Groves CJ, Saunders BP, Spigelman AD, et al. Duodenal cancer in patients with familial adenomatous polyposis (FAP): results of a 10 year prospective study. Gut 2002;50(5):636.
35. Thiruvengadam SS, Lopez R, O'Malley M, et al. Spigelman stage IV duodenal polyposis does not precede most duodenal cancer cases in patients with familial adenomatous polyposis. Gastrointest Endosc 2019;89(2):345–354 e2.
36. Kashiwagi H, Spigelman AD, Debinski HS, et al. Surveillance of ampullary adenomas in familial adenomatous polyposis. Lancet 1994;344(8936):1582.
37. Yoon JY, Mehta N, Burke CA, et al. The prevalence and significance of jejunal and duodenal bulb polyposis after duodenectomy in familial adenomatous polyposis: retrospective cohort study. Ann Surg 2019.
38. Ma T, Jang EJ, Zukerberg LR, et al. Recurrences are common after endoscopic ampullectomy for adenoma in the familial adenomatous polyposis (FAP) syndrome. Surg Endosc 2014;28(8):2349–56.
39. Huneburg R, Heling D, Kaczmarek DJ, et al. Dye chromoendoscopy leads to a higher adenoma detection in the duodenum and stomach in patients with familial adenomatous polyposis. Endosc Int Open 2020;8(10):E1308–14.
40. Lami G, Galli A, Macri G, et al. Gastric and duodenal polyps in familial adenomatous polyposis patients: conventional endoscopy vs virtual chromoendoscopy (fujinon intelligent color enhancement) in dysplasia evaluation. World J Clin Oncol 2017;8(2):168–77.
41. Abdelhafez M, Phillip V, Hapfelmeier A, et al. Comparison of cap-assisted endoscopy vs. side-viewing endoscopy for examination of the major duodenal papilla: a randomized, controlled, noninferiority crossover study. Endoscopy 2019;51(5):419–26.
42. Mehta NA, Shah RS, Yoon J, et al. Risks, benefits, and effects on management for biopsy of the papilla in patients with familial adenomatous polyposis. Clin Gastroenterol Hepatol 2021;19(4):760–7.
43. Matsumoto T, Iida M, Nakamura S, et al. Natural history of ampullary adenoma in familial adenomatous polyposis: reconfirmation of benign nature during extended surveillance. Am J Gastroenterol 2000;95(6):1557–62.
44. Gluck N, Strul H, Rozner G, et al. Endoscopy and EUS are key for effective surveillance and management of duodenal adenomas in familial adenomatous polyposis. Gastrointest Endosc 2015;81(4):960–6.
45. Labib PL, Goodchild G, Turbett JP, et al. Endoscopic ultrasound in the assessment of advanced duodenal adenomatosis in familial adenomatous polyposis. BMJ Open Gastroenterol 2019;6(1):e000336.
46. Bianchi LK, Burke CA, Bennett AE, et al. Fundic gland polyp dysplasia is common in familial adenomatous polyposis. Clin Gastroenterol Hepatol 2008;6(2):180–5.
47. Arnason T, Liang WY, Alfaro E, et al. Morphology and natural history of familial adenomatous polyposis-associated dysplastic fundic gland polyps. Histopathology 2014;65(3):353–62.
48. Hofgartner WT, Thorp M, Ramus MW, et al. Gastric adenocarcinoma associated with fundic gland polyps in a patient with attenuated familial adenomatous polyposis. Am J Gastroenterol 1999;94(8):2275–81.

49. Leone PJ, Mankaney G, Sarvapelli S, et al. Endoscopic and histologic features associated with gastric cancer in familial adenomatous polyposis. Gastrointest Endosc 2019;89(5):961–8.
50. Mankaney G, Leone P, Cruise M, et al. Gastric cancer in FAP: a concerning rise in incidence. Fam Cancer 2017;16(3):371–6.
51. Walton SJ, Frayling IM, Clark SK, et al. Gastric tumours in FAP. Fam Cancer 2017; 16(3):363–9.
52. Mankaney GN, Cruise M, Sarvepalli S, et al. Surveillance for pathology associated with cancer on endoscopy (SPACE): criteria to identify high-risk gastric polyps in familial adenomatous polyposis. Gastrointest Endosc 2020;92(3): 755–62.
53. Ruys AT, Alderlieste YA, Gouma DJ, et al. Jejunal cancer in patients with familial adenomatous polyposis. Clin Gastroenterol Hepatol 2010;8(8):731–3.
54. Church JM, McGannon E, Burke C, et al. Teenagers with familial adenomatous polyposis: what is their risk for colorectal cancer? Dis Colon Rectum 2002; 45(7):887–9.
55. Olsen KO, Juul S, Bulow S, et al. Female fecundity before and after operation for familial adenomatous polyposis. Br J Surg 2003;90(2):227–31.
56. Warrier SK, Kalady MF. Familial adenomatous polyposis: challenges and pitfalls of surgical treatment. Clin Colon Rectal Surg 2012;25(2):83–9.
57. Church J, Burke C, McGannon E, et al. Predicting polyposis severity by proctoscopy: how reliable is it? Dis Colon Rectum 2001;44(9):1249–54.
58. Sommavilla J, Liska D, Kalady M, et al. Ileal pouch-anal anastomosis is more "desmoidogenic" than ileorectal anastomosis in familial adenomatous polyposis. Dis Colon Rectum 2021. in press.
59. Wu JS, Paul P, McGannon EA, et al. APC genotype, polyp number, and surgical options in familial adenomatous polyposis. Ann Surg 1998;227(1):57–62.
60. Remzi FH, Church JM, Bast J, et al. Mucosectomy vs. stapled ileal pouch-anal anastomosis in patients with familial adenomatous polyposis: functional outcome and neoplasia control. Dis Colon Rectum 2001;44(11):1590–6.
61. Lovegrove RE, Constantinides VA, Heriot AG, et al. A comparison of hand-sewn versus stapled ileal pouch anal anastomosis (IPAA) following proctocolectomy: a meta-analysis of 4183 patients. Ann Surg 2006;244(1):18–26.
62. Bulow S, Bulow C, Vasen H, et al. Colectomy and ileorectal anastomosis is still an option for selected patients with familial adenomatous polyposis. Dis Colon Rectum 2008;51(9):1318–23.
63. Slors FJ, van Zuijlen PP, van Dijk GJ. Sexual and bladder dysfunction after total mesorectal excision for benign diseases. Scand J Gastroenterol Suppl 2000;(232):48–51.
64. Campos FG, Sulbaran M, Safatle-Ribeiro AV, et al. Duodenal adenoma surveillance in patients with familial adenomatous polyposis. World J Gastrointest Endosc 2015;7(10):950–9.
65. Walsh RM, Augustin T, Aleassa EM, et al. Comparison of pancreas-sparing duodenectomy (PSD) and pancreatoduodenectomy (PD) for the management of duodenal polyposis syndromes. Surgery 2019;166(4):496–502.
66. Komori S, Kawai M, Nitta T, et al. A case of carcinoma of the papilla of Vater in a young man after subtotal colectomy for familial adenomatous polyposis. World J Surg Oncol 2016;14(1):47.
67. Sabol M, Donat R, Kajo K, et al. Ampullary cancer in a patient with familial adenomatous polyposis – a rare case report and current status of management. Bratislava Med J 2019;120(12):908–11.

68. Mamidanna R, Ni Z, Anderson O, et al. Surgeon volume and cancer esophagectomy, gastrectomy, and pancreatectomy. Ann Surg 2016;263(4):727–32.
69. Augustin T, Moslim MA, Tang A, et al. Tailored surgical treatment of duodenal polyposis in familial adenomatous polyposis syndrome. Surgery 2018;163(3):594–9.
70. Brosens LAA, Keller JJ, Offerhaus GJA, et al. Prevention and management of duodenal polyps in familial adenomatous polyposis. Gut 2005;54(7):1034.
71. Mackey R, Walsh RM, Chung R, et al. Pancreas-sparing duodenectomy is effective management for familial adenomatous polyposis. J Gastrointest Surg 2005;9(8):1088–93.
72. Naples R, Simon R, Moslim M, et al. Long-term outcomes of pancreas-sparing duodenectomy for duodenal polyposis in familial adenomatous polyposis syndrome. J Gastrointest Surg 2020;1–8.
73. de Castro SMM, van Eijck CHJ, Rutten JP, et al. Pancreas-preserving total duodenectomy versus standard pancreatoduodenectomy for patients with familial adenomatous polyposis and polyps in the duodenum. Br J Surg 2008;95(11):1380–6.
74. Chung RS, Church JM, vanStolk R. Pancreas-sparing duodenectomy: indications, surgical technique, and results. Surgery 1995;117(3):254–9.
75. van Heumen BWH, Nieuwenhuis MH, van Goor H, et al. Surgical management for advanced duodenal adenomatosis and duodenal cancer in Dutch patients with familial adenomatous polyposis: a nationwide retrospective cohort study. Surgery 2012;151(5):681–90.
76. Offerhaus GJA, Giardiello FM, Krush AJ, et al. The risk of upper gastrointestinal cancer in familial adenomatous polyposis. Gastroenterology 1992;102(6):1980–2.
77. Ravoire A, Faivre L, Degrolard-Courcet E, et al. Gastric adenocarcinoma in familial adenomatous polyposis can occur without previous lesions. J Gastrointest Cancer 2014;45(3):377–9.
78. Zuin M, Celotto F, Pucciarelli S, et al. Isoperistaltic jejunal loop interposition after total gastrectomy for gastric cancer in patients with familial adenomatous polyposis. J Gastric Cancer 2020;20(2):225.
79. Otsuka R, Hayashi H, Hanari N, et al. Laparoscopic double-tract reconstruction after total gastrectomy for postoperative duodenal surveillance: case series. Ann Med Surg 2017;21:105–8.
80. Martin AN, Das D, Turrentine FE, et al. Morbidity and Mortality After Gastrectomy: Identification of Modifiable Risk Factors. J Gastrointest Surg 2016;20(9):1554–64.
81. Tran TB, Worhunsky DJ, Squires MH, et al. To Roux or not to Roux: a comparison between Roux-en-Y and Billroth II reconstruction following partial gastrectomy for gastric cancer. Gastric Cancer 2016;19(3):994–1001.

Chemoprevention Considerations in Patients with Hereditary Colorectal Cancer Syndromes

Check for updates

Carole Macaron, MD[a], Gautam N. Mankaney, MD[b],
Mahnur Haider, MD[c], Mohamad Mouchli, MD[a,d],
Karen Hurley, PhD[e], Carol A. Burke, MD[a,f],*

KEYWORDS

- Chemoprevention • Hereditary colon cancer syndromes
- Familial adenomatous polyposis • Lynch syndrome
- Hamartomatous polyposis syndromes

KEY POINTS

- Nonsteroidal anti-inflammatory medications are the most widely studied chemoprevention agents in hereditary colorectal cancer syndromes, although novel agents influencing non-COX pathways are being evaluated in human trials.
- Chemoprevention has been shown to be efficacious for colorectal polyposis and duodenal polyposis in patients with familial adenomatous polyposis and for cancer reduction in Lynch syndrome.
- Chemoprevention can be considered for use in select patients as an adjunct to standard of care in patients with hereditary gastrointestinal cancer syndromes.
- The goals, risks, and benefits of chemoprevention therapy should be carefully considered before embarking on their clinical use.

[a] Department of Gastroenterology, Hepatology and Nutrition, Desk A 30, 9500 Euclid Avenue, Cleveland, OH 44195, USA; [b] Department of Gastroenterology and Hepatology, Virginia Mason Franciscan Health, 1100 9th Avenue, Seattle, WA 98101, USA; [c] John W. Deming Department of Medicine, Tulane University School of Medicine, 1430 Tulane Avenue, #8016, New Orleans, LA 70112, USA; [d] Department of Gastroenterology, Hepatology, and Nutrition, Digestive Disease and Surgical Institute, Cleveland Clinic, Cleveland, OH, USA; [e] Center for Behavioral Health, Desk P57, 9500 Euclid Avenue, Cleveland, OH 44195, USA; [f] Department of Colorectal Surgery, Sanford R. Weiss MD Center for Hereditary Gastrointestinal Neoplasia, Digestive Disease and Surgical Institute, Cleveland Clinic, Cleveland, OH, USA
* Corresponding author. Department of Gastroenterology, Hepatology and Nutrition, Desk A-30, 9500 Euclid Avenue, Cleveland, OH 44195.
E-mail address: burkec1@ccf.org

Gastrointest Endoscopy Clin N Am 32 (2022) 131–146
https://doi.org/10.1016/j.giec.2021.08.005
1052-5157/22/© 2021 Elsevier Inc. All rights reserved.

giendo.theclinics.com

INTRODUCTION

Hereditary colorectal cancer syndromes (HCCS) are associated with benign and malignant tumors within and outside of the intestinal tract (**Table 1**). Their onset occurs in childhood or young adult life, and in familial adenomatous polyposis (FAP), will lead to colorectal cancer (CRC) unless colectomy is performed.[1] Endoscopic management, often beginning at a young age, is standard, although surgery may be required. Disease reduction with chemoprevention in HCCS targets enzymatic pathways of carcinogenesis (**Table 2**) and is an area of investigation. Chemoprevention use outside of a clinical trial requires appropriate patient selection (**Table 3**), establishment of treatment goals, and knowledge of the efficacy and safety of the agent.

FAMILIAL ADENOMATOUS POLYPOSIS

Most chemoprevention research in FAP has focused on inhibition of the cyclooxygenase (COX) pathway through the use of nonsteroidal anti-inflammatory medications (NSAIDs) with adenoma reduction as the clinical end point. Although some agents have shown success in preventing or reducing adenomas in the intestinal tract, none reduce the incidence of or mortality from cancer. Major cancer risks in FAP include the colorectum, duodenum, stomach, and thyroid. Desmoid tumors, although nonneoplastic, contribute to significant morbidity and mortality in FAP and may impact surgical approaches to disease management. Effective chemoprevention has the potential to mitigate the impact of FAP directly through reduced disease manifestations or symptom burden (eg, pain) and/or indirectly by averting or postponing surgery. Life-altering surgeries figure prominently in the management of FAP and can thwart attainment of important life goals in education, work, relationships, and family.[2] Delaying surgery by polyp control may be particularly important in adolescents and young adults who are still in the process of defining and establishing goals that will be central to their identities.[3]

Colorectal Polyposis

Colorectal polyposis control has been the primary target of most chemoprevention studies in FAP because CRC is the greatest health threat to these patients.

Early trials assessed the efficacy of chemoprevention by the impact on findings on flexible sigmoidoscopy (FS) rather than colonoscopy. One of the first randomized controlled trials (RCT) was a 9-month study of 22 participants with rectosigmoid polyps (18 of whom had not previously undergone colon surgery) assessing the efficacy of sulindac, a nonspecific COX inhibitor, at a dose of 150 mg twice daily compared with placebo.[4] Significant reductions in both polyp number (by 44%) and diameter (by 35%) were observed in the sulindac arm. Notably, 3 months after sulindac discontinuation, the size and number of polyps increased but was still lower than at baseline. No side effects were attributed to sulindac, but the investigators stated that sulindac is unlikely to replace colectomy as primary therapy for colorectal polyposis. Another placebo-controlled RCT assessed the utility of sulindac for the prevention of rectosigmoid polyp development over 4 years in 41 young individuals with a pathogenic variant (PV) in *APC* and no polyps on baseline FS.[5] Sulindac was dosed at 75 mg or 150 mg twice daily based on weight. No significant difference in polyp occurrence was noted between the study arms. Importantly, 11 patients (27%) were withdrawn from the study for polyposis progression, 6 in the sulindac and 5 in the placebo arm. Of 34 patients completing at least 40 months of treatment, the mean number and size of adenomas in the sulindac and placebo arms were 5.9 versus 7.5 and 0.70 mm versus 1.2 mm, respectively. Adverse events did not differ significantly

Table 1
Hereditary colorectal cancer syndromes, associated genes, and frequent clinical features

Syndrome	Genes	Features
Lynch syndrome	MLH1, MSH2, MSH6, PMS2, EPCAM	Colorectal, gynecologic, urothelial, brain, gastric, small bowel, skin carcinoma
Familial adenomatous polyposis	APC	Colorectal, gastric and duodenal adenomas; colorectal, duodenal, gastric, thyroid, and brain cancers; osteomas; Congenital Hypertrophy of the Retinal Pigment Epithelium (CHRPE); soft tissue tumors; desmoid tumors
MutYH-associated polyposis	MUTYH	Colorectal and duodenal adenomas; colorectal, duodenal, thyroid cancer; desmoid tumors
NTHL1-associated polyposis	NTHL1*	Colorectal and duodenal adenomas; breast, endometrial, urothelial, brain, and colorectal cancers
Polymerase proofreading associated polyposis	POLE, POLD1	Colorectal adenomas; endometrial, colorectal, and brain cancers
Peutz-Jeghers syndrome	STK11	Mucocutaneous pigmentation, panintestinal hamartomatous polyps, breast, gastric, small bowel, colorectal, pancreatic, lung, and gynecologic/testicular cancers
PTEN hamartoma tumor syndrome	PTEN	Panintestinal hamartomatous polyps, esophageal glycogen acanthosis, skin lesions, macrocephaly, breast, thyroid, renal, endometrial, and colorectal cancers
Juvenile polyposis syndrome	BMPR1A, SMAD4	Gastric and colorectal hamartomatous polyposis, gastric and colon cancer; SMAD4: hereditary hemorrhagic telangiectasia overlap syndrome

Table 2
Molecular targets for chemoprevention in hereditary colorectal cancer syndromes

Medication	Classification
Sulindac	Nonselective COX inhibitor
Celecoxib	Selective COX-2 inhibitor
Rofecoxib	Selective COX-2 inhibitor
Aspirin	Nonselective COX inhibitor
Eicosapentaenoic acid	Anti-inflammatory
Difluoromethylornithine	Ornithine decarboxylase inhibitor
Rapamycin/sirolimus/everolimus	mTOR inhibitor
Erlotinib	EGFR inhibitor
Guselkumab	Immune modulation
Erlotinib-sulindac	
Rapamycin/sirolimus	
Frameshift peptide vaccines	
Nivolumab and other checkpoint inhibitors	

Abbreviations: COX, cyclooxygenase; EGFR, epidermal growth factor receptor; mTOR, mammalian target of rapamycin.

between the arms, and sulindac was reported to be well tolerated. Mucosal prostaglandin and thromboxane B2 levels were significantly lower than baseline in the sulindac arm at the end of treatment.

A 6-month RCT of celecoxib, a selective COX-2 inhibitor, at 400 mg, 100 mg, or placebo, twice daily demonstrated a significantly reduced number of colorectal polyps (by 28%) and burden (by 31%) on colonoscopy in the 400-mg arm, compared with reductions of 4.5% and 4.9% in the placebo arm.[6] No significant difference was noted between the placebo and celecoxib 100-mg arm. Both celecoxib doses were reported to be well tolerated, and adverse event did not differ between the celecoxib groups and the placebo group. In 1999, under US Food and Drug Administration (FDA)

Table 3
Potential benefits of chemoprevention in patients with hereditary colorectal cancer syndromes

FAP	LS	Hamartomatous Polyposis Syndromes
Delay colectomy • Children and young adults • Desmoid prone individuals	Decrease cancer risk • Colorectal • Endometrial	Decrease extraintestinal manifestations • Soft tissue • Vascular • Neurologic
Prevent or delay duodenectomy • Individuals with advanced-stage duodenal polyposis		Modulate polyposis burden • Gastric • Small bowel • Colorectal
Prevent secondary surgery • Individuals with advanced-stage rectal or pouch polyposis		Decrease symptoms from polyposis and improve quality of life • Protein losing enteropathy • Gastrointestinal bleeding • Diarrhea

Abbreviation: LS, Lynch syndrome.

accelerated approval regulations, 21 CFR part 314, subpart H, celecoxib was approved at 400 mg twice daily as an adjunct to endoscopy for colorectal polyposis in adults with FAP. In 2011, the study sponsor voluntarily withdrew the FAP indication for celecoxib because the FDA required a postmarketing study as a condition of approval under subpart H, which was not completed as planned.

In a phase 1, 3-month, dose escalation trial of celecoxib in 18 children aged 10 to 14 years, no clinically meaningful differences in adverse events were seen between placebo and the 3 weight-based celecoxib doses.[7] Compared with baseline, the end of treatment number of polyps increased by 39% in the placebo arm, whereas a significant reduction of 44% was observed in the highest dose group, 16 mg/kg/ d, which corresponds to the adult dose of 400 mg twice daily. A 5-year, international, pediatric, placebo-controlled RCT designed to study the effectiveness of 16 mg/kg/ d of celecoxib in reducing the progression of colorectal polyposis defined as the occurrence of 20 or more polyps, more than 2 mm in size after excision of all baseline colorectal polyps greater than 2 mm in size, was performed.[8] The trial was halted due to low enrollment. Of the 106 children randomized, the number of patients with progression of polyposis (12.7% vs 25.5%) and the time to progression (2 vs 1.1 years) favored the celecoxib group.

A previously available selective COX-2 inhibitor, rofecoxib, showed promise in a series of 8 Israeli patients treated with 25 mg daily for a mean of 16 months.[9] The drug was well tolerated without significant adverse events, and the rate of polyp formation was lowered between 70% and 100% versus baseline polyp counts. The same dose of rofecoxib was studied in a 9-month, placebo-controlled, RCT in 21 Japanese adults.[10] A significant reduction in both the number and size of polyps was observed in the rofecoxib arm without differences in adverse events between treatment arms.

Aspirin irreversibly inhibits both COX-1 and COX-2 isoenzymes. The impact of aspirin at 600 mg/d with or without resistant starch at 30 g/d versus placebo on the number of rectosigmoid polyps was evaluated in an international RCT in children and young adults between ages 10 and 21 years in the Colorectal Adenoma/Carcinoma Prevention Programme (CAPP) 1 study.[11] Of the 206 randomized patients 33 had at least 1 follow-up annual endoscopy and were included in the primary analysis. At a median of 17 months of treatment no significant reduction in the number of polyps was noted in any arm. A trend for a smaller mean size of the largest polyp, 3.8 mm versus 5.5 mm, was observed in patients who were treated for 1 or more year in the aspirin versus nonaspirin arms, and 3 mm versus 6 mm for patients treated for more than 1 year. The investigators posit that the effect of aspirin may be on disease progression rather than on inhibition of initiation. No serious adverse events were noted in the trial participants.

Aspirin 100 mg daily, mesalazine 2 g daily, or both together were compared versus placebo in an 8-month RCT of 104 Japanese patients aged 16 to 70 years with intact colons.[12] Polyps 5 mm or more in size were removed at baseline colonoscopy. The primary end point was the proportion of patients with polyps 5 mm or more at the end of treatment. Thirty percent of patients exposed to aspirin versus 50% of patients not on aspirin met the end point (for an adjusted odds ratio of 0.37 [95% confidence interval [CI],0.16 to 0.86]). No benefit was seen with mesalazine. No serious drug-related adverse events occurred, and grade 1 to 2 upper gastrointestinal symptoms were seen in 12% of patients who received aspirin plus mesalazine, and in 4% of those who received aspirin or mesalazine.

Levels of polyamines and the key enzyme that regulates their production, ornithine decarboxylase (ODC), are elevated in polyps in patients with FAP.[13]

Diflouromethylornithine (DFMO), also known as eflornithine, is an irreversible inhibitor of ODC and has been studied in combination with other agents in FAP to assess for any synergistic effect.

In a 6-month RCT the effect of DMFO (at a dose of 0.5 g/m^2/d rounded down to the nearest 250 mg) plus celecoxib 400 mg twice daily versus celecoxib alone on the number of adenomas in a defined area in the intact colon or rectum (in patients with prior colectomy) was compared in 112 adults with FAP.[14] No significant difference in the polyp count (−13.0% for celecoxib + DFMO vs −1.0% for celecoxib, P = .69) or secondarily in polyp burden (−40% for celecoxib + DFMO vs −27% for celecoxib, P = .13) was demonstrated. The video-based, blinded, assessment of global polyp change favored combination therapy (−0.80 vs −0.33, P = .03) over celecoxib alone. No DFMO-related ototoxicity, adverse cardiovascular outcomes, or significant increase in adverse events in the combination arm was noted. The investigators attributed the lack of added benefit with DMFO to the low baseline burden of polyps and use of still images to capture the primary end point, which were hard to standardize between examinations and may have inaccurately represented true disease burden.

A recent international RCT in 171 adult patients compared eflornithine 750 mg daily in combination with sulindac 150 mg daily to either agent alone on first FAP-related disease progression in the duodenum, in intact colon, or in the postcolectomy rectum or ileal pouch.[15] Patients were stratified on the basis of polyp burden and surgical status (precolectomy, rectal or ileal pouch polyposis, or duodenal polyposis). Disease progression was defined as need for surgery, advanced adenoma requiring excision by endoscopy, the occurrence of high-grade dysplasia, or duodenal polyposis stage progression. No difference was noted for the primarily end point or in adverse events between study arms. In the preplanned secondary efficacy analysis stratified by subgroup, disease progression in patients with an intact colon occurred in 17%, 46%, and 42% (for a hazard ratio [HR], 0.30; 95% CI, 0.07–1.32 for combination vs sulindac, and HR, 0.20; 95% CI, 0.03–1.32 for combination vs eflornithine). The mean time to progression was 39.3 months (95% CI, 37.1–41.6), 25.2 months (95% CI, 24.2–26.1), and 19.7 months (95% CI, 18.2–21.1) in the combination, sulindac, and eflornithine arms, respectively. No differences were noted in the secondary analysis in the postcolectomy or duodenal polyposis arms. The results of combination treatment in the 37 patients in the precolectomy arm are compelling, and additional trials in this population are warranted.

Adenomatous Polyposis Coli (APC) inactivation and epidermal growth factor receptor (EGFR) signaling promotes COX expression and intestinal polyps. Murine models of FAP demonstrated that a combination of sulindac and an EGFR inhibitor decreased intestinal adenomas by 87%.[16] In a prespecified secondary analysis[17] of a single-center, 6-month RCT of 92 adult patients with FAP comparing sulindac 150 mg twice daily plus erlotinib 75 mg daily versus placebo on duodenal polyposis,[18] the change in number of polyps in the intact colorectum, ileal pouch, and rectum was assessed.[17] Eighty-two patients had lower gastrointestinal data available. The number of polyps was significantly lower in the sulindac-erlotinib compared with placebo arm in patients with an intact colon (−69.4% [95% CI, −28.8%–109.2%]) and an ileal pouch (−121.7% [95% CI, −280% to −71.6%]). No difference was noted between arms in patients with an ileorectal anastomosis. Grade 2 and 3 adverse events were reported twice as common in the treatment than (44%) in the placebo group (22%). Most common was an erlotinib-induced acneiformlike rash, which occurred in 68% of the treatment group and 22% of the placebo group (P<.001). Rash treatment included topical cortisone and/or clindamycin. Although the effectiveness of the combination was shown, the toxicity as demonstrated in this trial limits its clinical potential in FAP at doses studied.

Foods or plant derivatives have also been studied in patients with FAP. The minimal side effect profile of naturally occurring compounds provides an advantage if effective for chemoprophylaxis and safe. Curcumin and quercetin are plant-derived polyphenols with antioxidant and anti-inflammatory properties. The effectiveness of a combination of both compounds at a dose of 480 mg and 20 mg both 3 times daily, respectively, for 6 months was studied in 5 adults postcolectomy and showed a significant decrease in the number (60.4%) and size of polyps (50.9%).[19] In a follow-up trial, 44 adults with an intact colon, ileorectal anastomosis, or ileal anal pouch, and 5 or more polyps, were randomized to curcumin 1.5 g twice per day or placebo for 12 months. The primary outcome was the number of polyps on FS. In contrast to the pilot study, no significant difference in the number or size of polyps was observed.[20]

Limited data suggest that long-term use of ascorbic acid, an antioxidant, induces regression of rectal adenomas in FAP. In a single-center RCT, 49 patients with an ileorectal anastomosis received 3 g/d ascorbic acid or placebo; 36 patients were evaluable. Over 18 months, a significant reduction in the number of polyps as assessed by 3 monthly sigmoidoscopies was noted in the ascorbic acid group at 9 months only versus in the placebo group.[21] A trial randomized 58 patients to 4 g/d of ascorbic acid plus 400 mg of alpha-tocopherol per day, a wheat fiber supplement at 22.5 g/d, or placebo.[22] No effect on rectal polyps was noted in any treatment arm.

Eicosapentaenoic acid (EPA), an omega-3 polyunsaturated fatty acid, has been shown to have antineoplastic activity in a 6-month RCT, of 55 European adults with a history of ileorectal anastomosis and at least 3 rectal polyps.[23] Treatment included EPA free fatty acid at 2 g daily or placebo, and the primary end point was the number of polyps in a tattooed area in the rectum. Secondary end points included the sum of the polyp diameters in the photographed area and global rectal polyp burden score by blinded video review. EPA resulted in a significant decrease in all parameters with a 22.4% reduction in polyp number compared with placebo wherein all parameters worsened. Currently, a phase 3, multicenter, 2-year, European RCT study is underway to determine whether EPA-FFA can reduce the number of rectal polypectomies compared with placebo in adults with FAP and previous colectomy with ileorectal anastomosis.

Black raspberries (BRBs) contain multiple compounds including calcium; vitamins A, C, and E; selenium; folic acid; quercetin; b-sitosterol; ellagic acid; ferulic acid; and anthocyanins. These substances have demonstrated chemopreventive activity in vitro and in murine models of FAP. In a phase 1b study, 14 adult patients with at least 5, 2-mm rectal polyps were treated with BRB suppositories (each containing 720 mg BRB powder) administered at bedtime and randomized to either 20 g of BRB placebo powder administered orally as a slurry (60 g/d total) or 20 g of placebo BRB powder slurry 3 times daily for 9 months.[24] A reduction in rectal polyp number (-3.5, $P = .069$) and burden (-8.5, $P = .036$) was observed. No additional benefit was noted on adenoma end points in patients randomized to oral BRB powder. BRBs significantly decreased proliferation, DNA methylation methyl transferase 1 protein expression, and p16 promoter methylation in adenomas from responders but not from the 3 nonresponders.

Agents with novel mechanisms of controlling polyposis in FAP are being studied. In murine models of FAP, the mechanistic target of rapamycin (mTORC1) pathway is activated and is associated with an increased expression of mTOR protein in intestinal polyps, whereas inhibition of the mTOR pathway has been shown to decrease mTOR activity and suppress both the number and size of polyps, and prolong mouse survival.[25]

The effect of the mTOR inhibition by sirolimus, a rapalogue of rapamycin, on rectal or pouch polyps was reported in a case series of 4 adult patients with InSiGHT Polyposis Stage 3.[26] Sirolimus was initiated at a dose of 2 mg once daily and adjusted to achieve a target sirolimus blood level range of 5 to 8 µg/L; 18 adverse events, related to both drug dose and blood level, with toxicity grades 1 to 3 were noted, and 1 patient withdrew due to adverse events. The size of 5 marked polyps decreased in 80% of polyps evaluated. An increase in apoptosis and decrease in proliferation was seen in 3 of 4 patients. The investigators suggested that sirolimus was promising for polyposis in the rectal remnant and ileal pouch but associated with numerous adverse events likely due to the narrow therapeutic window of classical mTOR inhibitors. A new formulation of rapamycin with drug particles embedded in a pH-sensitive methacrylic acid copolymer (eRapa) was found to produce consistent blood concentrations in a phase Ib trial of men with low-grade prostate cancer undergoing surveillance.[27] At present, a phase IIa, dose escalation, 12-month trial with eRapa is underway in the United States to assess the safety and effect of eRapa on colorectal polyp burden in patients with FAP.

Inflammatory features associated with activation of the interleukin (IL) 23/IL-17/JAK/STAT3 pathway have been demonstrated in polyps from patients with FAP and linked to growth and progression of CRC. An FDA-approved human monoclonal antibody known as guselkumab that inhibits IL-23-specific intracellular signaling and downstream pathways is currently being evaluated in a 24-week, placebo-controlled RCT to determine if monthly administration of subcutaneous guselkumab can reduce polyp burden in the duodenum, rectum or ileal pouch.

Duodenal Polyposis

Duodenal polyposis affects nearly 100% of patients with FAP, and advanced-stage duodenal polyposis may require duodenectomy to prevent duodenal cancer. Duodenal cancer is a leading cause of cancer and cancer deaths in patients with FAP once colectomy has been performed. The duodenum with its intimate association with the pancreatic-biliary duct complex and associated organs make duodenectomy a technically demanding surgery associated with substantial morbidity. Studies on extracolonic risk management and quality of life after duodenal surgery[28,29] are sparse, but one recent report on pancreatico-duodenectomy (PD) in patients who had previously undergone IPAA for FAP provides evidence that avoidance of PD through management of adenomas may confer clear benefits.[29] Results of that study showed that one-quarter of the patients undergoing PD developed diabetes, with a resulting drop in quality-of-life scores. Therefore, there is a compelling need for chemoprevention in the duodenum.

Sulindac has not convincingly been shown to reduce duodenal polyposis. In an RCT, 24 patients with Spigelman stage III or IV duodenal polyposis received either sulindac 200 mg twice daily or placebo for 6 months.[30] No difference in polyposis was noted between arms by blinded review of pretreatment and posttreatment videotape recordings. Duodenal mucosal epithelial cell proliferation was significantly reduced in patients in the sulindac arm. In a secondary analysis of this trial, a significantly greater number of patients exposed to sulindac versus placebo had regression of duodenal polyps less than 3 mm (9 of 11, 82% vs 2 of 11, 38%) and fewer new polyps (2 of 11, 18%, vs 5 of 12, 42%).[31]

In a 6-month RCT, celecoxib, when compared with placebo, led to an improvement of duodenal polyposis as assessed by blinded video review at a dose of 400 mg twice daily ($P = .03$), but no effect was noted at 100 mg twice daily.[32] Compared with patients on placebo, those on celecoxib 400 mg twice daily had a 14.5% reduction in the involved duodenum versus 1.4% ($P = .436$), and in a subanalysis those with greater than 5% of the duodenum covered by polyps at baseline showed a 31% reduction in involved areas compared with 8% on placebo ($P = .049$). Baseline or end-of-treatment polyp characteristics such as polyp size, number, and Spigelman stage were not reported.

FAP mouse models have shown a pronounced effect of sulindac in combination with erlotinib, an inhibitor of EGFR tyrosine kinase activity on duodenal polyps. In a single-center, 6-month RCT, the combination of erlotinib 75 mg daily with sulindac 150 mg twice daily was compared with placebo and reduced the duodenal polyp burden (19 mm between-group difference, $P<.001$) and number of polyps (8 mm between-group difference, $P<.001$).[18] Adverse events were more common in patients in the combination versus the placebo arm including an acneiformlike rash (87% vs 20%, $P<.001$) managed with topical cortisone and/or clindamycin therapy. Notably, 73% of patients in the combination arm required erlotinib dose reduction versus 28% in the placebo arm. Results are pending from an open-label study in the United States using erlotinib 350 mg once weekly on duodenal polyp burden in FAP.

The RCT comparing eflornithine 750 mg daily in combination with sulindac 150 mg daily, to either agent alone, on FAP-related disease progression demonstrated an increase in Spigelman stage or excision of duodenal polyps in 27% (15 of 56) in the combination arm, 19% (11 of 58) in the sulindac arm, and 21% (12 of 57) in the eflornithine arm without obvious benefit on duodenal polyposis in any of the study arms.[15]

LYNCH SYNDROME

Lynch syndrome (LS) the commonest hereditary cause of CRC is the genesis of 3% to 5% of CRC[33] and 10% of endometrial cancer (EC) in women younger than 50 years.[34] Colonoscopy and polypectomy reduce CRC incidence and mortality in LS.[35,36] Despite recommended surveillance colonoscopy every 1 to 2 years in LS,[37] a recent study showed that CRC occurred in 8.4% at 10 years and was independent of whether colonoscopy was performed at 1- to 3-year intervals.[38] The heightened cancer risk and accelerated CRC pathway make LS an attractive target for chemoprevention.

Colorectal Neoplasia

The RCT, CAPP-2 randomized 861 individuals with LS to aspirin 600 mg/d, resistant starch 30 mg/d, or both.[39] After a mean treatment of 25 months, no difference in the incidence of adenoma or CRC was observed between arms. In longer-term follow-up, resistant starch had no effect on CRC incidence,[40] but over 10 years of observation, patients who received aspirin for 2 years had a substantial reduction in CRC (HR, 0.65; 95% CI, 0.43–0.97) with a relatively low-risk safety profile.[41] The aspirin effect was apparent after 5 years of initiating aspirin and sustained for up to 20 years. This "legacy effect"[42] suggests that initiating aspirin for at least 2 years in younger patients, when the risk of aspirin-related adverse effects such as major bleeding are less common, may be more effective and safer than incepting it in older patients. A subgroup analysis of CAPP-2 identified obesity as an independent risk factor for CRC, which was mitigated with aspirin,[43] suggesting that aspirin might be most beneficial in obese patients with LS. An RCT, "CAPP-3," is underway to assess the efficacy of 100 mg, 300 mg, or 600 mg of daily aspirin on CRC incidence. Based on current evidence, guidelines suggest consideration of aspirin for CRC prevention in LS, but the optimal dose is unknown.[37,44]

Observational data in LS showed an association between CRC risk and use of aspirin and/or ibuprofen (HR, 0.41; 0.28–0.61), multivitamins (HR, 0.55; 0.40–0.75), or calcium (HR, 0.46; 0.30–0.71) compared with nonusers, and appeared stronger for longer duration of exposure.[45,46]

The impact of NSAIDs on biomarkers in LS was tested in a 4-week study in 22 patients with LS or meeting the Amsterdam criteria and found that sulindac 150 mg twice daily increased proximal, but not distal, colon epithelial cell proliferation and had no effect on apoptosis compared with placebo.[47] A phase Ib, 6-month study randomized 80 patients with LS and Lynch-like syndrome to daily naproxen 220 mg versus 440 mg versus placebo and found no difference in adverse events between arms.[48] Mucosal prostaglandin E_2 levels were significantly reduced with naproxen compared with placebo. Naproxen downregulated genes in cell cycle dynamics and upregulated immune genes with a dose-dependent effect, thus playing a role in the activation of the immune system of the colorectum. A phase 1, nonrandomized trial of atorvastatin 20 mg with or without aspirin 325 mg is currently underway to assess any synergistic effects of these agents on colorectal biomarkers in LS.

Preclinical studies suggest an association between tumor neoantigens and the immune microenvironment in the DNA mismatch repair (MMR)-deficient adenoma-carcinoma pathway.[49] These findings are key to understanding why tumor vaccines or immune checkpoint inhibitors may work in LS. MMR-deficient crypts seem to be the earliest epithelial abnormality identified in colorectal mucosa in LS. MMR-deficient cells generate immunogenic frameshift peptide (FSP) neoantigens and can elicit host immune responses.[50] Checkpoint blockade therapies targeting PD-1/PD-L1 are highly effective for treatment of advanced MMR-deficient CRC[51] and are being studied as immunopreventive agents in LS. A phase 2, 3-month, study of nivolumab in adults with LS and a personal history of advanced neoplasia will assess its impact on the incidence of adenomas, LS-related cancers, and biomarkers of immunologic activity. Vaccines are a promising strategy in LS, and work has shown strong immunogenicity in animal models.[52] A phase 1/2a study of an FSP vaccine was conducted in 22 patients with advanced MMR-deficient CRC.[53] Of 19 analyzed patients, all showed FSP-specific immune humoral and cellular immune responses after vaccination. Three patients had grade 2 local injection site reactions, and no severe adverse events occurred. Another phase 1/2 vaccine study is underway testing frameshift-derived neoantigen-loaded dendritic cells in patients with LS.

Endometrial Cancer

Little data on chemoprevention on non-CRC in LS are available. Epidemiologic studies have shown that progestin-containing contraceptive pills reduce EC in average risk women. A phase 2 biomarker study of progestin-containing OCP or depo-medroxyprogesterone acetate (depoMPA) demonstrated that both agents significantly decreased endometrial epithelial proliferation and induced microscopic endometrial changes characteristic of progestin effect after 3 months of treatment in 51 women with LS or hereditary non-polyposis colorectal cancer (HNPCC).[54] The long-term CAPP-2 results noted a trend toward fewer EC among women in the aspirin than placebo arm (HR, 0.50; 95% CI, 0·22–1·11).[41] Findings from both studies suggest benefit in EC but warrant further study in LS.

Hamartomatous Polyposis Syndromes

The phosphatase and tensin homolog (PTEN) hamartoma tumor syndrome, Peutz-Jeghers syndrome (PJS), and juvenile polyposis syndrome (JPS) are rare intestinal hamartomatous polyposis syndromes associated with benign and malignant intestinal and extraintestinal cancers. Cancers develop through hamartoma-carcinoma pathway or transformation of the adjacent epithelium of the abnormal stromal environment.[55] Data on chemoprevention are limited in these syndromes.

Patients with a PV in *PTEN* have abnormal PI3K-AKT-mTOR signaling, and targeting P13K, AKT1, mTOR, or PDK1 could be a means for chemoprevention.[56] The mTOR inhibitor sirolimus was found to regress mucocutaneous lesions in mice with *PTEN* gene deletion[57] and, in case reports in children, to attenuate abdominal lipomatosis and thymus volume,[58] soft tissue vascular lesions in forearm,[59] and hamartomas of the chest, mediastinum, abdomen, and pelvis.[60]

An open-label study with sirolimus 2 mg daily for 56 days in 18 patients with *PTEN* PVs showed regression of gastrointestinal and skin lesions with favorable modulation of mTOR pathways on immunohistochemistry, improved cerebellar function, and was well tolerated.[61] An open-label, 12-month, 10-patient study of sirolimus 2 mg daily on colorectal polyposis is underway in individuals with a PV in *PTEN*.

The intestinal hamartomatous polyposis syndromes PJS, due to a germline PV in *STK11* (also known as *LKB1*), and JPS, due to PVs in either *BMRPR1A* or *SMAD4*, are associated with increased risks of CRC and gastric cancer, and in the case of PJS, breast, pancreas, lung, gonadal, and gynecologic cancers.

Polyps in patients with PJS and in LKB1 knockout mice models have elevated COX-2 levels.[62,63] Initiation of celecoxib before and after the development of polyposis led to a reduction in murine tumor burden and vascularity of polyps.[63] Celecoxib 400 mg daily was administered to 8 patients with PJS for 6 months to determine the effects on gastric polyps. Based on video recordings from EGDs, 2 of 6 patients had a significant reduction in gastric polyps at end of treatment.[63]

LKB1 is a serine/threonine protein kinase with mTOR as its major downstream effector. Sirolimus also has been shown to decrease polyp size and vascularity and tumor burden in murine models of PJS.[64,65] An open-label, phase 2,12-month study of the mTOR inhibitor everolimus at 10 mg daily to assess its effect on large gastrointestinal polyps was terminated before completion. Three patients completed therapy, and all developed stomatitis causing dose reductions, but no other serious adverse events were noted. Unfortunately, there was insufficient polyp burden to draw any conclusions.[66] At present, a trial assessing the safety and efficacy of sirolimus in decreasing polyp burden in children and adults with PJS is enrolling.

No chemoprevention studies in JPS exist. Juvenile polyposis of infancy (JPI) caused by the combined loss of function of *PTEN* and *BMPR1A* presents in the first 2 years of life and has a severe phenotype characterized by gastrointestinal bleeding, diarrhea, protein-losing enteropathy, and early mortality. Sirolimus has been shown successful in case reports in patients with JPI in improving gastrointestinal bleeding, protein-losing enteropathy, patient growth, and reducing intestinal polyp burden.[67,68]

A multicenter cohort of 25 patients with JPI at mean age of 13 months reported the effect of mTOR inhibition on adverse events, disease progression, time to colectomy, and mortality in 7 patients compared with children who received standard-of-care treatment.[69] The risk of colectomy (HR, 0.27; 95% CI, 0.07–0.95), change in serum albumin (mean increase = 16.3 g/L), and hemoglobin (mean increase = 2.68 g/dL), and mortality (0% vs 22%) favored the sirolimus group. The investigators report that mTOR inhibitor therapy was well tolerated over a follow-up of 30 patient-years, and no serious adverse events were reported.

SUMMARY

No chemoprevention agents for the HCCS are FDA approved. A variety of studies demonstrate modest efficacy of NSAIDs including sulindac, selective COX-2 inhibitors, and aspirin on reducing colorectal polyps in adults with FAP and preventing CRC in LS. Celecoxib regresses colorectal polyposis in children and may have a modest effect in duodenal polyposis in adults. Combination chemoprevention holds promise for more effectiveness than single agents for polyposis, but daily erlotinib and sulindac benefits occur at the expense of toxicity. RCT data for nutraceutical benefit exist only for EPA in FAP. The mTOR pathway seems important in polyposis because animal models and descriptive studies using mTOR inhibitors have suggested benefit and more RCT evidence is being generated. Immunopreventative strategies may prove highly effective in LS. The long-term durability and safety of many agents is unknown and will not substitute for endoscopic and surgical management of HCCS.

CLINICS CARE POINTS

- There are no FDA-approved agents for chemoprevention for patients with HCCS.
- Chemoprevention use for patients with HCCS is adjunctive to standard of care, including endoscopy and surgery.
- Chemoprevention may blunt polyposis burden and progression in familial adenomatous polyposis and the typical endoscopic features of polyps.
- Chemopreventive agents have toxicity, and the long-term benefit and risk of chemoprevention is unknown.

AUTHOR CONTRIBUTIONS

C.A. Burke: concept, design, drafting, critical revision, final approval, and accountability for work; C. Macaron, G.N. Mankaney, M. Haider, M. Mouchli, K. Hurley: drafting, critical revision, final approval, and accountability for work.

REFERENCES

1. Attard TT, Burke CA, Hyer W, et al. ACG clinical report and recommendations on transition of care in children and adolescents with hereditary polyposis syndromes. Am J Gastroenterol 2021;116:638–46.
2. Duncan R, Gillam L, Savulescu J, et al. "You're one of us now": young people describe their experiences of predictive genetic testing for huntington disease (hd) and familial adenomatous polyposis (FAP). Am J Med Genet C Semin Med Genet 2008;148C:47–55.
3. Schulenberg J, Bryant A, O'Malley P. Taking hold of some kind of life: how developmental tasks relate to trajectories of well-being during the transition to adulthood. Dev Psychopathol 2004;16:1119–40.
4. Giardiello FM, Hamilton SR, Krush AJ, et al. Treatment of colonic and rectal adenomas with sulindac in familial adenomatous polyposis. N Engl J Med 1993; 328(18):1313–6.
5. Giardiello FM, Yang VW, Hylind LM, et al. Primary chemoprevention of familial adenomatous polyposis with sulindac. N Engl J Med 2002;346:1054–9.
6. Steinbach G, Lynch PM, Phillips RKS, et al. The effect of celecoxib, a cyclooxygenase-2 inhibitor, in familial adenomatous polyposis. N Engl J Med 2000;342:1946–52.
7. Lynch PM, Ayers GD, Hawk E, et al. The safety and efficacy of celecoxib in children with familial adenomatous polyposis. Am J Gastroenterol 2010;105:1437–43.

8. Burke CA, Phillips R, Berger MF, et al. Children's International Polyposis (CHIP) study: a randomized, double-blind, placebo-controlled study of celecoxib in children with familial adenomatous polyposis. Clin Exp Gastroenterol 2017;10: 177–85.

9. Hallak A, Alon-Baron L, Shamir R, et al. Rofecoxib reduces polyp recurrence in familial polyposis. Dig Dis Sci 2003;48(10):1998–2002.

10. Higuchi T, Iwama T, Toyooka KYM, et al. A randomized, double-blind, placebo-controlled trial of the effects of rofecoxib, a selective cyclooxygenase-2 inhibitor, on rectal polyps in familial adenomatous polyposis patients. Clin Cancer Res 2003;9(13):4756–60.

11. Burn J, Bishop DT, Chapman PD, et al. A randomized placebo-controlled prevention trial of aspirin and/or resistant starch in young people with familial adenomatous polyposis. Cancer Prev Res 2011;4(5):655–65.

12. Ishikawa H, Mutoh M, Sato Y, et al. Chemoprevention with low-dose aspirin, mesalazine, or both in patients with familial adenomatous polyposis without previous colectomy (J-FAPP Study IV): a multicentre, double-blind, randomised, two-by-two factorial design trial. Lancet Gastroenterol Hepatol 2021;6:474–81.

13. Kemp Bohan PM, Mankaney G, Vreeland TJ, et al. Chemoprevention in familial adenomatous polyposis: past, present and future. Fam Cancer 2021;20(1): 23–33.

14. Lynch PM, Burke CA, Phillips R, et al. An international randomised trial of celecoxib versus celecoxib plus difluoromethylornithine in patients with familial adenomatous polyposis. Gut 2016;65:286–95.

15. Burke CA, Dekker E, Lynch P, et al. Eflornithine plus sulindac for prevention of progression in familial adenomatous polyposis. N Engl J Med 2020;383(11): 1028–39.

16. Roberts RB, Min L, Washington MK, et al. Importance of epidermal growth factor receptor signaling in establishment of adenomas and maintenance of carcinomas during intestinal tumorigenesis. Proc Natl Acad Sci U S A 2002;99(3): 1521–6.

17. Samadder NJ, Kuwada SK, Bouche KM, et al. Association of sulindac and erlotinib vs placebo with colorectal neoplasia in familial adenomatous polyposis secondary analysis of a randomized clinical trial. JAMA Oncol 2018;4(5):671–7.

18. Samadder NJ, Neklason DW, Boucher KM, et al. Effect of sulindac and erlotinib vs placebo on duodenal neoplasia in familial adenomatouspolyposis: a randomized clinical trial. JAMA 2016;315(12):1266–75.

19. Cruz-Correa M, Shoskes DA, Sanchez P, et al. Combination treatment with curcumin and quercetin of adenomas in familial adenomatous polyposis. Clin Gastroenterol Hepatol 2006;4(8):1035–8.

20. Cruz-Correa M, Hylind LM, Hernandez Marrero J, et al. Efficacy and safety of curcumin in treatment of intestinal adenomas in patients with familial adenomatous polyposis. Gastroenterology 2018;155(3):668–73.

21. Bussey HJR, DeCosse JJ, Deschnera EE, et al. Randomized trial of ascorbic acid in polyposis coli. Cancer 1982;50:1434–9.

22. DeCosse JJ, Miller HH, Lesser ML. Effect of wheat fiber and vitamins C and E on rectal polyps in patients with familial adenomatous polyposis. J Natl Cancer Inst 1989;81(17):1290–7.

23. West NJ, Clark SK, Phillips RK, et al. Eicosapentaenoic acid reduces rectal polyp number and size in familial adenomatous polyposis. Gut 2010;59(7):918–25.

24. Wang L-S, Burke CA, Hasson H, et al. A Phase Ib study of the effects of black raspberries on rectal polyps in patients with familial adenomatous polyposis. Cancer Prev Res 2014;7(7):666–74.
25. Parihar M, Dodds SG, Hubbard G, et al. Rapamycin extends life span in Apc Min/ + colon cancer FAP Model. Clin Colorectal Cancer 2021;20(1):e61–70.
26. Roos VH, Meijer BJ, Kallenberg FGJ, et al. Sirolimus for the treatment of polyposis of the rectal remnant and ileal pouch in four patients with familial adenomatous polyposis: a pilot study. BMJ Open Gastro 2020;7:e000497.
27. Kemp Bohan PM, Chick RC, O'Shea AE, et al. Phase I trial of encapsulated rapamycin in patients with prostate cancer under active surveillance to prevent progression. Cancer Prev Res (Phila) 2021;14(5):551–62.
28. Ganschow P, Hackert T, Biegler M, et al. Post-operative outcome and quality of life after surgery for FAP-associated duodenal polyposis. Langenbecks Arch Surg 2018;403:93–102.
29. Collard M, Lefevre J, Ahmed O, et al. Ten-year impact of pancreaticoduodenectomy on bowel function and quality of life of patients with ileal pouch-anal anastomosis for familial adenomatous polyposis. HPB (Oxford) 2020;22:1402–10.
30. Nugent KP, Farmer KC, Spigelman AD, et al. Randomized controlled trial of the effect of sulindac on duodenal and rectal polyposis and cell proliferation in patients with familial adenomatous polyposis. Br J Surg 1993;80(12):1618–9.
31. Debinski HS, Trojan J, Nugent KP, et al. Effect of sulindac on small polyps in familial adenomatous polyposis. Lancet 1995;345(8953):855–6.
32. Phillips RK, Wallace MH, Lynch PM, et al. A randomised, double blind, placebo controlled study of celecoxib, a selective cyclooxygenase 2 inhibitor, on duodenal polyposis in familial adenomatous polyposis. Gut 2002;50(6):857–60.
33. Hampel H, Frankel WL, Martin E, et al. Feasibility of screening for Lynch syndrome among patients with colorectal cancer. J Clin Oncol 2008;26(35):5783–8.
34. Lu KH, Schorge JO, Rodabaugh KJ, et al. Prospective determination of prevalence of lynch syndrome in young women with endometrial cancer. J Clin Oncol 2007;25(33):5158–64.
35. Järvinen HJ, Aarnio M, Mustonen H, et al. Controlled 15-year trial on screening for colorectal cancer in families with hereditary nonpolyposis colorectal cancer. Gastroenterology 2000;118(5):829–34.
36. de Jong AE, Hendriks YM, Kleibeuker JH, et al. Decrease in mortality in Lynch syndrome families because of surveillance. Gastroenterology 2006;130(3): 665–71.
37. NCCN Guidelines Version 1.2020 genetic/familial high-risk assessment: colorectal NCCN guidelines version 1.2020 genetic/familial high-risk assessment: colorectal NCCN guidelines index table of contents discussion NCCN guidelines panel disclosures continue. Available at: https://www.nccn.org/professionals/physician_gls/pdf/genetics_colon.pdf. Accessed September 10, 2021.
38. Engel C, Vasen HF, Seppälä T, et al. No difference in colorectal cancer incidence or stage at detection by colonoscopy among 3 countries with different lynch syndrome surveillance policies. Gastroenterology 2018;155:1400–9.
39. Burn J, Bishop DT, Mecklin J-P, et al. Effect of aspirin or resistant starch on colorectal neoplasia in the lynch syndrome. N Engl J Med 2008;359(24):2567–78.
40. Mathers JC, Movahedi M, Macrae F, et al. Long-term effect of resistant starch on cancer risk in carriers of hereditary colorectal cancer: an analysis from the CAPP2 randomised controlled trial. Lancet Oncol 2012;13(12):1242–9.
41. Burn J, Sheth H, Elliott F, et al. Cancer prevention with aspirin in hereditary colorectal cancer (Lynch Syndrome), 10-year follow-up and registry-based 20-year

data in the CAPP2 study: a double-blind, randomised, placebo-controlled trial. Lancet 2020;395:1855–63.
42. Yurgelun MB, Chan AT. Aspirin for Lynch syndrome: a legacy of prevention. Lancet 2020;395(10240):1817–8.
43. Movahedi M, Bishop DT, Macrae F, et al. Obesity, aspirin, and risk of colorectal cancer in carriers of hereditary colorectal cancer: a prospective investigation in the CAPP2 study. J Clin Oncol 2015;33(31):3591–7.
44. Monahan KJ, Bradshaw N, Dolwani S, et al. Guidelines for the management of hereditary colorectal cancer from the British Society of Gastroenterology (BSG)/ Association of Coloproctology of Great Britain and Ireland (ACPGBI)/United Kingdom Cancer Genetics Group (UKCGG). Gut 2020;69(3):411–44.
45. Ait Ouakrim DA, Dashti SG, Chau R, et al. Aspirin, ibuprofen, and the risk for colorectal cancer in lynch syndrome. J Natl Cancer Inst 2015;107(9):djv170.
46. Chau R, Dashti SG, Ait Ouakrim D, et al. Multivitamin, calcium and folic acid supplements and the risk of colorectal cancer in Lynch syndrome. Int J Epidemiol 2016;45:940–53.
47. Rijcken FEM, Hollema H, van der Zee AGJ, et al. Sulindac treatment in hereditary non-polyposis colorectal cancer. Eur J Cancer 2007;43(8):1251–6.
48. Reyes-Uribe L, Wu W, Gelincik O, et al. Naproxen chemoprevention promotes immune activation in Lynch syndrome colorectal mucosa. Gut 2021;70(3):555–66.
49. Willis JA, Reyes-Uribe L, Chang K, et al. Immune activation in mismatch repair-deficient carcinogenesis: more than just mutational rate. Clin Cancer Res 2020; 26:11–7.
50. Von Knebel Doeberitz M, Kloor M. Towards a vaccine to prevent cancer in Lynch syndrome patients. Fam Cancer 2013;12(2):307–12.
51. Le DT, Uram JN, Wang H, et al. PD-1 blockade in tumors with mismatch-repair deficiency. N Engl J Med 2015;372(26):2509–20.
52. Leoni G, D'Alise AM, Cotugno G, et al. A genetic vaccine encoding shared cancer neoantigens to treat tumors with microsatellite instability. Cancer Res 2020; 80(18):3972–82.
53. Kloor M, Reuschenbach M, Pauligk C, et al. A frameshift peptide neoantigen-based vaccine for mismatch repair-deficient cancers: a phase I/IIa clinical trial. Clin Cancer Res 2020;26(17):4503–10.
54. Lu KH, Loose DS, Yates MS, et al. Prospective multicenter randomized intermediate biomarker study of oral contraceptive versus depo-provera for prevention of endometrial cancer in women with Lynch syndrome. Cancer Prev Res (Phila) 2013;6(8):774–81.
55. Kinzler KW, Vogelstein B. Landscaping the cancer terrain. Science 1998; 280(5366):1036–7.
56. Laukaitis CM, Erdman SH, Gerner EW. Chemoprevention in patients with genetic risk of colorectal cancers. Colorectal Cancer 2012;1(3):225–40.
57. Squarize CH, Castilho RM, Gutkind JS. Chemoprevention and treatment of experimental Cowden's disease by mTOR inhibition with rapamycin. Cancer Res 2008; 68(17):7066–72.
58. Schmid G, Kässner F, Uhlig H, et al. Sirolimus treatment of severe PTEN hamartoma tumor syndrome: case report and in vitro studies. Pediatr Res 2014;75: 527–34.
59. Iacobas I, Burrows PE, Adams DM, et al. Oral rapamycin in the treatment of patients with hamartoma syndromes and PTEN mutation. Pediatr Blood Cancer 2011;57(2):321–3.

60. Marsh DJ, Trahair TN, Martin JL, et al. Rapamycin treatment for a child with germ-line PTEN mutation. Nat Clin Pract Oncol 2008;5:357–61.
61. Komiya T, Blumenthal GM, DeChowdhury R, et al. A pilot study of sirolimus in subjects with cowden syndrome or other syndromes characterized by germline mutations in PTEN. Oncologist 2019;24(12):1510.
62. McGarrity TJ, Peiffer LP, Amos CI, et al. Overexpression of cyclooxygenase 2 in hamartomatous polyps of Peutz-Jeghers syndrome. Am J Gastroenterol 2003; 98(3):671–8.
63. Udd L, Katajisto P, Rossi DJ, et al. Suppression of Peutz-Jeghers polyposis by inhibition of cyclooxygenase-2. Gastroenterology 2004;127(4):1030–7.
64. Wei C, Amos CI, Zhang N, et al. Suppression of peutz-jeghers polyposis by targeting mammalian target of rapamycin signaling. Clin Cancer Res 2008;14: 1167–71.
65. Robinson J, Lai C, Martin A, et al. Oral rapamycin reduces tumour burden and vascularization in Lkb1(+/-) mice. J Pathol 2009;219:35–40.
66. Kuwada SK, Burt RA. Rationale for mTOR inhibitors as chemoprevention agents in Peutz-Jeghers syndrome. Fam Cancer 2011;10:469–72.
67. Busoni VB, Orsi M, Lobos PA, et al. Successful treatment of juvenile polyposis of infancy with sirolimus. Pediatrics 2019;144(2):e20182922.
68. Quaranta M, Laborde N, Ferrand A, et al. Sustainable positive response to sirolimus in juvenile polyposis of infancy. J Pediatr Gastroenterol Nutr 2019;68(2): e38–40.
69. Taylor H, Yerlioglu D, Phen C, et al. mTOR inhibitors reduce enteropathy, intestinal bleeding and colectomy rate in juvenile polyposis of infancy due to PTEN-BMPR1A deletion syndrome. Hum Mol Genet 2021;30(14):1273–82.

Genetic Syndromes Associated with Gastric Cancer

Woojin Kim, MD, Trilokesh Kidambi, MD, James Lin, MD, MPH,
Gregory Idos, MD, MS*

KEYWORDS

- Gastric cancer • Familial polyposis • Lynch syndrome • GAPPS
- Li-Fraumeni syndrome • Peutz–Jeghers syndrome • Juvenile polyposis syndrome

KEY POINTS

- Pathogenic germline variants in certain genes are associated with an increased risk of gastric cancer.
- Genetic cancer risk assessment and multigene panel testing is helpful in identifying patients with gastric cancer predisposition.
- There is emerging evidence about new genes that may be associated with an increased risk of gastric cancer.
- Identification of high-risk individuals may prompt gastric cancer surveillance and risk reducing surgery.
- Discussion with a cancer genetics professional or referral to an academic center of expertise may help inform appropriate prevention strategies.

INTRODUCTION

Although the incidence of gastric cancer (GC) continues to decrease in the United States, it remains a highly prevalent and deadly disease around the world, accounting for the fifth most diagnosed cancer and the third most deadly cancer worldwide.[1] Outcomes are poor with a 5-year survival of 5% for metastatic disease. Environmental factors, such as *Helicobacter pylori* infection, dietary factors including high salt intake, and tobacco use, are strong risk factors. However, 5% to 10% of GC cases are thought to be due to germline pathogenic variants. Although hereditary diffuse gastric cancer (HDGC) caused by germline pathogenic variants in the CDH1 gene is the principal familial GC syndrome, several well-established hereditary cancer syndromes have been associated with GC (**Table 1**). The syndromes include Lynch syndrome

Journal: Gastrointestinal Endoscopy Clinics of North America Inherited GI Cancers: Identification, Management and the Role of Genetic Evaluation and Testing.
City of Hope National Medical Center, 1500 East Duarte Road, Duarte, CA 91010, USA
* Corresponding author. City of Hope National Medical Center, 1500 East Duarte Road, Duarte, CA 91010.
E-mail address: gidos@coh.org

Gastrointest Endoscopy Clin N Am 32 (2022) 147–162
https://doi.org/10.1016/j.giec.2021.08.004
giendo.theclinics.com

Table 1
Hereditary cancer syndromes associated with gastric cancer

Syndrome	Gene	Lifetime Gastric Cancer Risk	Gastric Cancer Histology	Surveillance	Ref
Lynch Syndrome	MLH1 MSH2 MSH6 PMS2 EPCAM	MLH1 – 9% MSH2-10% MSH6-7% PMS2-0% EPCAM-0%	Intestinal GC	Upper Endoscopy every 3–5 y	3-6,8,15,67
Familial Adenomatous Polyposis	APC	4%-7%	Intestinal Type	Upper endoscopy based on Spigelman Criteria	5,34,42,43,67
MUTYH Polyposis	MYH	2%-5%	Intestinal GC	Upper endoscopy based on Spigelman Criteria	5,39,67
GAPPS	APC 1B Promoter	13%	Intestinal and mixed GC arising in the context of fundic gland polyposis of the proximal stomach	No consensus guidelines at this time	33,44,47,50
Li-Fraumeni	TP53	2%-5%	Intestinal or Diffuse GC	Upper Endoscopy every 2–5 y	5,58-60,62,67
Peutz–Jeghers Syndrome (PJS)	STK11	29%	Intestinal GC	Upper Endoscopy every 2-3 y	5,63,66,67
Juvenile Polyposis Syndrome (JPS)	SMAD4 or BMPR1A	5%-21%	Intestinal or Diffuse GC	Upper Endoscopy every 1-3 y	5,67,70,72
Emerging Syndromes: Hereditary Breast and Ovarian	BRCA1/BRCA2	2%	Intestinal GC	No recommendations	81

Abbreviation: GC, gastric cancer.

(LS), familial adenomatous polyposis (FAP), Li-Fraumeni syndrome (LFS), and hamartomatous polyposis syndromes [Peutz–Jeghers (PJ) and juvenile polyposis] have been associated with GC and will be discussed here. Gastric adenocarcinoma and proximal polyposis of the stomach (GAPPS), a subset of FAP[2], will also be reviewed in this article. Also, we will discuss emerging germline genetic association with GC from pathogenic variants in the homologous recombination pathway including *BRCA1* and *BRCA2*. Given that GC presents in advanced stages, it is important to identify carriers early via genetic testing to tailor risk stratification and offer the possibility of early detection through surveillance.

LYNCH SYNDROME

LS is the most common hereditary gastrointestinal cancer predisposition syndrome and is caused by autosomal dominant heterozygous germline mutations in the mismatch repair (MMR) genes *MLH1, MSH2, MSH6 or PMS2,* and *EPCAM* (which leads to epigenetic inactivation of *MSH2*).[3–6] Pathogenic variants result in the loss of function of the MMR protein, whose normal function is postreplicative proofreading and editing, explaining the hallmark feature of high tumor mutational burden. This manifests as an alteration in the length of tandem repeats within microsatellite repeat regions termed microsatellite instability (MSI) seen in LS-associated tumors.[3,4] The most common cancers associated with LS are colorectal and endometrial, whereby LS accounts for 3% and 2% of cases, respectively[4]; however, LS is associated with a spectrum of extracolonic cancers including ovarian, gastric, duodenal, genitourinary, and prostate.[5]

Historical context

The initial report of Warthin,[7] a pathologist at the University of Michigan, documenting the pedigree of Family G and 2 other cancer-prone families identified colorectal, endometrial, and GCs among others within the family—these reports along with those of Dr Henry Lynch[3] laid the foundation for the discovery of the genetic basis of LS. When the *MSH2* germline variant was found and Family G was followed for 7 generations, GC was noted to be the third most common cancer in the family.[8] As such, an association with GC and LS has been suggested from the beginning of our understanding of the disease, though the implications for management and surveillance remain controversial.

LS-associated gastric cancer risk

Several studies have shown that LS is associated with an increased risk of GC.[9–12] One of the most meaningful studies to date[9] examining the risk of cancers in patients with LS was carried out prospectively, using the Colon Cancer Family Registry. The study followed patients with LS without a cancer diagnosis (with germline mutations in the MMR genes but unaffected by cancer) as well as their family members without the germline mutations (noncarriers). This study design was the first prospective study on the topic and eliminated the biases of previous retrospective study designs.[10] In addition to confirming the strong association of LS with colorectal and endometrial cancer, the study also found an increased risk of extracolonic cancers, including GC, which had a greater than 9-fold increased risk in patients with LS than their unaffected family members.

Prospective data examining the cumulative lifetime incidence of different cancers in LS have also been reported[11] from the Prospective LS Database. Patients in this cohort were adults with germline mutations in MMR genes consistent with LS and were recruited at the time of their first surveillance colonoscopy and followed. The results confirmed an increased incidence of any cancer with increasing age and showed different lifetime risks depending on the specific MMR gene, with the highest risk in patients with mutations in *MSH2*, followed by *MLH1* and lowest risk in those with mutations in *MSH6*. Due to low rates of cancer development in LS patients with *PMS2* mutations, firm conclusions regarding risks associated with this mutation could not be drawn. Among upper gastrointestinal cancers, the cumulative risk of GC was the greatest at 7% to 8%. For comparison, the cumulative risks of colorectal cancer (CRC) ranged from 60% to 80%, endometrial cancer ranged from 43% to 46%, and ovarian cancer ranged from 10% to 17%. The conclusion from this study was that although the lifetime risk of GC was elevated in patients with LS, the absolute risk was considerably less than that associated with colorectal and endometrial cancers and roughly half that associated with ovarian cancer.

A recent case–control study[12] specifically examined clinical risk factors for the development of GC in patients with LS by analyzing data from more than 50,000 patients who underwent genetic testing through a commercial laboratory. In this study, 266 patients with GC were identified, of which 41 had LS (1.1% with LS has GC, than 0.5% without LS with GC). On multivariable analysis, male sex, increasing age, and pathogenic germline mutations in the *MLH1 and MSH2* genes well as the number of first-degree relatives with GC were all associated with GC. Similar to other studies looking at GC incidence overall, older age and male gender were associated with higher rates of GC.[13] This study confirmed the increased risk of GC in LS, but more importantly provided a rationale for a personalized, risk-stratified approach to GC surveillance in patients with LS.

Molecular pathways and histologic features of LS-associated gastric cancer

Most (60%–80%) of the GCs in LS are intestinal type, whereas 20% to 30% are of the diffuse or poorly differentiated type,[8] though data are limited. The tumors can occur anywhere in the stomach. There is an association with *H. pylori* infection reported in an Italian LS registry, in which 3 of the 4 patients with LS and GC had *H. pylori* infection.[14] However, in a more recent study[15] of esophagogastroduodenoscopy (EGD) for the surveillance of upper gastrointestinal cancers in patients with LS, none of the 6 GC cases occurred in patients with *H. pylori* infection.[8] Given the small number of cases published, it is difficult to draw definitive conclusions about the role of *H. pylori* infection in the development of LS-associated gastric cancers.

Autoimmune, including atrophic, gastritis[16,17] is a common histologic finding in LS-associated GCs. In a retrospective analysis of 255 patients with LS followed in a hereditary gastrointestinal cancer program,[16] 7 cases of GC were identified and underwent full histopathological review. In 5 (71%) of these cases, chronic immune gastritis was identified with 4 cases showing chronic atrophic gastritis and 1 showing lymphocytic gastritis. In another retrospective review of LS-associated GC in patients in a Japanese LS registry,[17] of the 49 available GC specimens, all were associated with intestinal metaplasia gastric atrophy.

Current surveillance guidelines

Given the increased risk of LS-associated upper gastrointestinal cancers including gastric and duodenal cancers, surveillance with EGD is recommended by consensus guidelines.[5,18,19] The guidelines recommend beginning EGD between 30 and 35 years with surveillance at every 2 to 5-year intervals; all guidelines also recommend testing for *H. pylori* and eradicating if positive. However, consensus guidelines acknowledge that data demonstrating the yield and efficacy of EGD surveillance are lacking.

Recent studies[15,20] have examined the yield of EGD for surveillance in patients with LS. In a single-center study[15] of more than 200 patients with LS undergoing EGD, 11 upper gastrointestinal cancers were identified, of which 6 were GCs. Of note, half of these cancers were identified on surveillance examination, whereas the others were identified as part of diagnostic evaluation for symptoms; 80% of the surveillance detected cancers were stage I versus just 30% in those undergoing workup for symptoms. The authors concluded[21] that surveillance EGD was indicated given the ability to detect early cancers and that the current short surveillance intervals were justified as cancer was detected on surveillance in patients who were up to date with their surveillance examinations. A large, multi-center study of patients with LS in the German Consortium for Familial Intestinal Cancer registry undergoing EGD also supported regular EGD for the surveillance of upper gastrointestinal cancer.[20] Data from more than 5000 EGDs in more than 1100 patients were analyzed and 49 GCs were identified. Roughly 25% of these patients with GC were less than 45 years and GC identified through surveillance was more likely to be early stage (85%) than cancer identified due to diagnostic evaluation for symptoms (25%). This study also concluded that EGD was warranted for surveillance.

FAMILIAL ADENOMATOUS POLYPOSIS

FAP syndrome (FAP) is the second most common hereditary CRC predisposition syndrome after LS.[22] It is an autosomal dominant disease caused by germline mutations in the tumor suppressor gene, *Adenomatous polyposis coli* (APC), located on chromosome 5q21[23–26]

Populations registries have shown the disease to affect one in 10,000 individuals[27,28] FAP is characterized by the development of hundreds to thousands of adenomatous polyps distributed throughout the colon and rectum. The incidence of CRC starts by the second decade of life with a 100% lifetime risk of CRC in classic FAP when no interventions are performed.[22] FAP is associated with other extracolonic malignancies including duodenal, gastric, thyroid, liver (hepatoblastoma), biliary, pancreas, and central nervous system (medulloblastoma)[22]

FAP-associated gastric cancer

Historically GC was not acknowledged as a significant risk factor in Western FAP patients as the reported lifetime risk of 0.6% was comparable to the general population.[29] Several studies have shown variable rates of GC in patients with FAP from 1.3% to 7.1% with differences seen between Eastern (Korea and Japan) and Western FAP patients.[30–32] In a large US-based registry of patients with FAP who underwent 1 or more upper endoscopies, there was a total of 10 cases of GC out of 767 patients with FAP (1.3%), resulting in a standardized incidence ratio of 140. All cases of GC were presented in the proximal stomach with 60% presenting with metastatic disease at diagnosis.[33] Interestingly, since the inception of the registry in 1979 to 2006, there were no reported cases of GC with all 10 cases diagnosed within a 10-year span (2006–2016). This increase in GC in the phenotypic presentation of the Western FAP cohort is a concerning development. The largest European polyposis registry is from the international FAP database curated by the International Society for Gastrointestinal Hereditary Tumors' (InSiGHT) group.[34] In this study, they found a total of 8 patients who developed GC (adenocarcinoma) and 21 with adenoma (median age 52 and 44 years, respectively). GCs were located proximally in 63%, whereas gastric adenomas were evenly distributed between the proximal and distal stomach. Three-quarters of patients with GC had nodal or metastatic disease on presentation. There was an association noted between GC and gastric adenoma with a personal or family history of desmoid.[34]

In Eastern FAP patients, GC incidence rates are higher than that reported in Western patients ranging from 2.6% to 7.1%.[30–32,35,36] Eastern FAP patients with GC are diagnosed at an earlier stage, found to be multicentric, and located distally.[31,32,37] The largest series of Eastern FAP patients is from a Japanese polyposis registry of 1050 patients with FAP. In this series, there were 27 cases of GC (2.6%) with the mean age of diagnosis at 49.[32] The relative risk of GC was found to be 2.4 times higher in men and 4.7 times higher in women compared with the general population.[32] The higher rates of GC in Eastern FAP patients are possibly related to the higher incidence of gastric adenomas and *H. pylori* infections[30,38,39]

FAP-gastric cancer precursor lesion

In FAP-associated GC, the precursor lesion leading to cancer is still unknown. It has been postulated to occur from both fundic gland polyposis or from gastric adenomas which maybe hidden under a carpet of gastric polyposis. Fundic gland polyps (FGPs) are found in most patients with FAP. These small sessile polyps are primarily found proximal to the incisura, with low-grade dysplasia occurring in 38% of patients with FAP.[40] In a study of 41 FGPs in 17 patients with FAP, an inactivating somatic APC gene mutation was identified in 51% of the polyps and no mutations in the sporadic comparison group.[41] This second hit somatic APC gene alteration in addition to the germline APC mutation could potentially account for the neoplastic potential of FGPs in FAP.[42] Gastric adenomas in patients with FAP have been reported in upwards of 35% in Asia and as low as 10% in Western populations.[30,38] Foveolar-type adenoma (85%) is the most common followed by pyloric gland adenoma (15%) and intestinal-type adenomas (1%–2%).[39] FAP-associated pyloric gland adenomas have been reported to have a high prevalence of GNAS and KRAS mutations, also supporting a second hit model to the neoplastic potential of these lesions.[33]

Current surveillance guidelines

Upper gastrointestinal tract surveillance recommendations in FAP are primarily driven by the risk of duodenal cancer. Screening for gastric and proximal small bowel tumors should be conducted using both a gastroscope and a duodenoscope starting at the age of 25 to 30 years, whereas obtaining random samples of FGPs in the stomach[5] surveillance is repeated based on the Spigelman stage of duodenal polyposis: 4 years for stage 0, 1 to 2 years for stage I, 1 to 3 years for stage II, 6 to 12 months in stage III, and surgical evaluation in stage IV.[5] These current surveillance recommendations do not reflect the emerging risk of GC in patients with FAP. A study examining 10 patients with FAP with GC and 40 age-matched FAP control subjects identified 3 endoscopic features associated with GC which include carpeting of gastric polyps, solitary polyps greater than 20 mm, and a polypoid mound of polyps.[43] In addition, patients with FAP with GC had a higher prevalence of gastric adenomas, polyps with high-grade dysplasia, and pyloric gland adenomas.[43] Taking into consideration these findings, an expert opinion on surveillance for proximal gastric polyposis is summarized in **Table 2**. Given the varying surveillance recommendations for gastric polyposis and duodenal polyposis in patients with FAP, the upper gastrointestinal tract surveillance interval should ultimately be based on the segment of the gastrointestinal tract with the severe disease presentation.

GASTRIC ADENOCARCINOMA AND PROXIMAL POLYPOSIS OF THE STOMACH

GAPPS (GAPPS) is a recently described autosomal dominant gastric polyposis syndrome with a significant risk for gastric adenocarcinoma. The clinical pathologic

Table 2
Recommended surveillance for gastric polyposis

Polyp Number, Size of Solitary Polyp, Presence of Polypoid Mounds	Histology	Surveillance Strategy
Numerous, <10 mm	FGP with or without foveolar LGD	EGD according to SS duodenal polyposis or 3 y
Numerous or Carpeted, <10 mm	PGA or TA	1 y
Numerous or Carpeted, >10 mm	FGP with or without foveolar LGD, TA, PGA	6–12 mo
Numerous, Any size, No Polypoid Mounds	FGP-HGD, PGA-HGD, or TA-HGD	3–6 mo or offer gastrectomy
Any Proximal Polypoid Mounds	FGP with or without foveolar LGD, PGA, TA	3–6 mo, baseline EUS, consider CT or MRI abdomen
Any Proximal Polypoid Mounds	FGP-HGD, PGA-HGD, or TA-HGD	Prophylactic gastrectomy
Any Size or Number	Intramucosal or invasive adenocarcinoma	Gastrectomy

Abbreviations: FGP, fundic gland polyp; HGD, high-grade dysplasia; LGD, low-grade dysplasia; PGA, pyloric gland adenoma; SS, Spigelman stage; TA, tubular adenoma.

Adapted from Mankaney G, Leone P, Cruise M, et al. Gastric cancer in FAP: a concerning rise in incidence. Fam Cancer 2017;16:371-376.

features of GAPPS were first described in 2012 in a large Australian family and 2 smaller families in the US and Canada. The affected family members had fundic gland polyposis (>100) carpeting the fundus and body while sparing the antrum and lesser curvature, with the development of intestinal-type gastric adenocarcinoma arising in areas of fundal gland polyposis with high-grade dysplasia and adenomatous polyps and an autosomal dominant pattern of inheritance.[44] Diagnostic criteria for GAPPS were developed based on endoscopic and pathologic criteria (**Box 1**). The genetic underpinnings of GAPPS were elucidated in 2016 whereby a germline point mutation in promoter 1B of *APC* was identified.[45] Point mutations in the *APC* 1B promoter significantly reduce the binding of the transcription factor Yin Yang 1 and

Box 1
Diagnostic criteria for GAPPS

1. Gastric polyps restricted to the body and fundus with no evidence of colorectal or duodenal polyposis

2. Greater than 100 polyps carpeting the proximal stomach in the index case or greater than 30 polyps in a first-degree relative of another case

3. Predominantly FGPs, some having regions of dysplasia (or a family member with either dysplastic FGPs or gastric adenocarcinoma)

4. Autosomal dominant pattern of inheritance

5. Exclusion of other heritable gastric polyposis syndromes and use of PPIs[a].

[a]In patients on PPIs, recommend repeating upper endoscopy while off therapy.[1]

Adapted from Rudloff U. Gastric adenocarcinoma and proximal polyposis of the stomach: diagnosis and clinical perspectives. Clin Exp Gastroenterol 2018;11:447-459.

transcriptional activity of the *APC* promoter.[45] On histopathology, a characteristic finding in GAPPS is hyperproliferative aberrant pits (HPAP), which correspond to hyperproliferative and disorganized oxyntic glands around gastric pits and are felt to be precursor lesions of dysplastic FGPs and adenomas.[46] It has been postulated that HPAP is the incipient dysplasia awaiting a second hit mutation which then leads to gastric dysplasia and subsequent carcinoma.[46]

The clinical course of GAPPS is highly variable with several phenotypic variations noted in the age of onset, penetrance, and degree of dysplasia. The overall risk for GC in GAPPS is high with the reported incidence ranging from 12% to 25%[44,47] In a recent report from the Czech Republic on 24 carriers with the promoter 1B *APC* gene mutation: c.-191T > C, there were 6 cases (25%) of GC ranging in age from 29 to 64 years.[47] There was incomplete penetrance with obligate carriers at age 31 and 65 showing no signs of disease. The earliest reported age of onset is in a 10 year old from the original large Australian GAPPS family whereby there was evidence of fundic gland polyposis with multiple areas of focal dysplasia.[44] Diagnosing GC presents a challenge in GAPPS as the proximal stomach is carpeted with FGPs which frequently harbor a heterogeneous mix of dysplastic and adenomatous changes.[48] There have been cases whereby GC was diagnosed on a prophylactic gastrectomy, despite the patients undergoing multiple endoscopic examinations[49] bringing to question the role of prolonged endoscopic surveillance similar to HDGC syndrome.

Due to limited data on GAPPS, current guidelines on endoscopic surveillance or timing of prophylactic gastrectomies are based on expert opinions[48,50] Patients who meet current diagnostic criteria for GAPPS are advised to get genetic testing for point mutations in the *APC* 1B promoter. Upper endoscopy should be performed starting at the age of 15 or earlier with dyspeptic symptoms, with a detailed examination of gastric polyps and surrounding mucosa with multiple biopsies performed from the suspected areas.[50] A colonoscopy should be performed in all cases of suspected GAPPS to exclude colonic polyposis.[50] The recommendations for surveillance interval between upper endoscopies have varied with some advocating for an upper endoscopy every 6 to 12 months,[47] whereas others recommend surveillance intervals based on the degree of polyposis: 5-year interval for no polyps, 3-year interval for any FGPs without dysplasia, and individualized decision on patients with greater than 100 FGPs.[50] For patients with GAPPS with fundic gland polyposis and the presence of any dysplasia, a prophylactic gastrectomy is recommended.[48,50] Given the significant interindividual heterogeneity within GAPPS, an individual approach to the affected and at-risk GAPPS family members should be taken by a multidisciplinary team of genetics, gastroenterology, and surgery.

LI-FRAUMENI SYNDROME

LFS is a rare hereditary cancer predisposition syndrome caused by autosomal dominant germline mutations in the *TP53* gene.[51–54] *TP53* is a tumor suppressor gene that encodes a protein involved in controlling cell proliferation and homeostasis; thus, loss of function suppresses protection against the accumulation of genetic alterations leading to cancer formation.[52,53] LFS is characterized by the familial clustering of tumors in patients less than 45 years with a predominance of sarcomas, breast cancer, brain tumors, and adrenal carcinomas; however, LFS is also associated with GC, leukemia, lung cancer, and skin cancers.[51,52,54]

Historical context

The clinical syndrome of LFS was first described in 1969[55] in 4 families with young-onset sarcomas, breast cancer, and other cancers and a larger, follow-up description was published nearly 20 years later in 1988[56] by searching the Cancer Family Registry of the National Cancer Institute and identifying 24 families with 151 patients with cancer. These studies laid the initial foundation for the clinical criteria used to identify LFS until 1990[53] when the *TP53* gene mutation was identified as the cause of LFS after sequencing identified germline missense mutations in 5 classic LFS families. This has been subsequently confirmed in numerous follow-up studies.[57]

LFS-associated gastric cancer risk

Studies have described the risk of GC in patients with LFS.[58,59] The largest study examining this association was a case series from the Dana Farber Cancer Institute/ National Cancer Institute LFS registry.[58] In 62 families with 429 patients, GC was identified in nearly 5% of probands with a median and mean age at diagnosis 36 and 43 years, respectively. GC was found in 14 (22.6%) of the families. This study was the largest series published and showed high rates of GC in LFS. A subsequent review article[59] summarized the rates of GC seen in smaller published studies and the percent of tumors with GC in the smaller studies ranged from 1.3% to 4.7%. However, case series of LFS families have not shown a risk of GC in small reports.[14] GC in LFS have both diffuse-type and intestinal-type histology.[59]

Current surveillance guidelines

Surveillance guidelines for LFS-GC detection are based on consensus opinion due to limited data.[60,61] The recommendation is for EGD beginning at the age of 25 years, or 10 years younger than earliest onset GC in the family (whichever is younger) and to repeat every 2 to 5 years. A recent publication[62] examined the prevalence of GC as well as the yield and update of EGD in patients with LFS by examining patients with LFS in the International Agency for Research on Cancer (IARC) database as well as from the University of Pennsylvania database. The IARC database search confirmed the presence of GC in 6% of families and 3% of patients. Using chart review of the University of Pennsylvania database, 40 EGD reports were reviewed from 48 EGD procedures on 35 patients and no upper gastrointestinal cancers were identified in this small subset, though low-grade dysplasia and a duodenal adenoma were found. Interestingly, 65% of patients had not undergone EGD surveillance as recommended by guidelines. The authors concluded that longer longitudinal data were required and that an emphasis on adherence to surveillance recommendations was a potential future point of emphasis.

PEUTZ–JEGHERS SYNDROME

Peutz–Jeghers syndrome (PJS) is an autosomal dominant condition characterized by the association of gastrointestinal polyposis, mucocutaneous pigmentation, and cancer predisposition. The syndrome is caused by germline pathogenic variants in the *STK11* gene. The diagnostic clinical features of PJS include the presence of: (a) 2 or more histologically confirmed PJ polyps; or (b) any number of PJ polyps in an individual who has a family history of PJS in a first-degree relative; (c) characteristic mucocutaneous pigmentation in a person with a family history of PJS; or (d) any number of PJ polyps in a person with the characteristic mucocutaneous pigmentation of PJS.[63]

PJ-type hamartomatous polyps can vary from one to hundreds and most commonly occur in the small intestine but also frequently in the colon and stomach. There have been several studies evaluating cancer risks in PJS.[64–66] In a meta-analysis of 210 cases reported in 6 retrospective studies with kindred-based ascertainment from the US, UK, and Netherlands, the relative risk for GC was 213 and cumulative risk of 29%. Based on these estimates, consensus guidelines recommend that PJ patients undergo a baseline upper endoscopy beginning at the age of 8, whereas some other recommend between the ages of 8 and 10. Surveillance is recommended every 2 to 3 years.[5,67]

JUVENILE POLYPOSIS SYNDROME

Juvenile polyposis syndrome (JPS) is a rare autosomal dominant disorder associated with an increased risk of gastrointestinal cancer. It is characterized by the presence of multiple juvenile-type hamartomatous polyps throughout the gastrointestinal tract. Two genes are currently known to cause JPS: *SMAD4* and *BMPR1A*. It is estimated that 60% of patients with JPS have a pathogenic variant in either gene.[5,67]

The diagnosis of JPS is made based on clinical criteria or the identification of a germline pathogenic variant in *SMAD4* or *BMPR1A*. The clinical diagnosis of JPS is made when a person has any one of the following: (1) 5 or more juvenile polyps of the colon or rectum; (2) any number of juvenile polyps in parts of the gastrointestinal tract other than the colon; or (3) any number of juvenile polyps and one or more first-degree relatives with JPS.

Colon and GC are the most commonly observed cancer in JPS. The first studies reporting an association of juvenile polyposis with GC appeared in the 1970s.[68,69] Although data remain limited in evaluating the stomachs of patients with JPS, the lifetime risk of GC for individuals with JPS ranges from 5% to 21%.[62,70–73] Studies suggest that the risk of GC is higher in carriers of *SMAD4* germline pathogenic variants than *BMPR1A* carriers. In a study of 80 unrelated patients with JPS, 16 patients with *SMAD4* pathogenic variants developed gastric polyposis than none in the 11 patients with *BMPR1A* pathogenic variants. In the same study, all 7 cases of GC occurred in *SMAD4* carriers.[72]

Based on the limited amount of studies, current guidelines and expert consensus statements recommend that patients with JPS undergo the assessment of the upper tract with upper endoscopy beginning between the ages of 12 and 15 with surveillance every 1 to 3 years.[5,67] It is still uncertain as to whether *BMPR1A* pathogenic variants are associated with GC risk, but upper endoscopy surveillance is suggested at intervals similar to those recommended for *SMAD4* carriers. In adults, partial or complete gastrectomy is indicated in patients with: GC, high-grade dysplasia, inability to adequately survey or endoscopically control polyposis, persistent anemia or GI bleeding from gastric polyposis or angioectasia, and/or symptoms of gastric outlet obstruction or protein-losing gastropathy.

EMERGING GERMLINE GENETIC ASSOCIATIONS WITH GASTRIC CANCER

HBOC syndrome affects both men and women and remains the most common form of hereditary breast and ovarian cancer in all racial-ethnic backgrounds (1 in 200–800 general population prevalence but significantly higher among Ashkenazi Jewish population; 1 in 40)[74] Over the last several years, there have emerged new data on the link between homologous recombination gene defects (HRD) and GC. HBOC syndrome and its association with GC is a prime example. HBOC syndrome is autosomal dominant inherited syndrome characterized by pathogenic variants in *BRCA1* and *BRCA2* genes leading to defects in the DNA repair pathway which increases the likelihood of not only developing breast cancer but also ovarian/fallopian tube cancer.[75] *BRCA1/BRCA2* increase the risk of developing other specific types of epithelial cancer including pancreatic cancer, melanoma, prostate cancer, and biliary/gallbladder as well as GC.[76,77] GC risk in BRCA1[78] and BRCA2[79] carriers were reported to be higher shortly after these genes were first discovered more than 25 years ago.

Further genetic analysis and pathology studies of BRCA1/2-associated breast cancer will likely add more clarification on hereditary components of GC as there have been mixed data on GC and BRCA2 associations[80] in 2 Northern European studies.[76] In a study from Japan, however, whereby the incidence of GC is very high, BRCA1/2 pathogenic variants were found to be a predisposing factor in the cohort of patients with GC family history; although those carrying BRCA1/2 mutation may need a "second hit" mutation from H. pylori infection which is also prevalent in Japan leading to the complete loss of BRCA 1/2 function. The authors also propose that the second hit may also explain the higher number of metachronous GC in Japan.[81] Additionally, in a large registry study of HDGC families (N = 3858 subjects from 75 families) without CDH1 mutations, BRCA2 carriers were identified.[82] Among 144 patients who met the HDGC criteria but were negative for CDH1, 16 (11%) were found to carry pathogenic variants in CTNNA1, BRCA2, STK11, SDHB, PRSS1, ATM, MRS1, and PALB2. Interestingly, a very rare case report of both familial breast cancer and diffuse GC co-occurrence has been reported with germline pathogenic variants in both BRCA1 and CDH1 genes.[83]

Poly adenosine diphosphate ribose polymerase (PARP) inhibitors target cancers with HRD that lead to dsDNA breaks.[84] BRCA1/2 breast and ovarian cancers respond to PARP inhibitors after initial platinum-based chemotherapy.[85] In a study from Korea, whereby GC prevalence is very high, patients with GC treated with paclitaxel plus the PARP inhibitor Olaparib demonstrated an overall survival benefit than placebo.[86] However, the authors noted that most patients with BRCA1/2 mutations will usually develop breast and/or ovarian cancer at earlier ages before GC, which develops at later ages. In another study from Northern Europe, men were found to have GC at a significantly higher rate than women while assessing families with ovarian, breast, and GC.[87]

Other moderately penetrant genes within the HRD pathway (PALB2, CHEK2, ATM, RAD51 C/D, and BARD1)[88] have also been associated with GC.[89,90] In a study looking at both diffuse and nondiffuse/intestinal-type GC, germline pathogenic variants in PALB2, BRCA1, and RAD51 C were identified.[91] The study was somewhat limited due to confounding including samples obtained from geographic areas whereby GC is more prevalent due to H. pylori infection and tobacco smoking.

SUMMARY

GC is still a common cancer worldwide and mainly related to H. pylori infection or other environmental exposures (including tobacco smoking and high salt intake) that trigger the Correa pathway[92] leading to chronic inflammation and the development of intestinal-type adenocarcinoma. However, genetic cancer risk assessment is a powerful tool in identifying carriers of germline pathogenic variants who are at increased risk for GC. Identification of these individuals can lead to tailored risk stratification and offer the possibility of early detection through surveillance. Although there is still a gap in our understanding of the germline genetic causes of GC, multigene panel testing is expanding our understanding of emerging germline genetic associations within the homologous recombination pathway genes and beyond.[93,94] Also, there seems to be a pronounced increase in the risk of GC in patients with a rare hereditary syndrome that comes from countries such as Korea and Japan than Western countries. Further studies examining the interaction between genes and the environment (eg, H. Pylori) may help us better understand these differences.

CLINICS CARE POINTS

- The worldwide prevalence of gastric cancer is high, particularly in Asia and Latin America.
- Patients with young onset gastric cancer or a strong family history of gastric cancer may warrant genetic cancer risk assessment and genetic testing.
- Patients with pathogenic variants in CDH1 are at highest risk of hereditary diffuse gastric cancer.
- There are other established hereditary cancer syndromes that are associated with an increased risk of gastric cancer.

DISCLOSURE

Gregory Idos was supported by National Institutes of Health Grants No. KL2-TR000131.

REFERENCES

1. Bray F, Ferlay J, Soerjomataram I, et al. Global cancer statistics 2018: GLOBO-CAN estimates of incidence and mortality worldwide for 36 cancers in 185 countries. CA Cancer J Clin 2018;68:394–424.
2. Molinaro E, Andrikou K, Casadei-Gardini A, et al. BRCA in gastrointestinal cancers: current treatments and future perspectives. Cancers (Basel) 2020;12:3346.
3. Lynch HT, Snyder CL, Shaw TG, et al. Milestones of Lynch syndrome: 1895-2015. Nat Rev Cancer 2015;15:181–94.
4. Boland PM, Yurgelun MB, Boland CR. Recent progress in Lynch syndrome and other familial colorectal cancer syndromes. CA Cancer J Clin 2018;68:217–31.
5. Syngal S, Brand RE, Church JM, et al. ACG clinical guideline: Genetic testing and management of hereditary gastrointestinal cancer syndromes. Am J Gastroenterol 2015;110:223–62 [quiz: 263].
6. Idos G, Valle L. Lynch Syndrome. In: Adam MP, Ardinger HH, Pagon RA, et al, eds GeneReviews((R)). Seattle (WA): University of Washington, Seattle Copyright a 1993- 2021, University of Washington, Seattle. GeneReviews is a registered trademark of the University of Washington, Seattle. All rights reserved.; 1993.
7. Classics in oncology. Heredity with reference to carcinoma as shown by the study of the cases examined in the pathological laboratory of the University of Michigan, 1895-1913. By Aldred Scott Warthin. 1913. CA Cancer J Clin 1985;35:348–59.
8. Boland CR, Yurgelun MB, Mraz KA, et al. Managing gastric cancer risk in lynch syndrome: controversies and recommendations. Fam Cancer 2021. https://doi.org/10.1007/s10689-021-00235-3.
9. Win AK, Young JP, Lindor NM, et al. Colorectal and other cancer risks for carriers and noncarriers from families with a DNA mismatch repair gene mutation: a prospective cohort study. J Clin Oncol 2012;30:958–64.
10. Capelle LG, Van Grieken NC, Lingsma HF, et al. Risk and epidemiological time trends of gastric cancer in Lynch syndrome carriers in the Netherlands. Gastroenterology 2010;138:487–92.
11. Møller P, Seppälä TT, Bernstein I, et al. Cancer risk and survival in path_MMR carriers by gene and gender up to 75 years of age: a report from the Prospective Lynch Syndrome Database. Gut 2018;67:1306–16.
12. Kim J, Braun D, Ukaegbu C, et al. Clinical Factors Associated With Gastric Cancer in Individuals With Lynch Syndrome. Clin Gastroenterol Hepatol 2020;18:830–7.e1.

13. Kumar S, Metz DC, Ellenberg S, et al. Risk Factors and Incidence of Gastric Cancer After Detection of Helicobacter pylori Infection: A Large Cohort Study. Gastroenterology 2020;158:527–36.e7.
14. Fornasarig M, Magris R, De Re V, et al. Molecular and pathological features of gastric cancer in lynch syndrome and familial adenomatous polyposis. Int J Mol Sci 2018;19:1682.
15. Kumar S, Dudzik CM, Reed M, et al. Upper endoscopic surveillance in lynch syndrome detects gastric and duodenal adenocarcinomas. Cancer Prev Res (Phila) 2020;13:1047–54.
16. Adar T, Friedman M, Rodgers LH, et al. Gastric cancer in Lynch syndrome is associated with underlying immune gastritis. J Med Genet 2019;56:844–5.
17. Cho H, Yamada M, Sekine S, et al. Gastric cancer is highly prevalent in Lynch syndrome patients with atrophic gastritis. Gastric Cancer 2021;24:283–91.
18. Stoffel EM, Mangu PB, Gruber SB, et al. Hereditary colorectal cancer syndromes: American Society of Clinical Oncology Clinical Practice Guideline endorsement of the familial risk-colorectal cancer: European Society for Medical Oncology Clinical Practice Guidelines. J Clin Oncol 2015;33:209–17.
19. Giardiello FM, Allen JI, Axilbund JE, et al. Guidelines on genetic evaluation and management of Lynch syndrome: a consensus statement by the US Multi-Society Task Force on colorectal cancer. Gastroenterology 2014;147:502–26.
20. Ladigan-Badura S, Vangala DB, Engel C, et al. Value of upper gastrointestinal endoscopy for gastric cancer surveillance in patients with Lynch syndrome. Int J Cancer 2021;148:106–14.
21. Kumar S, Katona BW. Upper gastrointestinal cancers in Lynch syndrome: the time for surveillance is now. Oncoscience 2021;8:31–3.
22. Kanth P, Grimmett J, Champine M, et al. Hereditary Colorectal Polyposis and Cancer Syndromes: A Primer on Diagnosis and Management. Am J Gastroenterol 2017;112:1509–25.
23. Herrera L, Kakati S, Gibas L, et al. Gardner syndrome in a man with an interstitial deletion of 5q. Am J Med Genet 1986;25:473–6.
24. Groden J, Thliveris A, Samowitz W, et al. Identification and characterization of the familial adenomatous polyposis coli gene. Cell 1991;66:589–600.
25. Kinzler KW, Nilbert MC, Su LK, et al. Identification of FAP locus genes from chromosome 5q21. Science 1991;253:661–5.
26. Nishisho I, Nakamura Y, Miyoshi Y, et al. Mutations of chromosome 5q21 genes in FAP and colorectal cancer patients. Science 1991;253:665–9.
27. Bülow S, Faurschou Nielsen T, Bülow C, et al. The incidence rate of familial adenomatous polyposis. Results from the Danish Polyposis Register. Int J Colorectal Dis 1996;11:88–91.
28. Järvinen HJ. Epidemiology of familial adenomatous polyposis in Finland: impact of family screening on the colorectal cancer rate and survival. Gut 1992;33:357–60.
29. Jagelman DG, DeCosse JJ, Bussey HJ. Upper gastrointestinal cancer in familial adenomatous polyposis. Lancet 1988;1:1149–51.
30. Park SY, Ryu JK, Park JH, et al. Prevalence of gastric and duodenal polyps and risk factors for duodenal neoplasm in korean patients with familial adenomatous polyposis. Gut Liver 2011;5:46–51.
31. Shibata C, Ogawa H, Miura K, et al. Clinical characteristics of gastric cancer in patients with familial adenomatous polyposis. Tohoku J Exp Med 2013;229:143–6.
32. Iwama T, Mishima Y, Utsunomiya J. The impact of familial adenomatous polyposis on the tumorigenesis and mortality at the several organs. Its rational treatment. Ann Surg 1993;217:101–8.

33. Mankaney G, Leone P, Cruise M, et al. Gastric cancer in FAP: a concerning rise in incidence. Fam Cancer 2017;16:371–6.
34. Walton SJ, Frayling IM, Clark SK, et al. Gastric tumours in FAP. Fam Cancer 2017; 16:363–9.
35. Noh JH, Song EM, Ahn JY, et al. Prevalence and endoscopic treatment outcomes of upper gastrointestinal neoplasms in familial adenomatous polyposis. Surg Endosc 2021. https://doi.org/10.1007/s00464-021-08406-0.
36. Yamaguchi T, Ishida H, Ueno H, et al. Upper gastrointestinal tumours in Japanese familial adenomatous polyposis patients. Jpn J Clin Oncol 2016;46:310–5.
37. Park JG, Park KJ, Ahn YO, et al. Risk of gastric cancer among Korean familial adenomatous polyposis patients. Report of three cases. Dis Colon Rectum 1992;35:996–8.
38. Offerhaus GJ, Giardiello FM, Krush AJ, et al. The risk of upper gastrointestinal cancer in familial adenomatous polyposis. Gastroenterology 1992;102:1980–2.
39. Gullo I, van der Post RS, Carneiro F. Recent advances in the pathology of heritable gastric cancer syndromes. Histopathology 2021;78:125–47.
40. Bianchi LK, Burke CA, Bennett AE, et al. Fundic gland polyp dysplasia is common in familial adenomatous polyposis. Clin Gastroenterol Hepatol 2008;6:180–5.
41. Abraham SC, Nobukawa B, Giardiello FM, et al. Fundic gland polyps in familial adenomatous polyposis: neoplasms with frequent somatic adenomatous polyposis coli gene alterations. Am J Pathol 2000;157:747–54.
42. Galiatsatos P, Foulkes WD. Familial adenomatous polyposis. Am J Gastroenterol 2006;101:385–98.
43. Leone PJ, Mankaney G, Sarvapelli S, et al. Endoscopic and histologic features associated with gastric cancer in familial adenomatous polyposis. Gastrointest Endosc 2019;89:961–8.
44. Worthley DL, Phillips KD, Wayte N, et al. Gastric adenocarcinoma and proximal polyposis of the stomach (GAPPS): a new autosomal dominant syndrome. Gut 2012;61:774–9.
45. Li J, Woods SL, Healey S, et al. Point Mutations in Exon 1B of APC Reveal Gastric Adenocarcinoma and Proximal Polyposis of the Stomach as a Familial Adenomatous Polyposis Variant. Am J Hum Genet 2016;98:830–42.
46. de Boer WB, Ee H, Kumarasinghe MP. Neoplastic Lesions of Gastric Adenocarcinoma and Proximal Polyposis Syndrome (GAPPS) Are Gastric Phenotype. Am J Surg Pathol 2018;42:1–8.
47. Foretová L, Navrátilová M, Svoboda M, et al. GAPPS - Gastric Adenocarcinoma and Proximal Polyposis of the Stomach Syndrome in 8 Families Tested at Masaryk Memorial Cancer Institute - Prevention and Prophylactic Gastrectomies. Klin Onkol 2019;32:109–17.
48. Rudloff U. Gastric adenocarcinoma and proximal polyposis of the stomach: diagnosis and clinical perspectives. Clin Exp Gastroenterol 2018;11:447–59.
49. Repak R, Kohoutova D, Podhola M, et al. The first European family with gastric adenocarcinoma and proximal polyposis of the stomach: case report and review of the literature. Gastrointest Endosc 2016;84:718–25.
50. Tacheci I, Repak R, Podhola M, et al. Gastric adenocarcinoma and proximal polyposis of the stomach (GAPPS) - A Helicobacter-opposite point. Best Pract Res Clin Gastroenterol 2021;101728:50–1.
51. Birch JM, Alston RD, McNally RJ, et al. Relative frequency and morphology of cancers in carriers of germline TP53 mutations. Oncogene 2001;20:4621–8.
52. Olivier M, Goldgar DE, Sodha N, et al. Li-Fraumeni and related syndromes: correlation between tumor type, family structure, and TP53 genotype. Cancer Res 2003;63:6643–50.

53. Malkin D, Li FP, Strong LC, et al. Germ line p53 mutations in a familial syndrome of breast cancer, sarcomas, and other neoplasms. Science 1990;250:1233–8.
54. Corso G, Pedrazzani C, Marrelli D, et al. Familial gastric cancer and Li-Fraumeni syndrome. Eur J Cancer Care (Engl) 2010;19:377–81.
55. Li FP, Fraumeni JF Jr. Soft-tissue sarcomas, breast cancer, and other neoplasms. A familial syndrome? Ann Intern Med 1969;71:747–52.
56. Li FP, Fraumeni JF Jr, Mulvihill JJ, et al. A cancer family syndrome in twenty-four kindreds. Cancer Res 1988;48:5358–62.
57. Guha T, Malkin D. Inherited TP53 Mutations and the Li-Fraumeni Syndrome. Cold Spring Harb Perspect Med 2017;7.
58. Masciari S, Dewanwala A, Stoffel EM, et al. Gastric cancer in individuals with Li-Fraumeni syndrome. Genet Med 2011;13:651–7.
59. McBride KA, Ballinger ML, Killick E, et al. Li-Fraumeni syndrome: cancer risk assessment and clinical management. Nat Rev Clin Oncol 2014;11:260–71.
60. Kratz CP, Achatz MI, Brugières L, et al. Cancer Screening Recommendations for Individuals with Li-Fraumeni Syndrome. Clin Cancer Res 2017;23:e38–45.
61. Daly MB, Pilarski R, Yurgelun MB, et al. NCCN Guidelines Insights: Genetic/Familial High-Risk Assessment: Breast, Ovarian, and Pancreatic, Version 1.2020. J Natl Compr Canc Netw 2020;18:380–91.
62. Katona BW, Powers J, McKenna DB, et al. Upper Gastrointestinal Cancer Risk and Surveillance Outcomes in Li-Fraumeni Syndrome. Am J Gastroenterol 2020;115:2095–7.
63. Beggs AD, Latchford AR, Vasen HF, et al. Peutz-Jeghers syndrome: a systematic review and recommendations for management. Gut 2010;59:975–86.
64. Giardiello FM, Brensinger JD, Tersmette AC, et al. Very high risk of cancer in familial Peutz-Jeghers syndrome. Gastroenterology 2000;119:1447–53.
65. Hearle N, Schumacher V, Menko FH, et al. Frequency and spectrum of cancers in the Peutz-Jeghers syndrome. Clin Cancer Res 2006;12:3209–15.
66. van Lier MG, Westerman AM, Wagner A, et al. High cancer risk and increased mortality in patients with Peutz-Jeghers syndrome. Gut 2011;60:141–7.
67. Gupta S, Provenzale D, Llor X, et al. NCCN Guidelines Insights: Genetic/Familial High-Risk Assessment: Colorectal, Version 2.2019. J Natl Compr Canc Netw 2019;17:1032–41.
68. Watanabe A, Nagashima H, Motoi M, et al. Familial juvenile polyposis of the stomach. Gastroenterology 1979;77:148–51.
69. Stemper TJ, Kent TH, Summers RW. Juvenile polyposis and gastrointestinal carcinoma. A study of a kindred. Ann Intern Med 1975;83:639–46.
70. Latchford AR, Neale K, Phillips RK, et al. Juvenile polyposis syndrome: a study of genotype, phenotype, and long-term outcome. Dis Colon Rectum 2012;55:1038–43.
71. Aytac E, Sulu B, Heald B, et al. Genotype-defined cancer risk in juvenile polyposis syndrome. Br J Surg 2015;102:114–8.
72. Aretz S, Stienen D, Uhlhaas S, et al. High proportion of large genomic deletions and a genotype phenotype update in 80 unrelated families with juvenile polyposis syndrome. J Med Genet 2007;44:702–9.
73. Howe JR, Mitros FA, Summers RW. The risk of gastrointestinal carcinoma in familial juvenile polyposis. Ann Surg Oncol 1998;5:751–6.
74. Levy-Lahad E, Catane R, Eisenberg S, et al. Founder BRCA1 and BRCA2 mutations in Ashkenazi Jews in Israel: frequency and differential penetrance in ovarian cancer and in breast-ovarian cancer families. Am J Hum Genet 1997;60:1059–67.

75. Yoshida R. Hereditary breast and ovarian cancer (HBOC): review of its molecular characteristics, screening, treatment, and prognosis. Breast Cancer 2020. https://doi.org/10.1007/s12282-020-01148-2.
76. van Asperen CJ, Brohet RM, Meijers-Heijboer EJ, et al. Cancer risks in BRCA2 families: estimates for sites other than breast and ovary. J Med Genet 2005;42:711–9.
77. Petrucelli N, Daly MB, Pal T. BRCA1- and BRCA2-Associated Hereditary Breast and Ovarian Cancer. In: Adam MP, Ardinger HH, Pagon RA, et al, editors. GeneReviews(®). Seattle (WA): University of Washington, Seattle Copyright © 1993-2021, University of Washington, Seattle. GeneReviews is a registered trademark of the University of Washington, Seattle. All rights reserved.; 1993.
78. Cancer risks in BRCA2 mutation carriers. J Natl Cancer Inst 1999;91:1310–6.
79. Ford D, Easton DF, Bishop DT, et al. Risks of cancer in BRCA1-mutation carriers. Breast Cancer Linkage Consortium. Lancet 1994;343:692–5.
80. Tulinius H, Olafsdottir GH, Sigvaldason H, et al. The effect of a single BRCA2 mutation on cancer in Iceland. J Med Genet 2002;39:457–62.
81. Ichikawa H, Wakai T, Nagahashi M, et al. Pathogenic germline BRCA1/2 mutations and familial predisposition to gastric cancer. JCO Precis Oncol 2018;2. https://doi.org/10.1200/PO.18.00097.
82. Hansford S, Kaurah P, Li-Chang H, et al. Hereditary Diffuse Gastric Cancer Syndrome: CDH1 Mutations and Beyond. JAMA Oncol 2015;1:23–32.
83. Villy MC, Mouret-Fourme E, Golmard L, et al. Co-occurrence of germline BRCA1 and CDH1 pathogenic variants. J Med Genet 2021;58:357–61.
84. Prakash R, Zhang Y, Feng W, et al. Homologous recombination and human health: the roles of BRCA1, BRCA2, and associated proteins. Cold Spring Harb Perspect Biol 2015;7:a016600.
85. Robson M, Im SA, Senkus E, et al. Olaparib for Metastatic Breast Cancer in Patients with a Germline BRCA Mutation. N Engl J Med 2017;377:523–33.
86. Bang YJ, Im SA, Lee KW, et al. Randomized, Double-Blind Phase II Trial With Prospective Classification by ATM Protein Level to Evaluate the Efficacy and Tolerability of Olaparib Plus Paclitaxel in Patients With Recurrent or Metastatic Gastric Cancer. J Clin Oncol 2015;33:3858–65.
87. Bermejo JL, Pérez AG, Hemminki K. Contribution of the Defective BRCA1, BRCA2 and CHEK2 Genes to the Familial Aggregation of Breast Cancer: a Simulation Study Based on the Swedish Family-Cancer Database. Hered Cancer Clin Pract 2004;2:185–91.
88. Tung N, Domchek SM, Stadler Z, et al. Counselling framework for moderate-penetrance cancer-susceptibility mutations. Nat Rev Clin Oncol 2016;13:581–8.
89. Friedenson B. BRCA1 and BRCA2 pathways and the risk of cancers other than breast or ovarian. MedGenMed 2005;7:60.
90. Thompson D, Easton DF. Cancer Incidence in BRCA1 mutation carriers. J Natl Cancer Inst 2002;94:1358–65.
91. Sahasrabudhe R, Lott P, Bohorquez M, et al. Germline Mutations in PALB2, BRCA1, and RAD51C, Which Regulate DNA Recombination Repair, in Patients With Gastric Cancer. Gastroenterology 2017;152:983–6.e6.
92. Moss SF. The Clinical Evidence Linking Helicobacter pylori to Gastric Cancer. Cell Mol Gastroenterol Hepatol 2017;3:183–91.
93. Slavin TP, Weitzel JN, Neuhausen SL, et al. Genetics of gastric cancer: what do we know about the genetic risks? Transl Gastroenterol Hepatol 2019;4:55.
94. Lott PC, Carvajal-Carmona LG. Resolving gastric cancer aetiology: an update in genetic predisposition. Lancet Gastroenterol Hepatol 2018;3:874–83.

Surveillance and Surgical Considerations in Hereditary Diffuse Gastric Cancer

Lauren A. Gamble, MD, Jeremy L. Davis, MD*

KEYWORDS

- Hereditary diffuse gastric cancer • Endoscopic surveillance • Cancer screening
- Prophylactic total gastrectomy • Signet ring cells • CDH1

KEY POINTS

- Germline pathogenic *CDH1* gene variants increase the risk of diffuse-type gastric cancer and lobular breast cancer.
- Endoscopic screening and surveillance for gastric cancer in HDGC currently relies on careful inspection and nontargeted mucosal biopsies.
- Prophylactic total gastrectomy is a life-altering operation with both acute and chronic sequelae.

INTRODUCTION

The hereditary diffuse gastric cancer (HDGC) syndrome is most commonly attributed to inactivating germline variants in the *CDH1* (cadherin 1, OMIM 192090) tumor suppressor gene.[1] *CDH1* encodes the transmembrane protein E-cadherin located at epithelial adherens junctions and functions in cell-cell adhesion and signal transduction.[2,3] There are more than 150 pathogenic or likely pathogenic germline *CDH1* variants that are inherited in an autosomal-dominant pattern and associated with a spectrum of disease consisting of diffuse-type gastric adenocarcinoma, lobular breast cancer, and cleft lip and palate.[1,4]

IDENTIFICATION OF INDIVIDUALS AT RISK FOR HEREDITARY DIFFUSE GASTRIC CANCER

The identification of individuals at risk for HDGC based on clinical criteria has evolved over the last 20 years. Clinical criteria were originally developed based on the multiple cases of diffuse gastric cancer cases diagnosed within families, which were often

Center for Cancer Research, National Cancer Institute, National Institutes of Health, 10 Center Drive, Room 4-3742, Bethesda, MD 20892, USA
* Corresponding author.
E-mail address: Jeremy.Davis@nih.gov

Gastrointest Endoscopy Clin N Am 32 (2022) 163–175
https://doi.org/10.1016/j.giec.2021.08.009
1052-5157/22/© 2021 Elsevier Inc. All rights reserved.

diagnosed at young ages. However, fewer than 50% of individuals who fulfilled the original clinical criteria were identified as germline carriers of pathogenic variants in the *CDH1* gene.[5]

The International Gastric Cancer Linkage Consortium recently updated recommendations to help identify individuals eligible for germline genetic testing for HDGC based on a personal and family history of gastric cancer (**Box 1**).[6] In addition to gastric cancer, genetic testing was recommended in those patients with familial lobular breast cancer diagnosed before the age of 70, patients with diffuse gastric cancer and cleft lip/palate, and those with precursor lesions for signet ring cell (SRC) carcinoma.[7,8] Based on a Dutch study using registry data, the inclusion of the additional criteria beyond diffuse gastric cancer was shown to increase sensitivity to 89% in identifying patients with pathogenic germline *CDH1* variants.[8]

Individuals who are suspected to be at high risk for HDGC should be offered genetic counseling, which includes evaluation of a 3-generation family pedigree and confirmation of cancer diagnoses. Because *CDH1* variants seem to be associated only with lobular breast cancer and not ductal breast cancer, the confirmation of breast pathology is important. Similarly, intestinal-type gastric cancers should not be used in the evaluation of clinical criteria to guide genetic testing for *CDH1*-associated HDGC. Individuals who meet HDGC genetic testing criteria and are negative for a *CDH1* variant should be tested for additional germline variants, including *CTNNA1*.[9–12] A second germline truncating allele in *CTNNA1* has been described in families who meet the clinical criteria for genetic testing for HDGC, but without obvious mutation in the *CDH1* gene. This gene encodes alpha-E-catenin, which functions in the same transmembrane complex as E-cadherin.

Testing for germline variants of *CDH1* and *CTNNA1* should be performed in accredited laboratories certified by the Association for Molecular Pathology and the

---

Box 1
HDGC syndrome genetic testing criteria

Germline testing for CDH1 variants is recommended when one of the following criteria have been met. Individuals who meet criteria but are negative for a *CDH1* variant should be tested also for *CTNNA1* variants.

Individual criteria
- DGC in individuals less than 50 years of age[a]
- DGC at any age in individuals with a personal or family history of cleft lip or cleft palate
- History of DGC and LBC in individuals less than 70 years of age
- Bilateral LBC/LCIS in individuals less than 70 years of age
- Gastric biopsy with in situ SRCs and/or pagetoid spread of SRCs in individuals less than 50 years of age

Family criteria[b]
- Two or more cases of gastric cancer in family (any age), with at least 1 confirmed DGC
- Two or more cases of LBC in family members less than 50 years of age
- One or more case of DGC any age and 1 or more case of LBC less than 70 years of age in different family members

Abbreviations: DGC, diffuse gastric cancer; LBC, lobular breast cancer; LCIS, lobular carcinoma in situ.
[a] All diagnoses of DGC and LBC must be confirmed histologically.
[b] Family members must be first- or second-degree blood relatives of each other.
From Blair VR, McLeod M, Carneiro F, et al. Hereditary diffuse gastric cancer: updated clinical practice guidelines. The Lancet Oncology 2020;21(8):e386-e397. Reprinted with permission from Elsevier.

American College of Medical Genetics. Families without an identifiable *CDH1* or *CTNNA1* variant that have 2 or more cases of gastric cancer, one of which is confirmed diffuse type, or 1 case of diffuse gastric cancer and 1 lobular breast cancer, are classified as HDGC-like. These families should present to specialty care centers for further genetic counseling and possible undiscovered genetic variants.

FREQUENCY OF *CDH1* DETECTION AND ASSOCIATED GASTRIC CANCER RISK

Current availability and increased uptake of multigene panel testing, particularly among women and families with breast cancer, has led to an increased frequency in the detection of pathogenic variants in *CDH1*, even among families without gastric cancer. In a recent study of 26,936 patients who had undergone germline multigene panel testing, 20 patients were found to carry pathogenic *CDH1* variants where 13 did not meet prior International Gastric Cancer Linkage Consortium clinical criteria for *CDH1* testing.[13] Of those with pathogenic *CDH1* variants, 19 patients had a personal history of cancer, including breast cancer (both ductal and lobular), colon cancer, and gastric cancers. Three *CDH1* carriers underwent gastrectomy and had evidence of early (stage I, T1a) diffuse gastric cancer on resection, despite not meeting the diagnostic testing criteria.

An understanding of the associated gastric and breast cancer risks related to pathogenic *CDH1* variants is important when counseling affected patients. Earlier lifetime estimates of gastric cancer risk among *CDH1* carriers were as high as 67% for men and 83% for women, but were derived from families with an increased burden of diffuse gastric cancer who met the original, more stringent clinical criteria for HDGC and thereby subject to ascertainment bias. In addition, reports of *CDH1* associated gastric cancer risk were also overestimated owing to a common haplotype suggestive of a founder effect from Newfoundland; an associated 40% risk of gastric cancer was appreciated among *CDH1* male carriers by age 75 years and of 63% in females.[14]

In studies of *CDH1* carriers identified through multigene panel testing, the lifetime risk of gastric cancer by age 80 has lowered to 37.2% to 42.0% in men and approximately 33.0% for women; interestingly, only 33.0% of newly identified carriers met the clinical criteria for HDGC.[15,16] With respect to lobular breast cancer risk among female carriers, a recent study reported a lifetime risk of 42% by the age of 80 years and when female carriers are not ascertained by clinical criteria for HDGC, the lifetime risk of lobular breast cancer was 55%.[16,17]

CLINICAL MANAGEMENT OF CARRIERS WITH PATHOGENIC *CDH1* GENE VARIANTS

Upon diagnosis of a pathogenic germline *CDH1* (or *CTNNA1*) variant, patients should be referred to a center with expertise in the management of HDGC. To provide up-to-date and thorough care, evaluation and counseling by a multidisciplinary team that includes a genetic counselor, surgical oncologist, pathologist, dietitian, and gastroenterologist should be standard. Patients and families should be educated on consensus management guidelines and offered preoperative counseling that include alternatives to surgery. Clinicians caring for patients with HDGC and their families should be prepared to care for patients undergoing cancer surveillance and prophylactic surgery and be prepared to manage the consequences of both. In addition, reproductive counseling that incorporates birth control, in vitro fertilization, and preimplantation genetic testing, should be made available to carriers of pathogenic *CDH1* variants.

Current guidelines recommend that any individual carrying a pathogenic *CDH1* variant consider prophylactic total gastrectomy, especially when families have confirmed HDGC.[6] However, significant risks come with surgical resection of the stomach, including substantial postoperative risks as well as life-altering long-term morbidities. For carriers who choose to avoid or delay surgery, the recommendation is annual endoscopic surveillance.

GASTRIC CANCER SURVEILLANCE

Even though prophylactic total gastrectomy is recommended to *CDH1* variant carriers, it is prudent for patients to undergo upper endoscopy at the time of diagnosis. In cases where gastrectomy is planned, a preceding endoscopy may identify pathology such as hiatal hernia, Barrett's esophagus, or gastric metaplasia in the duodenum, which may impact operative planning. Additionally, screening endoscopy can identify clinically evident gastric cancer that would require adequate staging and possible multimodality treatment prior to surgical intervention.

There are circumstances when endoscopic surveillance is recommended over gastrectomy, at which time the goals and limitations of surveillance should be discussed. Predilection for surveillance over gastrectomy can be considered in *CDH1* carriers who have an absence of a family history of gastric cancer, as well as in patients with competing medical risks or those who wish to avoid surgery. A primary goal of surveillance endoscopy is early detection, and therefore potentially curative treatment, of localized gastric cancer. However, it has been shown that asymptomatic *CDH1* variant carriers will harbor occult (microscopic) foci of SRC carcinomas in their stomachs, which are often missed during surveillance endoscopy and only detected at the time of prophylactic total gastrectomy.[18,19] One of the largest studies of 41 *CDH1* carriers who underwent prophylactic gastrectomy found that 85% had 1 or more foci of SRC cancer.[20] Both positive and negative endoscopic surveillance and histologic findings are known to guide patients' decision-making. Barriers to undergoing surgery included patient age, positive beliefs about endoscopic surveillance, close relatives who had negative surgical experiences, and fertility concerns and life stress.[21]

For *CDH1* carriers who opt to undergo surveillance, annual endoscopy is recommended at an expert center. Surveillance should be performed using white-light, high-definition endoscopy with particular attention to the distensibility of the stomach and presence of mucosal abnormalities. The gastric mucosa should be washed with a mucolytic and any focal lesions or pale mucosa areas should be sampled to possibly identify microscopic foci of SRCs. In addition, a minimum of 28 to 30 random mucosal biopsies should be obtained from 5 distinct areas of the stomach. This approach is known as the Cambridge protocol where 3 to 5 biopsies are obtained from the cardia, 5 from the fundus, 10 from the body, 5 from the transition zone, and 5 from the antrum.[6,22] Pathologic specimens should be reviewed by a pathologist expert in upper gastrointestinal luminal disease and examined with both hematoxylin and eosin and periodic acid-Schiff to aid in the identification of SRCs. The progression of HDGC includes (a) in situ SRCC, with depolarized and disorganized SRCs; (2) pagetoid spread of SRCs with proliferation of SRCs between the preserved gastric epithelium and basal membrane (**Fig. 1A**); and (3) early intramucosal invasive SRCC where SRCs invade the lamina propria (Fig. 1B).

Limitations of Endoscopic Surveillance

Although conventional white light endoscopy is useful for the detection of gastric mucosal lesions, such as ulcers and polyps, its usefulness for the detection of early SRC carcinoma has limitations. SRCs, which are pathognomonic for HDGC, are typically located beneath the epithelial layer within the lamina propria and are therefore

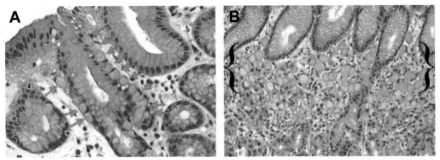

Fig. 1. Precursor and intramucosal lesions from a HDGC patient. Representative photomicrograph images of hematoxylin and eosin (H&E) staining showing (A) pagetoid progression of SRCs (arrows) (original magnification 400×), and (B) intramucosal SRCC (original magnification 100×). In (B), note the progressive enlargement of SRCs toward the luminal surface (curly brackets { }), conferring a layered structure. HDGC, hereditary diffuse gastric cancer; SRCs, signet ring cells. (*From* Gullo I, Oliveira C, van der Post, RS et al. Chapter 9: Updated perspective and directions on hereditary diffuse gastric cancer. In: Research and Clinical Applications of Targeting Gastric Neoplasms. 1st ed. AP Academic Press: 2021:217-258.)

detected at varying rates using random gastric sampling methods. A review of contemporary reports of endoscopic surveillance demonstrates a wide range of cancer detection with random gastric biopsies (**Table 1**). Based on these data, the likelihood of a positive cancer finding on random biopsy in patients with HDGC approximates 40% to 50% in most specialty centers.[23–25] The challenge with these cancer detection rates is the corresponding prevalence of occult SRC cancers in patients with HDGC who undergo prophylactic total gastrectomy, which ranges from 87% to 100%.[22,26–29] Thus, the absence of pathologic findings with random gastric biopsies may be falsely reassuring as it relates to the presence of occult gastric cancer.

Furthermore, unlike intestinal-type gastric adenocarcinoma, diffuse-type cancers even at late stages may not be obvious on endoscopy and this nature justifies the recommendation of random gastric biopsies at the time of gastroscopic cancer surveillance. The goals of surveillance are not only to detect occult cancer foci, but also to exclude more advanced and invasive lesions.[6]

In addition to random biopsies, targeted biopsies of visible abnormalities should be obtained during surveillance endoscopy. Abnormalities may include nodular-

Table 1
Occult cancer detection rates with random gastric biopsies

Author	Year	Cohort Size	Detection Rate (%)
Curtin et al,[19] 2020	2020	120	36
Friedman et al,[54] 2019	2019	32	22
Jacobs et al,[23] 2019	2019	20	40
Mi et al,[24] 2018	2018	54	50
Schueler et al,[26] 2021	2021	36	11
van Dieren et al,[25] 2020	2020	42	24
Vos et al,[41] 2020	2020	142	18

appearing mucosa, gastric polyps, focal or diffuse gastritis, mucosal ulceration, and pale areas. Discrete pale areas of gastric mucosa have been suggested as harbingers of occult SRC foci, and adjuncts to traditional white light endoscopy have been explored, including narrow band imaging and chromoendoscopy, to improve the detection of gastric mucosal pale areas.[22,25] However, a major limitation of chromoendoscopy is the inability to detect lesions less than 4 mm in size, which makes its application impractical, because most SRCs are frequently less than 1 mm.[26,30] Although narrow band imaging can detect pale areas and abnormal vasculature within the mucosa, biopsies from these areas infrequently harbor SRC foci.[22,25] Furthermore, it is important to note that SRC detection on targeted biopsy of any focal abnormality remains low around 11%.[26]

Additional Surveillance Strategies for the Early Detection of Hereditary Diffuse Gastric Cancer

Advanced endoscopic imaging modalities

Additional improvements to endoscopic surveillance in patients with HDGC, such as endoscopic ultrasound examination and confocal laser endomicroscopy (CLE), have been explored. Endoscopic ultrasound examination, which allows for visualization of the layers of the gastric wall to identify any disruptions suggestive of invasive neoplasia, has been evaluated for the detection of early stage gastric cancer without favorable results. CLE consists of a fiberoptic probe passed through the working channel of an endoscope, which provides histologic microstructure images of the gastric mucosa in real time.[31,32] CLE can visualize intramucosal capillaries and gastric gland architecture, such as the distraction of gastric pits. However, displacement of gastric pits on CLE seems to be a nonspecific finding that can be secondary to enlarging SRC clusters or infiltrating inflammatory cells and mucosal edema.[26] In the first registered prospective clinical trial of endoscopic surveillance in *CDH1* variant carriers, CLE demonstrated a small improvement in cancer detection when compared with the Cambridge Protocol method of obtaining random biopsies.[26] Even still, a better understanding of the limitations and possibilities of adjuncts to traditional endoscopy, such as artificial intelligence, is expected to improve early cancer detection.

Optical coherence tomography (OCT) is an adjunctive endoscopic imaging technique that allows visualization deep to the gastric epithelium to the level of the muscularis propria with a high resolution of 10 μm.[33] Unlike endoscopic ultrasound techniques, OCT uses light rather than acoustic signals.[34] In a small ex vivo study combining OCT with machine learning, this imaging technology demonstrated a high accuracy for the detection of gastric cancer.[35] OCT is studied widely for the detection of mucosal dysplasia and early neoplasia of the esophagus[36] and, although applications to the stomach may be limited, the development of this and other advanced imaging techniques is relevant to the future of cancer surveillance in HDGC.

Intensive mucosal evaluation

Ongoing research of different endoscopic surveillance techniques is aimed at exploring both improved sensitivity and specificity of microscopic, early gastric cancers in patients with HDGC. For example, Curtin and colleagues[19] have expanded the method of nontargeted, random sampling of gastric mucosa beyond the Cambridge Protocol and have developed a systematic method of mucosal evaluation. This method included a modest expansion of gastric biopsies from 30 to 88, and incorporates a stepwise evaluation of the entire stomach based on 22 anatomic locations.[19] This strategy yielded a higher cancer detection rate compared with the Cambridge method (62% from 20%) and a decrease in false-negative biopsies

(80% compared with 37%).[19] Refinements in endoscopic surveillance protocols hold promise for not only improving cancer detection, but also allowing for standardization across centers worldwide.

Biomarker discovery
Noninvasive strategies, such as biomarkers present in the blood, urine, or stool, could be useful for early detection and gastric cancer surveillance. For example, E-cadherin as a serum biomarker has demonstrated the potential for early detection of gastric cancer development, screening, and surveillance. E-cadherin has an extracellular domain that is cleaved at a homeostatic rate. The soluble fragment can be detected in peripheral serum at normal levels, but can be high in the serum in patients with gastric cancer. After gastric cancer resection, soluble E-cadherin levels have been shown to return to normal levels.[37,38] Biomarker development is important to the study of early cancer development in *CDH1* carriers and can potentially be applied to sporadic diffuse-type gastric cancer. In addition, gastric and fecal microbiome studies are currently underway in some centers and forthcoming results may prove useful.

SURGICAL MANAGEMENT

Prophylactic surgery to remove an at-risk organ is an effective method of cancer risk reduction. In HDGC, total gastrectomy affords complete removal of the gastric epithelium and effectively eliminates the future risk of cancer. Consensus guidelines recommend prophylactic total gastrectomy as early as age 20 years in individuals with HDGC who carry a pathogenic *CDH1* variant.[6] Total gastrectomy may be associated with major morbidity; therefore, consideration must be given not only to the alternative of annual endoscopic surveillance, but also the potential for long-term sequelae of life without a stomach. Consideration should be given to both the physiologic and psychological impacts of the operation, as well as the acute risks of surgery considering that total gastrectomy is a relatively infrequent and high-risk operation. The operative approach, whether minimally invasive versus open gastrectomy, should be based on the surgeon's experience and outcomes. To ensure complete removal of all gastric mucosa, esophageal and duodenal margins should be assessed via frozen section intraoperatively. A perigastric (D1) lymphadenectomy is considered sufficient because lymph node metastasis is uncommon, even in patients who harbor early (T1a) SRC. Comprehensive pathologic assessment using a total-embedding protocol is recommended to evaluate the entirety of the gastrectomy explant and identify cancer lesions, which are most often less than 1 mm in diameter and in multiple locations throughout the organ.[39]

Preoperative Considerations

Preoperative counseling should include the patient and their family with a specific discussion about the plan of care during the recovery period. It is imperative to assess for competing medical and psychosocial risk factors, such as alcohol dependence or food aversions, which would complicate recovery from gastrectomy.[6] It is the authors' experience that psychological screening and the availability of psychosocial support are as critical to patient outcomes as medical assessment of operative risk. Just as postgastrectomy monitoring by a registered dietitian is essential, a preoperative assessment of dietary habits, micronutrient levels, and baseline bone health should be evaluated. An upper endoscopy should be performed within 6 to 12 months before the planned operation on all patients undergoing prophylactic total gastrectomy. The decision to proceed to surgery need not be rushed, because some of the issues presented here may take additional time to address.

Acute Complications

Postoperative complications of total gastrectomy are well-documented for patients with advanced gastric cancer who have received multimodality therapy.[40] It is likely that otherwise healthy patients undergoing prophylactic total gastrectomy might experience an overall lower complications rate. The data supporting this assertion are limited; however, perioperative morbidity rates represent necessary information to be shared during preoperative counseling. Additionally, total gastrectomy remains a relatively infrequent operation in many European and North American centers; therefore, clinicians caring for patients after gastrectomy should be aware of the range of possible operative outcomes. A retrospective cohort study of patients with HDGC by Vos and colleagues[41] described an overall acute (<30 days postoperative) complication rate of 28%, which included 16% major complications (Clavien–Dindo grade $\geq$3).[42] The most concerning acute complication is esophago-jejunal anastomotic leak wherein the Roux limb (jejunum), which has been joined with the distal esophagus, does not heal properly owing to imperfect surgical technique or compromised tissue healing. Anastomotic leak has been reported to occur in approximately 4% to 6% of patients and frequently requires interventions such as endoscopy with esophageal stent placement, percutaneous drainage, total parenteral nutrition, or jejunostomy tube feeding.[20,43–45] Other postoperative complications during the acute phase of recovery from total gastrectomy include duodenal stump leakage, hemorrhage, deep vein thrombosis or pulmonary embolism, pneumonia, and superficial surgical site infection. The range and rates of complication from total gastrectomy for advanced cancer are similar and can be used as a guide, even though many patients selected for prophylactic gastrectomy may be expected to fare better.[46]

Chronic Sequelae

The long-term outcomes of total gastrectomy in patients with HDGC are better appreciated. Although total gastrectomy has been performed for several decades, patients most often had cancer at time of surgery, thereby limiting long-term follow up. Even so, the most frequent chronic complications are the postgastrectomy syndromes (**Table 2**)[47,48] that result from alterations in both the anatomy and function of the stomach and small intestine. The dumping syndrome is commonly associated with gastrectomy and results from the rapid emptying of hyperosmolar food contents into the proximal small intestine. Symptoms include diaphoresis, flushing, palpitations, crampy abdominal pain, nausea, and diarrhea.[48] Dumping syndrome is most effectively prevented and treated with dietary modifications. Other postgastrectomy syndromes include bile (alkaline) reflux and Roux stasis.

Weight loss and nutritional deficiencies are frequently encountered after gastrectomy. Because of both the restrictive (loss of gastric reservoir) and malabsorptive nature related to total gastrectomy, patients will experience weight loss where baseline body weight decreases most dramatically within the first month after total gastrectomy and often plateaus at 6 to 12 months postoperatively.[49] The median weight loss from baseline is approximately 20% of total body weight, but potentially greater for obese patients and less for normal weight patients.[41] Monitoring and supplementing specific nutritional deficiencies are necessary in patients after total gastrectomy and are similar in part to those evaluated in patients who have undergone bariatric surgeries. The most commonly monitored nutritional components include vitamins folate (B9), cobalamin (B_{12}), A, D, E, and K, and calcium, iron, zinc, and protein.[50] Therefore, access to a registered dietitian is considered crucial to successful postoperative recovery. It is important to note that newer, oral formulations of daily (bariatric)

Table 2
Postgastrectomy syndromes

Syndrome	First-Line Therapy	Second-Line Therapy
Dumping	Dietary modifications	Roux-en-Y gastrojejunostomy[a]
Bile reflux gastritis	Medical therapy (eg, cholestyramine)	Roux-en-Y gastrojejunostomy[a]; Braun enteroenterostomy; jejunal interposition
Small gastric remnant	Dietary modifications	Jejunal pouch
Postvagotomy diarrhea	Dietary modifications	Antiperistaltic jejunal segment
Delayed gastric emptying	Prokinetic medication	Completion gastrectomy, conversion to Roux-en-Y[a]
Afferent loop syndrome	Address obstruction based on cause	Roux-en-Y gastrojejunostomy[a]
Efferent loop syndrome	Assess obstruction based on cause	None
Roux stasis	Completion gastrectomy, Roux-en-Y gastrojejunostomy	Feeding jejunostomy

[a] For those status post Billroth-II.
Adapted from Davis JL, Ripley RT. Postgastrectomy Syndromes and Nutritional Considerations Following Gastric Surgery. Surg Clin North Am. 2017 Apr;97(2):277-293.

multivitamins provide sufficient B_{12}, which can negate the need for intramuscular supplementation. Iron deficiency leading to anemia can be a frequent complication, particularly in menstruating females. This complication is due to a lack of iron absorption resulting from lack of gastric acid, decreased intrinsic factor, and bypass of the duodenum.[51,52] Furthermore, iron deficiency is also exacerbated by vitamin C deficiency. Vitamin D and calcium homeostasis may impact bone health and supplementation and monitoring of these factors is also necessary.

Contemporary studies often use patient-reported outcomes to assess quality of life after total gastrectomy. Although studies have reported generally on quality of life after gastrectomy, it may be difficult to capture all potential sequelae of total gastrectomy, which also encompass the diagnosis of a hereditary cancer syndrome.[53] In addition, standardized questionnaires may not assess for the myriad of other symptoms reported by patients, such as the frequency and severity of bile reflux, dry mouth, functional dysphagia, and an inability to tolerate free water. Further studies are needed to understand the complexity of postgastrectomy life for patients with HDGC. Regret after deciding to undergo prophylactic total gastrectomy is being studied and could provide opportunities to improve preoperative counseling. The impact of varied phenotypic expression among *CDH1* carriers and the burden of gastric cancer among relatives, may also impact surgical decision-making and is an area of continued research.

SUMMARY

Pathogenic germline variants in the *CDH1* gene are associated with an elevated lifetime risk of diffuse-type gastric cancer and lobular breast cancer, resulting in the HDGC syndrome. The current expert consensus recommendation is for *CDH1* carriers to undergo prophylactic total gastrectomy, particularly when there is a family history of gastric cancer. However, removal of the entire stomach may not be a viable or desirable option for some patients, particularly those with poor existing comorbid conditions. In patients who wish to avoid surgery, or those with substantial contraindications to surgery, annual endoscopic surveillance with intensive mucosal evaluation and multiple nontargeted biopsies is recommended. Current cancer surveillance techniques using conventional white light endoscopy and its adjuncts carry low rates of sensitivity and specificity for the detection of SRCC; therefore, endoscopic surveillance is currently assigned an indeterminate safety profile that patients should be aware of and is the only potential nonoperative strategy until more reliable early gastric cancer detection or preventive strategies are elucidated. Although total gastrectomy carries known perioperative risks and considerable life-altering sequelae, it is currently the only definitive form of gastric cancer prevention in HDGC.

CLINICS CARE POINTS

- Patients with germline *CDH1* pathogenic variants should have a baseline upper gastrointestinal endoscopy at the time of diagnosis.
- Counseling of *CDH1* variant carriers includes a recommendation for total gastrectomy or annual endoscopic surveillance.
- Annual endoscopic surveillance incorporates multiple, nontargeted gastric biopsies and is associated with low sensitivity for occult cancer detection.
- Prophylactic total gastrectomy is associated with many physiologic and psychosocial changes that necessitate management by a multidisciplinary care team.
- Alternatives to total gastrectomy, including enhanced endoscopic surveillance techniques, are under investigation.

DISCLOSURE

The authors have no financial relationships to disclose.

REFERENCES

1. Guilford P, Hopkins J, Harraway J, et al. E-cadherin germline mutations in familial gastric cancer. Nature 1998;392(6674):402–5.
2. Hermann Aberle HS, Kemler R. Cadherin-catenin complex: protein interactions and their implications for cadherin function. J Cell Biochem 1996;61:514–23.
3. Caldeira J, Figueiredo J, Bras-Pereira C, et al. E-cadherin-defective gastric cancer cells depend on Laminin to survive and invade. Hum Mol Genet 2015;24(20): 5891–900.
4. Caldas C, Carneiro F, Lynch HT, et al. Familial gastric cancer: overview and guidelines for management. J Med Genet 1999;36(12):873–80.
5. Petrovchich I, Ford JM. Genetic predisposition to gastric cancer. Semin Oncol 2016;43(5):554–9.
6. Blair VR, McLeod M, Carneiro F, et al. Hereditary diffuse gastric cancer: updated clinical practice guidelines. Lancet Oncol 2020;21(8):e386–97.
7. Fitzgerald RC, Hardwick R, Huntsman D, et al. Hereditary diffuse gastric cancer: updated consensus guidelines for clinical management and directions for future research. J Med Genet 2010;47(7):436–44.
8. van der Post RS, Vogelaar IP, Carneiro F, et al. Hereditary diffuse gastric cancer: updated clinical guidelines with an emphasis on germline CDH1 mutation carriers. J Med Genet 2015;52(6):361–74.

9. Benusiglio PR, Colas C, Guillerm E, et al. Clinical implications of CTNNA1 germline mutations in asymptomatic carriers. Gastric Cancer 2019;22(4):899–903.
10. Clark DF, Michalski ST, Tondon R, et al. Loss-of-function variants in CTNNA1 detected on multigene panel testing in individuals with gastric or breast cancer. Genet Med 2020;22(5):840–6.
11. Carreno M, Pena-Couso L, Mercadillo F, et al. Investigation on the role of PALB2 Gene in CDH1-negative patients with hereditary diffuse gastric cancer. Clin Transl Gastroenterol 2020;11(12):e00280.
12. Fewings E, Larionov A, Redman J, et al. Germline pathogenic variants in PALB2 and other cancer-predisposing genes in families with hereditary diffuse gastric cancer without CDH1 mutation: a whole-exome sequencing study. Lancet Gastroenterol Hepatol 2018;3(7):489–98.
13. Lowstuter KEC, Sturgeon D, Ricker C, et al. Unexpected CDH1 mutations identified on multigene panels pose clinical management challenges. JCO precision Oncol 2017;(1):1–2.
14. Kaurah P, MacMillan A, Boyd N, et al. Founder and recurrent CDH1 mutations in families with hereditary diffuse gastric cancer. JAMA 2007;297(21):2360.
15. Xicola RM, Li S, Rodriguez N, et al. Clinical features and cancer risk in families with pathogenic CDH1 variants irrespective of clinical criteria. J Med Genet 2019;838–43.
16. Roberts ME, Ranola JMO, Marshall ML, et al. Comparison of CDH1 penetrance estimates in clinically ascertained families vs families ascertained for multiple gastric cancers. JAMA Oncol 2019;1325–31.
17. Hansford S, Kaurah P, Li-Chang H, et al. Hereditary diffuse gastric cancer syndrome: CDH1 mutations and beyond. JAMA Oncol 2015;1(1):23–32.
18. DiBrito SR, Blair AB, Prasath V, et al. Total gastrectomy for CDH-1 mutation carriers: an institutional experience. J Surg Res 2020;247:438–44.
19. Curtin BF, Gamble LA, Schueler SA, et al. Enhanced endoscopic detection of occult gastric cancer in carriers of pathogenic CDH1 variants. J Gastroenterol 2021;56(2):139–46.
20. Strong VE, Gholami S, Shah MA, et al. Total gastrectomy for hereditary diffuse gastric cancer at a single center: postsurgical outcomes in 41 patients. Ann Surg 2017;266(6):1006–12.
21. McGarragle KM, Hart TL, Swallow C, et al. Barriers and facilitators to CDH1 carriers contemplating or undergoing prophylactic total gastrectomy. Fam Cancer 2021;20(2):157–69.
22. Lim YC, di Pietro M, O'Donovan M, et al. Prospective cohort study assessing outcomes of patients from families fulfilling criteria for hereditary diffuse gastric cancer undergoing endoscopic surveillance. Gastrointest Endosc 2014;80(1):78–87.
23. Jacobs MF, Dust H, Koeppe E, et al. Outcomes of endoscopic surveillance in individuals with genetic predisposition to hereditary diffuse gastric cancer. Gastroenterology 2019;157(1):87–96.
24. Mi EZ, Mi EZ, di Pietro M, et al. Comparative study of endoscopic surveillance in hereditary diffuse gastric cancer according to CDH1 mutation status. Gastrointest Endosc 2018;87(2):408–18.
25. van Dieren JM, Kodach LL, den Hartog P, et al. Gastroscopic surveillance with targeted biopsies compared with random biopsies in CDH1 mutation carriers. Endoscopy 2020;52(10):839–46.
26. Schueler SA, Gamble LA, Curtin BF, et al. Evaluation of confocal laser endomicroscopy for detection of occult gastric carcinoma in CDH1 variant carriers. J Gastrointest Oncol 2021;12(2):216–25.

27. Chen Y, Kingham K, Ford JM, et al. A prospective study of total gastrectomy for CDH1-positive hereditary diffuse gastric cancer. Ann Surg Oncol 2011;18(9): 2594–8.

28. Norton JA, Ham CM, Van Dam J, et al. CDH1 truncating mutations in the E-cadherin gene: an indication for total gastrectomy to treat hereditary diffuse gastric cancer. Ann Surg 2007;245(6):873–9.

29. Rogers WM, Dobo E, Norton JA, et al. Risk-reducing total gastrectomy for germline mutations in E-cadherin (CDH1): pathologic findings with clinical implications. Am J Surg Pathol 2008;32(6):799–809.

30. Shaw D, Blair V, Framp A, et al. Chromoendoscopic surveillance in hereditary diffuse gastric cancer: an alternative to prophylactic gastrectomy? Gut 2005; 54(4):461–8.

31. Kitabatake S, Niwa Y, Miyahara R, et al. Confocal endomicroscopy for the diagnosis of gastric cancer in vivo. Endoscopy 2006;38(11):1110–4.

32. Kakeji Y, Yamaguchi S, Yoshida D, et al. Development and assessment of morphologic criteria for diagnosing gastric cancer using confocal endomicroscopy: an ex vivo and in vivo study. Endoscopy 2006;38(9):886–90.

33. Brett Bouma GT, Compton C, Nishioka N. High-resolution imaging of the human esophagus and stomach in vivo using optical coherence tomography. Gastrointest Endosc 2000;51(1):467–74.

34. Sivak MKK, Izatt J, Rollins A, et al. High-resolution endoscopic imaging of the GI tract using optical coherence tomography. Gastrointestingal Endosc 2000;51(1): 474–9.

35. Luo S, Fan Y, Chang W, et al. Classification of human stomach cancer using morphological feature analysis from optical coherence tomography images. Laser Phys Lett 2019;16(9):095602.

36. Poneros JM, Nishioka NS. Diagnosis of Barrett's esophagus using optical coherence tomography. Gastrointest Endosc Clin N Am 2003;13(2):309–23.

37. Gofuku J, Doki Y, Inoue M, et al. Characterization of soluble E-cadherin as a disease marker in gastric cancer patients. Br J Cancer 1998;78(8):1095–101.

38. Chan AO, Chu KM, Lam SK, et al. Early prediction of tumor recurrence after curative resection of gastric carcinoma by measuring soluble E-cadherin. Cancer 2005;104(4):740–6.

39. Gullo I, Devezas V, Baptista M, et al. Phenotypic heterogeneity of hereditary diffuse gastric cancer: report of a family with early-onset disease. Gastrointest Endosc 2018;87(6):1566–75.

40. Selby LV, Vertosick EA, Sjoberg DD, et al. Morbidity after total gastrectomy: analysis of 238 patients. J Am Coll Surg 2015;220(5):863–71, e862.

41. Vos EL, Salo-Mullen EE, Tang LH, et al. Indications for total gastrectomy in CDH1 mutation carriers and outcomes of risk-reducing minimally invasive and open gastrectomies. JAMA Surg 2020;155(11):1050–7.

42. Dindo D, Demartines N, Clavien PA. Classification of surgical complications: a new proposal with evaluation in a cohort of 6336 patients and results of a survey. Ann Surg 2004;240(2):205–13.

43. Hebbard PC, Macmillan A, Huntsman D, et al. Prophylactic total gastrectomy (PTG) for hereditary diffuse gastric cancer (HDGC): the Newfoundland experience with 23 patients. Ann Surg Oncol 2009;16(7):1890–5.

44. Pandalai PK, Lauwers GY, Chung DC, et al. Prophylactic total gastrectomy for individuals with germline CDH1 mutation. Surgery 2011;149(3):347–55.

45. van der Kaaij RT, van Kessel JP, van Dieren JM, et al. Outcomes after prophylactic gastrectomy for hereditary diffuse gastric cancer. Br J Surg 2018;105(2): e176–82.
46. Nakauchi M, Vos E, Janjigian YY, et al. Comparison of long- and short-term outcomes in 845 open and minimally invasive gastrectomies for gastric cancer in the United States. Ann Surg Oncol 2021;3532–44.
47. Brooke-Cowden GL, Braasch JW, Gibb SP, et al. Postgastrectomy syndromes. Am J Surg 1976;131(4):464–70.
48. Davis JL, Ripley RT. Postgastrectomy syndromes and nutritional considerations following gastric surgery. Surg Clin North Am 2017;97(2):277–93.
49. Davis JL, Selby LV, Chou JF, et al. Patterns and predictors of weight loss after gastrectomy for cancer. Ann Surg Oncol 2016;23(5):1639–45.
50. Allied Health Sciences Section Ad Hoc Nutrition C, Aills L, Blankenship J, Buffington C, et al. ASMBS allied health nutritional guidelines for the surgical weight loss patient. Surg Obes Relat Dis 2008;4(5 Suppl):S73–108.
51. Mimura EC, Bregano JW, Dichi JB, et al. Comparison of ferrous sulfate and ferrous glycinate chelate for the treatment of iron deficiency anemia in gastrectomized patients. Nutrition 2008;24(7–8):663–8.
52. Tovey FI, Clark CG. Anaemia after partial gastrectomy: a neglected curable condition. Lancet 1980;1(8175):956–8.
53. Hu Y, Vos EL, Baser RE, et al. Longitudinal analysis of quality-of-life recovery after gastrectomy for cancer. Ann Surg Oncol 2021;28(1):48–56.
54. Friedman M, Adar T, Patel D, et al. Surveillance endoscopy in the management of hereditary diffuse gastric cancer syndrome. Clin Gastroenterol Hepatol 2021; 19(1):189–91.

Moving?

Make sure your subscription moves with you!

To notify us of your new address, find your **Clinics Account Number** (located on your mailing label above your name), and contact customer service at:

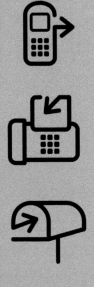

Email: journalscustomerservice-usa@elsevier.com

800-654-2452 (subscribers in the U.S. & Canada)
314-447-8871 (subscribers outside of the U.S. & Canada)

Fax number: 314-447-8029

Elsevier Health Sciences Division
Subscription Customer Service
3251 Riverport Lane
Maryland Heights, MO 63043

*To ensure uninterrupted delivery of your subscription, please notify us at least 4 weeks in advance of move.